Pharmacogenomics: The Personalized Approach to Patient Care

Pharmacogenomics: The Personalized Approach to Patient Care

Editor: Britney Jenner

AMERICAN
MEDICAL PUBLISHERS
www.americanmedicalpublishers.com

AMERICAN
MEDICAL PUBLISHERS
www.americanmedicalpublishers.com

Cataloging-in-Publication Data

Pharmacogenomics : the personalized approach to patient care / edited by Britney Jenner.
p. cm.
Includes bibliographical references and index.
ISBN 979-8-88740-374-8
1. Pharmacogenomics. 2. Pharmacogenetics. 3. Patients--Care. 4. Personalized medicine.
5. Medical care. I. Jenner, Britney.
RM301.3.G45 P43 2023
615.7--dc23

American Medical Publishers,
41 Flatbush Avenue,
1st Floor, New York,
NY 11217, USA

ISBN 979-8-88740-374-8 (Hardback)

Contents

Preface

The purpose of the book is to provide a glimpse into the dynamics and to present opinions and studies of some of the scientists engaged in the development of new ideas in the field from very different standpoints. This book will prove useful to students and researchers owing to its high content quality.

Pharmacogenomics is a field of research that studies the role of genome in drug response. It involves the study of how genes affect a person's response to drugs. This field integrates pharmacology with genomics to develop effective, safe medications that may be prescribed based on a person's genetic makeup. There are several factors such as a patient's age, weight, sex, and liver and kidney functions based on which the drugs are prescribed. Researchers have identified gene variants for a few drugs that affect the body's response to medications. These genetic variations are used to predict whether a medication will be effective for a particular person, and which dose will help in preventing adverse drug reactions. Pharmacogenomics may also be used to develop tailored drugs to treat a wide range of diseases such as cardiovascular disease, Alzheimer disease, cancer and asthma. This book contains some path-breaking studies in the field of pharmacogenomics. It will serve as a valuable resource for scientists, students, and clinicians engaged in pharmacogenomics research and therapeutic implementation.

At the end, I would like to appreciate all the efforts made by the authors in completing their chapters professionally. I express my deepest gratitude to all of them for contributing to this book by sharing their valuable works. A special thanks to my family and friends for their constant support in this journey.

Editor

1

Technologies for Pharmacogenomics

Maaike van der Lee [1,2], Marjolein Kriek [3], Henk-Jan Guchelaar [1,2] and Jesse J. Swen [1,2,*]

1 Department of Clinical Pharmacy and Toxicology, Leiden University Medical Center, 2333ZA Leiden, The Netherlands; m.vanderlee@lumc.nl (M.v.d.L.); h.j.guchelaar@lumc.nl (H.-J.G.)
2 Leiden Network of Personalized Therapeutics, 2333ZA Leiden, The Netherlands
3 Department of Clinical Genetics, Leiden University Medical Center, 2333ZA Leiden, The Netherlands; m.kriek@lumc.nl
* Correspondence: j.j.swen@lumc.nl

Abstract: The continuous development of new genotyping technologies requires awareness of their potential advantages and limitations concerning utility for pharmacogenomics (PGx). In this review, we provide an overview of technologies that can be applied in PGx research and clinical practice. Most commonly used are single nucleotide variant (SNV) panels which contain a pre-selected panel of genetic variants. SNV panels offer a short turnaround time and straightforward interpretation, making them suitable for clinical practice. However, they are limited in their ability to assess rare and structural variants. Next-generation sequencing (NGS) and long-read sequencing are promising technologies for the field of PGx research. Both NGS and long-read sequencing often provide more data and more options with regard to deciphering structural and rare variants compared to SNV panels—in particular, in regard to the number of variants that can be identified, as well as the option for haplotype phasing. Nonetheless, while useful for research, not all sequencing data can be applied to clinical practice yet. Ultimately, selecting the right technology is not a matter of fact but a matter of choosing the right technique for the right problem.

Keywords: pharmacogenomics; genotype; phenotype; next generation sequencing; long-read sequencing

1. Introduction

The field of pharmacogenomics (PGx) is developing rapidly. The first PGx dose recommendations for antidepressant and psychiatric drugs were published in 2001, even before the first human genome was sequenced [1]. An increase in available evidence and the ambition to implement PGx in clinical practice has led to the need for more comprehensive dosing guidelines and genotyping strategies. In 2005, the Dutch Pharmacogenetics Working Group (DPWG) was formed to develop evidence-based PGx guidelines [2]. In 2011, the Clinical Pharmacogenomics Implementation Consortium (CPIC) was founded [3]. Currently, CPIC and the DPWG combined have issued PGx dose recommendations covering more than 50 drugs and 21 genes (Table 1) [4,5].

In the last 20 years, there has not only been much progress in development of PGx guidelines, there has also been a significant technological advancement and rise of new technologies for assessing genetic variants. At the time of development of the first PGx guideline, only Sanger-based sequencing techniques and SNV (single nucleotide variant) arrays were available as methods for variant identification. To date, SNV panel testing remains the most commonly used technology in clinical practice. However, while it is efficient and comes at low costs, SNV panels cannot detect all important genetic variation such as rare and structural variants. Currently, multiple high throughput whole genome sequencing techniques are available, yielding an abundance of genetic information at a fraction of the costs of 20 years ago [6–10]. Nevertheless, these approaches are not yet routinely used in other clinical fields, despite their potential [11,12].

Table 1. Characteristics of pharmacogenes in CPIC and DPWG guidelines. Related drugs are all drugs with dose recommendations. A drug can be related to multiple genes and therefore counted more than once. The locus size and the number of known rare variants (the number of variants with a minor allele frequency < 1% in an aggregated population, including singletons) are extracted from Gnomad (GRCh38). Part of the locus defined as complex is the percentage of the locus defined as a repeat or segmental duplication extracted from UCSC browser (https://genome.ucsc.edu). CPIC: Clinical Pharmacogenetic Implementation Consortium, DPWG: Dutch Pharmacogenetics Working Group.

Protein	Gene	Related Drugs		Locus Size (bp)	Rare Variants, n (% of Known Variants)	Part of Locus Defined as Complex, %(bp)
		CPIC	DPWG			
CACNA1S	*CACNA1S*	7	-	73,055	2520 (98%)	33.3
CFTR	*CFTR*	1	-	250,187	1684 (99%)	42.2
CYP2B6	*CYP2B6*	1	1	27,149	761 (98%)	100.0
CYP2C9	*CYP2C9*	10	2	50,734	632 (98%)	72.0
CYP2C19	*CYP2C19*	15	10	90,525	712 (99%)	83.6
CYP2D6	*CYP2D6*	14	21	4408	992 (97%)	100.0
CYP3A5	*CYP3A5*	1	1	31,833	643 (98%)	49.4
CYP4F2	*CYP4F2*	1	-	20,098	766 (97%)	51.4
DPD	*DPYD*	2	4	917,258	1211 (98%)	40.0
FACT. V LEIDEN	*FACT. V LEIDEN*	-	1 *	72,423	1679 (97%)	41.9
G6PD	*G6PD*	1	-	16,183	465 (98%)	36.4
HLA-A	*HLA-A*	2	1	4625	423 (71%)	100.0
HLA-B	*HLA-B*	6	7	87,698	308 (78%)	62.1
IFNL3	*IFNL3*	2	-	1577	317 (95%)	100.0
IFNL4	*IFNL4*	2	-	3543	404 (97%)	100.0
NUDT15	*NUDT15*	3	3	9656	244 (99%)	64.7
RYR-1	*RYR1*	7	-	153,866	6584 (98%)	51.4
SLCO1B1	*SLCO1B1*	1	2	108,045	951 (96%)	69.6
TPMT	*TPMT*	3	3	26,764	346 (97%)	52.3
UGT1A1	*UGT1A1*	1	1	13,052	470 (99%)	40.3
VKORC1	*VKORC1*	1	3	5139	370 (98%)	41.8

* This interaction is aimed at the entire group of drugs classified as oral contraceptives with estrogen.

In this paper, we review the application of genotyping technologies for PGx. We first discuss the use of SNV panels, which are the most commonly used approach for clinical PGx. Next, we discuss the potential of next generation sequencing (NGS) and long-read sequencing and their current use in PGx. We review the challenges in PGx, both for clinical as well as research purposes, and the way PGx technologies can help in solving them. We mainly focus on germline variants and their role in PGx. Nonetheless, the outlined principles hold true for somatic mutations [13–15]. Additionally, implementation and adoption of PGx in clinical practice is outside the scope of this review and has been extensively discussed in previous publications [16–18].

2. SNV Panels: Current Clinical Practice

SNV panel testing is the most commonly used technology in PGx practice, either through commercially available micro-array platforms or with custom arrays. The arrays typically contain a preselected set of SNVs, which, depending on the array and platform, can range from a few variants in a single gene to thousands of variants genome wide. Commercially available PGx arrays typically contain variants that are linked to drug response in PGx guidelines or on PharmGKB [19]. The evidence underlying the selected variants can vary, from small arrays containing only the most strongly associated variants, to very large arrays containing all variants potentially or theoretically associated with drug response—for example, including all known drug-related genes. Almost all available arrays use PCR, sequencing by synthesis and nanospheres or beads, combined with a form of fluorescence or chemiluminescence detection to identify which variant is present at the site of interest [20–22]. Another technology is the use of mass spectrometry, relying on differences in mass between wildtype and mutant nucleotides [23]. Detailed descriptions of these techniques have been described previously [3,24–28]. The pre-selection of variants and the relatively low amount of data to process allow for a quick result at low costs (Table 2).

Table 2. Performance and applicability of available genotyping methods used for PGx. PGx: pharmacogenomics, WES: whole exome sequencing, WGS: whole genome sequencing. NA: not applicable, in this case due to a whole gene/genome coverage and therefore no need for imputation in this region. This table aims to serve as a guide to help select the best technology for the problem at hand. ++ indicates the best score on the parameter, + indicates a good score, - indicates a bad score, - - indicates the worst score on the parameters. Depending on the specific purpose, the weight of the parameters in the selection of the appropriate technology may vary.

		SNV Panel		**Short-Read Seq**			**Long-Read Seq**	
		PGx Panel	**Whole Genome Panel**	**PGx Panel**	**WES**	**WGS**	**PGx Panel**	**WGS**
Turnaround Time Wetlab *		++	+	+	+	+/-	-	- -
Haplotype phasing	Computational	-	+/-	+	+/-	+	++	++
	Direct	-	-	-	-	-	++	++
Imputation		-	+/-	+/-	+/-	NA	NA	NA
Coverage of PGx variation		+	+/-	++	+/-	++	++	++
Detection of rare variants †		+	+	++	+/-	++	++	++
Detection of variants outside the predefined gene/variant panel		- -	- -	-/+	-/+	++	++	++
Detection of structural and complex variants		- -	- -	+	+/-	+	++	++
Turnaround time data processing *		++	++	+	+	+/-	-	- -
Costs ‡ [29]	Investment	++	+	-	-	-	-	-
	Running costs per sample	+/-	++	+/-	+/-	-	+/-	-

† For SNV panels, it is assumed that the variants are present in the selected variant panel. * A short turnaround time is indicated by the +. ‡ Lower costs are indicated by the +.

2.1. Commercial Arrays

There are many arrays available that can be used for PGx; a full overview of these arrays is beyond the scope of this review. Two of the smaller commercial arrays are the VeraCode ADME core panel (Illumina Inc. San Diego, CA, USA) and the VeriDose core panel (Agena BioScience, San Diego, CA, USA). The VeraCode consists of 184 variants in 34 pharmacogenes [20] and the Veridose contains 68 variants in 20 genes and 5 copy number targets for CYP2D6 [30]. The ADME core variant list is based on an expert gene panel and contains the most biologically relevant variants within these genes [20,31]. For the VeriDose, genes with a known clinical impact and their common clinically actionable variants are selected. Additionally, it is possible to expand the panel if so desired [30]. Both panels provide sufficient coverage for clinical PGx by covering the most common variants in actionable pharmacogenes. More extensive panels are the pharmacofocus with (2000 variants in 150 genes including CNVs (Copy Number Variants) (ThermoFisher Scientific, Waltham, MA, USA) [32] and the pharmacoscan with 4627 variants in 1191 genes (ThermoFisher Scientific) [22]. The latter contain nearly all variants from the DMET and Illumina ADME core panel, in addition to all genes and variants with clinical annotations in CPIC and PharmGKB (Pharmacogenomics knowledge base), HLA genes and sample ID and tracking markers. These types of arrays are widely used in clinical PGx implementation studies. For example, the DMET array is used in the PG4KDS study from St. Jude's children's research hospital [3] and the VeraCode ADME core panel is used in the PREDICT study [33]. Both these studies use only a subset of the variants available on the panel for the clinical implementation part of the studies [3,33]. Only the variants in the genes of interest and the variants with sufficient data are reported for clinical practice. The remainder of the genetic data is, with informed consent permission, stored and can be used for research purposes or for later clinical use. For a full overview of studies using PGx panel approaches, we refer to previous publications providing such an overview [11,34].

2.2. Custom Arrays

Several of the commercial arrays contain a high number of variants, making a fast turnaround time and interpretation challenging. Additionally, these arrays will include variants which may not be of direct interest in a clinical setting as panels often include all known PGx variants regardless of the level of evidence supporting their clinical utility. This has driven many institutions to develop their own custom clinical array with a more focused set of clinically actionable variants. Typically, these custom arrays are performed using single gene-based testing covering only the variants with direct clinical applicability yet limiting broad applicability. To be able to test a broad set of variants while maintaining a rapid turnaround time, companies have developed customizable arrays. One example frequently used for clinical PGx is the OpenArray (Thermofisher scientific). This array can detect between 12 and 240 variants using standard TaqMan technology [35]. Selected TaqMan assays are spotted on a chip based on the clients need. Each chip contains wells for the patient samples; in each of these wells, through-holes are present which contain the assays desired. This format allows for a thorough characterization of a few genes as well as for a broader approach focused on a panel of common variants in multiple genes. This array has been used in clinical implementation studies as well. For example, in the INGENIOUS study it was used to interrogate a panel of 43 variants in 14 genes [36]. A similar approach was used by the Ubiquitous pharmacogenomics (U-PGx) consortium. The U-PGx consortium's initiated the PREPARE study aimed at collecting evidence of the clinical utility of a pre-emptive PGx panel consisting of 58 SNVs in 14 pharmacogenes [34]. The panel covers the most common variants in all actionable genes included in the DPWG guidelines [37] and is analyzed with KASP technology using the SNPline (LGC) [38].

2.3. Array Developments

The above-mentioned commercial and custom arrays are developed specifically for PGx. However, there are also multiple arrays with genome-wide coverage available. An added benefit of genome wide arrays is that they also allow for GWAS (Genome Wide Association Study) analysis in addition to providing PGx information. Examples of such arrays are the Illumina GSA (Global Screening Array) which contains over 600,000 SNVs genome-wide, including 17,750 PGx markers [39] and the Axiom arrays (Thermofisher scientific), which contain genome-wide coverage specifically for a certain population [40]. Nonetheless, these arrays often miss dense coverage of PGx regions and not all critical SNVs are available on the array. For example, in the case of the GSA v3.0, the SNVs for CYP2D6*4 and CYP2C19*9 and target CNV testing are not included. This is particularly concerning for the *CYP2D6* gene. The CYP2D6 enzyme is responsible for 25–30% of commonly prescribed drugs, making sufficient coverage on variants on the *CYP2D6* gene clinical important [41]. The *CYP2D6*4* allele is the most frequent null-allele in Caucasians, with the key SNV (rs3892097; NC_000022.11:g.42128945C>T) occurring in 19% of the European (non-Finnish) population [42,43]. Additionally, the GSA v3.0 does not contain probes for direct CNV detection.

3. Next Generation Sequencing

3.1. Next Generation Sequencing Technologies

NGS technologies are not yet routinely applied in clinical PGx. However, they are often used in PGx research and disease genetics. While SNV panels only cover a limited set of selected variants, sequencing data cover the full exome or genome. Technical details of NGS technologies have been extensively reviewed elsewhere [44–46]. In short, NGS technologies are capable of sequencing reads of 100–200 bp in a high throughput manner, allowing for the sequencing of a full genome in a matter of hours. These reads are aligned to the reference genome and variants are identified based on deviations from the reference.

NGS applications can be roughly categorized into three approaches. First, whole exome sequencing (WES) focusing on sequencing the coding regions of the genome, covering approximately 1–2% of the entire genome. Secondly, whole genome sequencing (WGS) which is aimed at sequencing the entire genome, both coding and non-coding regions. Lastly, targeted sequencing of a region or panel of genes of interest [44–46]. While NGS can be performed at relatively low costs, the large amount of data makes processing more challenging (Table 2).

3.2. Use of NGS for Pharmacogenomics

While NGS has become the standard for clinical diagnostics and in research, it is yet to be widely adopted for clinical PGx. Nonetheless, in a research setting NGS has been used for PGx for several years. Multiple studies have been conducted investigating the accuracy of NGS technologies in PGx as well as the applicability of an NGS sequencing panel or of the repurposing of clinical NGS data for PGx [9,10,47–51]. Yang et al. performed a three-way analysis with the DMET, WES and WGS, to investigate the concordance between PGx genotyping calls based on these different technologies. They showed a 94% concordance between the DMET and WES, and a 96% concordance between the DMET and WGS [47]. Similar results were reported by other groups, all of which report the superior results obtained from sequencing compared to orthogonal testing [49–53]. The difference in concordance between WES and the DMET array (94%), and WGS and the DMET array (96%) can be explained by the genomic coverage of each approach. WES only covers the exons and can therefore, by definition, not cover all relevant variants if they are located in the intronic or intergenic regions. WGS, on the other hand, also covers intronic regions leading to an expanded coverage. Nonetheless, intronic variants are of clinical importance in PGx. For example, one of the key *CYP2C19**17 variants (rs12248560; NC_000010.11:g.94761900C>T) is located upstream of the *CYP2C19* locus. Other examples are *CYP3A5**3 and *5 as well as *CYP2D6**4 and *41 [54]. A targeted sequencing approach can combine the lower costs of WES with the advances of WGS data. This type of panel only captures genes of interest, both intronic and exonic regions. This results in lower costs while maintaining the accuracy and abundance of data of WGS. One such approach is the PGRNseq panel [52]. This panel is based on full-gene sequencing of a panel of 84 pharmacogenes using NGS, it has also been used in clinical implementation studies showing promising results [49,55]. Another approach is the PGxSeq panel described by Gulilat et al., which covers 100 pharmacogenes [56].

3.3. Repurposing of Clinical Genetics Data

The abovementioned approaches are aimed at generating novel sequencing data with the goal of providing PGx results, whether it be panel, WES or WGS-based. However, in clinical diagnostics, the use of NGS is already standard practice in many centers leading to vast amounts of sequencing data. Several groups have investigated the feasibility of repurposing these data for PGx, by extracting a panel of evidence-based PGx variants from the data and translating this into a clinically applicable result [9,10]. The same type of analysis is performed for large populations studies, such as the Estonian biobank [8], the University of Colorado [57], SWEDEGENE [7] and the AllofUs initiative [58,59]. Unfortunately, the utility of the repurposing of data is dependent on the capture panel used in the original sequencing. This is particularly a problem in the use of WES data, as mentioned above, several important PGx variants are located in intronic regions which are not included in WES capture kits [54]. Nonetheless, even with these limitations, high percentages (>85%) of individuals with actionable phenotypes are identified [9,10,60], but one should bear in mind that important variants are missing.

4. Long-Read Sequencing

4.1. Long-Read Sequencing

Long-read sequencing technologies have emerged in the playing field and are slowly gaining ground over the short-read approaches in the field of research [46,61]. Both Pacific Bioscience (PacBio) technology as well as Oxford Nanopore Technologies (ONT) are becoming an integrated part of genetic approaches [12]. PacBio uses SMRT (single molecule real-time)-sequencing to be able to sequence reads up to 45 kB. SMRT cells make use of microwells, each of which contains one single strand of DNA which is then sequenced by assembly and recorded in real time [62]. Oxford Nanopore Technologies uses nanopores through which the DNA strand is pulled, the disruption in the current is specific to a codon, allowing for the full assembly of the DNA sequence [63]. By correcting for the randomly distributed errors in single cell sequencing, the consensus reads can obtain very high accuracy [12,62,64]. While an abundance of data can be generated by long-read sequencing, the processing is significantly more intensive compared to SNV panels and NGS (Table 2).

4.2. Long-Read Sequencing for PGx

Long-read sequencing has been shown to be capable of solving complex loci genome wide [12,64]. Current disease diagnostics already use long-read sequencing for complex genetic diseases such as the *ATXN10* repeats in Parkinson's disease [65] and tandem repeats in the *FMR1* gene associated with Fragile X syndrome [66]. Nonetheless, only a few long-read sequencing studies for pharmacogenes have been conducted. The most thoroughly investigated complex locus in PGx is the *CYP2D6* gene, which contains both SNVs and SVs. (Structural Variants) It has been shown that with long-read sequencing, the *CYP2D6* locus (~6.6 kbp) can be sequenced in one full read and be fully resolved into phased haplotypes, including structural variants [67,68]. The same has been observed for the notoriously complex HLA genes [12,64]. Long-read sequencing in PGx is currently, to our knowledge, limited to single gene studies and no large-scale studies applying long-read sequencing for clinical PGx to a panel of genes have been conducted.

5. Challenges

5.1. Drug Metabolizer Phenotype Inference

Prior to application in clinical practice, SNV data are translated into predicted drug metabolizer phenotypes. Many of the arrays mentioned above are developed based on the SNVs which are present in the genotype nomenclature. For CYP enzymes, haplotypes are named with the star (*) nomenclature [42,69]. All variants making up a *-allele are described by the Pharmacogene variation Consortium (PharmVar, https://www.pharmvar.org). The combination of the two *-alleles present in an individual is subsequently translated into a predicted drug metabolizer phenotype. For most pharmacogenes, there are four metabolizer phenotypes: normal metabolizers (NMs) displaying full protein function, intermediate metabolizers (IMs) associated with decreased protein function, poor metabolizers (PMs) indicating absence of protein function and ultra-rapid metabolizers (UMs), which are associated with increased enzyme function.

Depending on the number of variants and the presence of the variants in translation guidelines, the interpretation is relatively straightforward. However, if there are many variants leading to *-haplotypes of unknown function present on the array, the interpretation is challenging. Furthermore, PharmVar describes the *-haplotypes extensively, defining large numbers haplotypes and sub haplotypes which are constantly increasing. In theory, all variants defined by PharmVar at a certain point in time could be included on an SNV panel. Nonetheless, with over 2000 variants known in CYP2D6 alone, this would quickly grow to a very large panel which is difficult to apply and interpret in clinical practice [42]. As there is no standardization in regard to the variants which need to be tested in a clinical setting, every array contains its own set of variants. This can lead to differences in regard to assigned haplotypes when testing the same DNA in different laboratories [49]. For example, results from the pharmacoscan (4627 variants) will be much more extensive and detailed compared to the VeriDose Core panel (68 variants) [22,30]. The pharmacoscan analysis might also result in more variants and haplotypes of unknown effect while, on the other hand, the VeriDose core panel might miss variants with a known effect.

The use of sequencing data enables the inclusion of almost every known variant in the *-haplotype assignments and subsequently into predicted phenotypes. However, with this abundance of variant data comes an increased difficulty in haplotype assignments. Several tools have been developed to assign *-allele haplotypes based on sequencing data, incorporating all variants in the assignment. Yet, as Caspar et al. have shown, these tools are not performing perfectly with errors in the assigned haplotypes compared to the consensus genotype from GeT-RM [60]. An error is here defined as a haplotype assignment which differs from the consensus. The best performing tool was Aldy [70] with 2 out of 21 errors. Astrolab [71] and Stargazer [72] both performed worse with 9 and 10 errors, respectively. Similar results were reported by Twesigomwe et al. in a CYP2D6 specific study [73]. All tools use the variants and *-allele translation in PharmVar as their database. However, PharmVar is updated continuously leading to potential differences in assignments if not every tool is updated at the same time. Additionally, depending on the data on which the tools are trained and tested, they might be more sensitive for specific variants and alleles [60]. Even the most extensive tools in regard to *-haplotype calling might not be suitable for clinical practice as they contain variants of which the effect is unknown. Furthermore, for clinical implementation only, the variants of known functional effect are relevant, resulting in a need for translation tools focused on clinical implementation only. However, selecting which variants are of direct clinical relevance remains challenging and requires attention and standardization [37,74]. SNV panels are usually designed to contain known variants, often with known clinical effect. This makes them easy to implement in clinical practice with standardized variant to haplotype translations. Sequencing data, on the other hand, contain more variant information and allow for the extraction of additional variants should they become of interest. Therefore, sequencing based translations can be updated with the development of more guidelines and insights into variant effects. Nonetheless, this does come with more intense data processing.

5.2. Imputation

To expand the number of interrogated SNVs, imputation can be used for technologies that do not cover the entire genome (Table 2). Imputation is predominantly used in GWAS analysis and to expand the PGx panel in genome wide arrays [8]. With imputation, the presence of a genomic variant is inferred based on the absence or presence of a linked SNV. These predictions all come with a probability for the occurrence of the SNV of interest. Often only imputations with a high probability are included (e.g., >90%) to avoid inaccurate assignments. Reisberg et al. have shown that imputation accuracies as high as 99% can be reached for PGx variants [8]. Nevertheless, a probability of 90% also means that there is a 10% change that the imputed variant is not correct. While this is certainly acceptable for population studies, it is not sufficient for tailoring drug treatment in an individual patient. Furthermore, to reach high imputation accuracy, an imputation dataset specific to each patient's ethnical background is needed as the level of linkage disequilibrium (LD) between two SNVs can differ between different populations [8,75]. One clear example of the differences in LD between populations is the HLA tagging SNVs; to identify the HLA-A*3101 allele, associated with carbamazepine toxicity, a linked SNV is used. In Caucasians, the rs1061235 (NC_000006.12:g.29945521A>T) variant is in full LD with the *3101 haplotype, therefore the presence of the HLA-A*3101 allele can be inferred based on the presence of the rs1061235 variant [76]. However, in the Asian population, this variant is not in LD with the *3101 allele. For individuals of Asian descent, the rs1633021 (NC_000006.12:g.29779092T>C) variant can be used as a linked SNV as this variant is in LD with HLA-A*3101 in this population [77]. Using the Caucasian-linked SNV in the wrong population can lead to errors in the inferred haplotype, phenotype and ultimately lead to treatment errors. Therefore, the application of imputation should be limited to research purposes until the reliability for an individual patient has been proven.

5.3. Haplotype Phasing

In addition to variant expansion, imputation can also be used for haplotype phasing (Table 2). With haplotype phasing it can be determined if variants are located on the same allele or if they are on different alleles, potentially leading to differences in phenotype assignment [10,75,78]. The problem of phasing only exists when >1 heterozygous variant is present. However, given the polymorphic nature of many pharmacogenes, the likelihood of identifying multiple heterozygous variants within the gene locus of interest is highly likely [79]. The *-nomenclature is designed to describe only the variants in one allele, assuming that the variants have been phased into two separate alleles. Nonetheless, there are no clear guidelines available describing in what manner variants should be assigned to either one of the alleles. Both CPIC and the DPWG report which diplotypes translate into which phenotypes and occasionally which variants are needed to assign a specific haplotype but not on the phasing of variants. Haplotype phasing can, however, make the difference between a Poor Metabolizer (two loss-of-function variants on different alleles) and an Intermediate Metabolizer (two loss-of-function variants on the same allele and no variants on the other allele). Especially since many pharmacogenomic haplotypes are characterized by multiple variants, in theory all of them can have an impact on protein function. Including phasing in pharmacogenomics can, in some patients, improve haplotype assignments and therefore phenotype prediction. One example is the *CYP2B6* gene for which phasing has been shown to be relevant [10]. When the rs3745274 (NC_000019.10:g.41006936G>T) and the rs2279343 (NC_000019.10:g.41009358A>G) variant are both detected, conventional methods assume they are located on the same allele based on linkage disequilibrium and assign a *6 haplotype (Figure 1). Additionally, *CYP2B6**6 is the more common haplotype in most populations. The *CYP2B6**6 haplotype occurs around 10% in Asians and up to 40% in the African population. *CYP2B6**4 and *9 occur between 0 and 5% in all populations [80]. Clinical data show that in 1.5% of the individuals who carry both these variants, they are located on different alleles, resulting in a *4/*9 haplotype. In this case, both a *CYP2B6**1/*6 and a *CYP2B6**4/*9 call result in the same phenotype making the clinical impact limited [5]. However, for other variants, this might not be the case. Imputation could be used to infer haplotype phasing, by using the linkage between two observed SNVs to predict if they are located on the same allele or on different alleles. Nevertheless, the same limitations to imputation as described above apply [10].

With NGS, it is possible to phase read to their allele of origin without the need for pedigree information or computational phasing. For NGS, linked reads can be used for this purpose. Linked-read sequencing is based on partitioning the DNA with barcoded gel beads resulting in barcoded short fragments which can then be sequenced with conventional short-read methods. Due to the barcodes, every read can be linked back to the original position and artificial long input DNA can be reconstructed [81]. For long-read sequencing, the length of the reads in itself can be utilized for haplotype phasing. By overlapping the long-reads, large haploblocks can be formed. Nonetheless, large regions which are homozygous can cause an inability to phase large haploblocks [64].

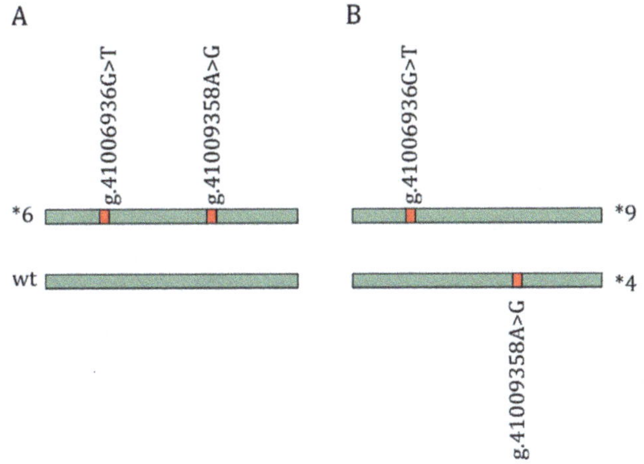

Figure 1. Haplotype phasing in CYP2B6. Inability to phase the rs3745274 (NC_000019.10:g.41006936G>T) and the rs2279343 (NC_000019.10:g.41009358A>G) to the correct allele can result in differences in *-haplotype assignment. Panel (**A**) shows the most common situation in individuals who are heterozygous for both variants, the CYP2B6*1/*6 diplotype. Panel (**B**) shows the alternative conformation where variants are located on opposing alleles leading to a CYP2B6*4/*9 diplotype. Both situations result in the same predicted CYP2B6 metabolizer phenotype (intermediate metabolizer). Conventional methods using linkage disequilibrium assume the variants to be located on the same allele, resulting in a CYP2B6*6 assignment. wt: Wild type.

5.4. Structural Variants

It has been shown that the majority of pharmacogenes is largely characterized by complex regions, such as CNVs, structural rearrangements and repetitive sections (Table 1) [82]. Full gene deletions or duplications of *CYP2D6* occur in 5–10% of the population [83]. Nonetheless, not all arrays contain probes that can directly detect CNVs. To still be able to obtain CNV data from microarrays, several tools are available. Examples of these types of tools are PennCNV [84], QuantiSNP [85], GenoCN [86] and Nexus [87]. These tools make use of the B allele frequency and the log R ratio which are extracted from the array data. SNP array make use of common SNPs indicated by an A or B (allele) variant. In a normal situation of two copies, there is either an AA, AB or BB at a specific locus. The presence of a deletion or a duplication can be derived from an aberrant number of either an A or a B allele frequency, which is reflected in the B allele frequency parameter. The log R ratio is the log of the ratio between observed and expected intensity values at each variant. It reflects the intensity of the signal at each variant site, a deviation from the expected intensity signal. [88,89]. While results seem promising [8], full validation of these tools for PGx is still needed.

NGS data can resolve all SNVs in the sequenced region, nevertheless, it is difficult to assess CNVs based on sequencing data alone. To aid CNV calling with NGS, several tools have been developed; XHMM [90], CoNIFER [91], Varseq [92] and CNVnator [93], all of which use sequencing depth as an indication of a gene deletion or duplication. These tools do require large datasets and a sufficient range in depth to identify CNVs; details of the use of sequencing depth for CNV calling have been reviewed previously [90,94,95]. Yao et al. tested these three tools on their performance on CNVs of different sizes. Unfortunately, the agreement between the methods was low and there was a bias towards the smaller CNVs as opposed to large CNVs, potentially caused by the limitations of read length [94]. Nonetheless, the advancements in this field evolve rapidly, leading to several laboratories which are now able to reliably identify CNV based on short-read sequencing data. Efforts of using sequencing based CNV calling for *CYP2D6* have shown mixed results [51,56]. Cohn et al. were able to accurately determine CNV status for 87 out of 98 patients. For nine, the CNV calls were inconclusive, and for a further two, there was a discrepant call between sequencing-based CNV calling and a targeted panel [51]. Gulilat et al., including 235 subjects, were able to confirm all sequencing-based CNV variants with panel-based testing [56].

The distinction between a pharmacogene and a pseudogene can be even more challenging. For example, *CYP2D6* and *CYP2D7* share >98% of their sequence, making it difficult to determine from which gene a sequencing read originates [67,96,97]. Due to the relatively short reads (100–200 bp), these complex regions cannot always be well characterized by NGS as reads are not long enough to distinguish between different locations in the complex region [98]. Long-read sequencing, on the other hand, allows for unambiguous mapping of a sequence to the gene of origin without interference of pseudogenes. Additionally, complex regions can be solved in one long read. Indels (deletions or duplications of 1–1000 base pairs) cannot always be accurately determined with short reads as the indel length might surpass the maximum read length. With a read length around 10 kbp in long-read sequencing any structural variants within this maximum length can be covered in one read [64,67,68].

The detection of CNVs in *CYP2D6* is routine in clinical practice. However, the full characterization of the complexity of pharmacogenes is still in the research phase, relying on the further development of long-read sequencing and bioinformatic tools.

5.5. Variants of Unknown Effect

A clear benefit of sequencing over SNV panels is the increase in the number of variants that can be identified. While SNV-panel approaches remain limited to the pre-selected variants, sequencing data can help identify variants in the entire sequenced region, including rare variants (Table 2). As mentioned previously, over 90% of the identified variants in pharmacogenes are classified as a rare variant [99–101] (Table 1). Additionally, rare variants are expected to be more deleterious than common variants resulting in a potential higher impact on protein function [82]. To collect the most data on rare and novel variants, a WGS or targeted whole gene sequencing approach would be most suitable. Nevertheless, due to a lack of knowledge regarding the impact of these variants, they cannot yet be applied in clinical practice [83,98,101–103]. As they are by definition not commonly observed, it is difficult to assign a functional effect. Several strategies have been proposed to detect the impact of rare variants, of which the most common options are the use of cell-line models, in silico predictions or by studying patients displaying the most extreme phenotypes [104]. For clinical application, in vivo studies are most suitable. However, due to the low frequency of these variants, it is nearly impossible to have an appropriate sample size to study these variants [99,105]. In vitro analyses are more easily accessible and generally show a good indication of the effect of a particular variant. Nonetheless, in vitro findings can deviate from the in vivo situation and can still be too laborious for high throughput analyses. Therefore, for high throughput variant predictions, the in silico approach is most desirable. In silico models are based on sequence conservation, the physiochemical and crystal structure of the protein, or on evolutionary scores [102,106]. One, or a combination, of these factors is used to predict the impact the variant will have on enzyme function. To assess the applicability of in silico tools in pharmacogenetics, Han et al. conducted a study to test the accuracy of these tools. They showed that for 10 selected SNPs, the best models accurately predicted the functionality of 80% of the SNPs [107]. In addition, Hao et al. showed that 68% of non-synonymous SNPs in phase II enzyme genes were correctly predicted to be damaging [108]. These results indicate that the applicability of these assays is still limited. Ultimately, collecting more genetic, accompanying clinical data and better prediction models can help us understand the role of these rare variants to be able to use them in clinical practice.

5.6. Pharmacogenomics and Disease Genes

Moreover, variants that are disease predictors can be encountered. Complex examples of this are genes which are both pharmacogenes as well as disease-causing genes. *RYR1* is linked to an increased risk of malignant hyperthermia which could classify it as a disease gene and, as such, it is included in the ACMG guidelines [109]. However, one of the factors that could cause the MH in susceptible patients is volatile anesthetics which could classify *RYR1* as a pharmacogene, as well as it interacting with drugs [110].

In summary, the number of available genotyping technologies for PGx has evolved rapidly in recent years and continues to expand. Ultimately, selecting the right technology is not a matter of fact but a matter of choosing the right technique for the right problem.

Author Contributions: Writing—original draft preparation, M.v.d.L. and J.J.S.; writing—review and editing, H.-J.G. and M.K. All authors have read and agreed to the published version of the manuscript.

References

1. Kirchheiner, J.; Brøsen, K.; Dahl, M.L.; Gram, L.F.; Kasper, S.; Roots, I.; Sjöqvist, F.; Spina, E.; Brockmöller, J. CYP2D6 and CYP2C19 genotype-based dose recommendations for antidepressants: A first step towards subpopulation-specific dosages. *Acta Psychiatr. Scand.* **2001**, *104*, 173–192. [CrossRef] [PubMed]
2. Swen, J.J.; Wilting, I.; de Goede, A.L.; Grandia, L.; Mulder, H.; Touw, D.J.; de Boer, A.; Conemans, J.M.; Egberts, T.C.; Klungel, O.H.; et al. Pharmacogenetics: From bench to byte. *Clin. Pharmacol. Ther.* **2008**, *83*, 781–787. [CrossRef] [PubMed]
3. Hoffman, J.M.; Haidar, C.E.; Wilkinson, M.R.; Crews, K.R.; Baker, D.K.; Kornegay, N.M.; Yang, W.; Pui, C.H.; Reiss, U.M.; Gaur, A.H.; et al. PG4KDS: A model for the clinical implementation of pre-emptive pharmacogenetics. *Am. J. Med. Genet. C Semin. Med. Genet.* **2014**, *166c*, 45–55. [CrossRef]
4. Dutch Pharmacogenetics Working group. *Pharmacogenetics Guidelines*; Royal Dutch Pharmacists Association (KNMP Kennisbank): The Hague, The Netherlands, 2020.
5. Clinical Pharmacogenetics Implementation Consortium. CPIC-guidelines. Available online: https://cpicpgx.org/ (accessed on 16 October 2020).
6. National Human Genome Research Institute. DNA Sequencing Costs: Data. Available online: https://www.genome.gov/about-genomics/fact-sheets/DNA-Sequencing-Costs-Data (accessed on 16 October 2020).
7. Hallberg, P.; Yue, Q.Y.; Eliasson, E.; Melhus, H.; Ås, J.; Wadelius, M. SWEDEGENE-a Swedish nation-wide DNA sample collection for pharmacogenomic studies of serious adverse drug reactions. *Pharm. J.* **2020**, *20*, 579–585. [CrossRef] [PubMed]
8. Reisberg, S.; Krebs, K.; Kals, M.; Magi, R.; Metsalu, K.; Lauschke, V.M.; Vilo, J.; Milani, L. Translating genotype data of 44,000 biobank participants into clinical pharmacogenetic recommendations: Challenges and solutions. *Genet. Med.* **2019**, *21*, 1345–1354. [CrossRef]
9. Cousin, M.A.; Matey, E.T.; Blackburn, P.R.; Boczek, N.J.; McAllister, T.M.; Kruisselbrink, T.M.; Babovic-Vuksanovic, D.; Lazaridis, K.N.; Klee, E.W. Pharmacogenomic findings from clinical whole exome sequencing of diagnostic odyssey patients. *Mol. Genet. Genom. Med.* **2017**, *5*, 269–279. [CrossRef]
10. Van der Lee, M.; Allard, W.G.; Bollen, S.; Santen, G.W.E.; Ruivenkamp, C.A.L.; Hoffer, M.J.V.; Kriek, M.; Guchelaar, H.J.; Anvar, S.Y.; Swen, J.J. Repurposing of Diagnostic Whole Exome Sequencing Data of 1,583 Individuals for Clinical Pharmacogenetics. *Clin. Pharmacol. Ther.* **2020**, *107*, 617–627. [CrossRef]
11. Krebs, K.; Milani, L. Translating pharmacogenomics into clinical decisions: Do not let the perfect be the enemy of the good. *Hum. Genom.* **2019**, *13*, 39. [CrossRef]
12. Ameur, A.; Kloosterman, W.P.; Hestand, M.S. Single-molecule sequencing: Towards clinical applications. *Trends Biotechnol.* **2019**, *37*, 72–85. [CrossRef]
13. Sakamoto, Y.; Sereewattanawoot, S.; Suzuki, A. A new era of long-read sequencing for cancer genomics. *J Hum. Genet.* **2020**, *65*, 3–10. [CrossRef]
14. Aganezov, S.; Goodwin, S.; Sherman, R.M.; Sedlazeck, F.J.; Arun, G.; Bhatia, S.; Lee, I.; Kirsche, M.; Wappel, R.; Kramer, M.; et al. Comprehensive analysis of structural variants in breast cancer genomes using single-molecule sequencing. *Genome Res.* **2020**, *30*, 1258–1273. [CrossRef] [PubMed]
15. Sakamoto, Y.; Xu, L.; Seki, M.; Yokoyama, T.T.; Kasahara, M.; Kashima, Y.; Ohashi, A.; Shimada, Y.; Motoi, N.; Tsuchihara, K.; et al. Long-read sequencing for non-small-cell lung cancer genomes. *Genome Res.* **2020**, *30*, 1243–1257. [CrossRef] [PubMed]

16. Just, K.S.; Steffens, M.; Swen, J.J.; Patrinos, G.P.; Guchelaar, H.J.; Stingl, J.C. Medical education in pharmacogenomics-results from a survey on pharmacogenetic knowledge in healthcare professionals within the European pharmacogenomics clinical implementation project Ubiquitous Pharmacogenomics (U-PGx). *Eur. J. Clin. Pharmacol.* **2017**, *73*, 1247–1252. [CrossRef] [PubMed]
17. Rollinson, V.; Turner, R.; Pirmohamed, M. Pharmacogenomics for Primary Care: An Overview. *Genes* **2020**, *11*, 1337. [CrossRef]
18. Bank, P.C.D.; Swen, J.J.; Guchelaar, H.J. Implementation of Pharmacogenomics in Everyday Clinical Settings. *Stud. Surf. Sci. Catal.* **2018**, *83*, 219–246. [CrossRef]
19. PharmGKB. DPWG: Dutch Pharmacogenetics Working Group. Available online: https://www.pharmgkb.org/page/dpwg (accessed on 23 June 2020).
20. Illumina Inc. VeraCode ADME Core Panel. Available online: https://www.illumina.com/documents/products/datasheets/datasheet_veracode_adme_core_panel.pdf (accessed on 21 July 2020).
21. Arbitrio, M.; Di Martino, M.T.; Scionti, F.; Agapito, G.; Guzzi, P.H.; Cannataro, M.; Tassone, P.; Tagliaferri, P. DMET™ (Drug Metabolism Enzymes and Transporters): A pharmacogenomic platform for precision medicine. *Oncotarget* **2016**, *7*, 54028–54050. [CrossRef]
22. ThermoFisher Scientific. Pharmacoscan Assay. Available online: https://www.thermofisher.com/order/catalog/product/903010TS (accessed on 16 October 2020).
23. Gabriel, S.; Ziaugra, L.; Tabbaa, D. SNP genotyping using the Sequenom MassARRAY iPLEX platform. *Curr. Protoc. Hum. Genet.* **2009**. [CrossRef]
24. Spierings, G.; Dunbar, S.A. Pharmacogenetics using Luminex(R) xMAP(R) technology: A method for developing a custom multiplex single nucleotide polymorphism mutation assay. *Methods Mol. Biol.* **2013**, *1015*, 115–126. [CrossRef]
25. Chen, C.; Li, S.; Lu, X.; Tan, B.; Huang, C.; Qin, L. High resolution melting method to detect single nucleotide polymorphism of VKORC1 and CYP2C9. *Int. J. Clin. Exp. Pathol.* **2014**, *7*, 2558–2564.
26. Jannetto, P.J.; Laleli-Sahin, E.; Wong, S.H. Pharmacogenomic genotyping methodologies. *Clin. Chem. Lab. Med.* **2004**, *42*, 1256–1264. [CrossRef]
27. Ghasemi, Z.; Hashemi, M.; Ejabati, M.; Ebrahimi, S.M.; Kheiri Manjili, H.; Sharafi, A.; Ramazani, A. Development of a High-Resolution Melting Analysis Method for CYP2C19*17 Genotyping in Healthy Volunteers. *Avicenna J. Med. Biotechnol.* **2016**, *8*, 193–199. [PubMed]
28. Mukerjee, G.; Huston, A.; Kabakchiev, B.; Piquette-Miller, M.; van Schaik, R.; Dorfman, R. User considerations in assessing pharmacogenomic tests and their clinical support tools. *NPJ Genom. Med.* **2018**, *3*, 26. [CrossRef] [PubMed]
29. Vilella, A. Next-Generation-Sequencing, v1.5.7. Available online: https://docs.google.com/spreadsheets/d/1GMMfhyLK0-q8XkIo3YxlWaZA5vVMuhU1kg41g4xLkXc/htmlview?hl=en_GB (accessed on 27 October 2020).
30. Agenda Bioscience. VeriDose Core Panel. Available online: https://agenabio.com/products/panel/veridose-core-panel/ (accessed on 2 November 2020).
31. Huang, S.M.; Goodsaid, F.; Rahman, A.; Frueh, F.; Lesko, L.J. Application of pharmacogenomics in clinical pharmacology. *Toxicol. Mech. Methods.* **2006**, *16*, 89–99. [CrossRef] [PubMed]
32. ThermoFisher Scientifuic. Axiom Pharmacofocus. Available online: https://www.thermofisher.com/order/catalog/product/952425?SID=srch-hj-952425#/952425?SID=srch-hj-952425 (accessed on 3 November 2020).
33. Pulley, J.M.; Denny, J.C.; Peterson, J.F.; Bernard, G.R.; Vnencak-Jones, C.L.; Ramirez, A.H.; Delaney, J.T.; Bowton, E.; Brothers, K.; Johnson, K.; et al. Operational implementation of prospective genotyping for personalized medicine: The design of the Vanderbilt PREDICT project. *Clin. Pharmacol. Ther.* **2012**, *92*, 87–95. [CrossRef]
34. Van der Wouden, C.H.; Cambon-Thomsen, A.; Cecchin, E.; Cheung, K.C.; Davila-Fajardo, C.L.; Deneer, V.H.; Dolzan, V.; Ingelman-Sundberg, M.; Jonsson, S.; Karlsson, M.O.; et al. Implementing Pharmacogenomics in Europe: Design and Implementation Strategy of the Ubiquitous Pharmacogenomics Consortium. *Clin. Pharmacol. Ther.* **2017**, *101*, 341–358. [CrossRef]
35. ThermoFisher Scientific. Open Array Technology Overview. Available online: https://www.thermofisher.com/nl/en/home/life-science/pcr/real-time-pcr/real-time-openarray/open-array-technology.html (accessed on 3 November 2020).

36. Eadon, M.T.; Desta, Z.; Levy, K.D.; Decker, B.S.; Pierson, R.C.; Pratt, V.M.; Callaghan, J.T.; Rosenman, M.B.; Carpenter, J.S.; Holmes, A.M.; et al. Implementation of a pharmacogenomics consult service to support the INGENIOUS trial. *Clin. Pharmacol. Ther.* **2016**, *100*, 63–66. [CrossRef]
37. van der Wouden, C.H.; van Rhenen, M.H.; Jama, W.O.M.; Ingelman-Sundberg, M.; Lauschke, V.M.; Konta, L.; Schwab, M.; Swen, J.J.; Guchelaar, H.J. Development of the PGx-Passport: A Panel of Actionable Germline Genetic Variants for Pre-emptive Pharmacogenetic Testing. *Clin. Pharmacol. Ther.* **2019**, *106*, 866–873. [CrossRef]
38. Biosearch Technologies. SNPline Genotyping Automation. Available online: https://www.biosearchtech.com/products/instruments-and-consumables/genotyping-instruments/snpline-genotyping-automation (accessed on 3 November 2020).
39. Illumina Inc. Illumina Global Screening Array. Available online: https://emea.illumina.com/products/by-type/microarray-kits/infinium-global-screening.html (accessed on 23 June 2020).
40. ThermoFisher Scientific. Axiom Genotyping Solutions. Available online: https://assets.thermofisher.com/TFS-Assets/LSG/brochures/axiom_solution_brochure.pdf (accessed on 3 November 2020).
41. Ingelman-Sundberg, M. Pharmacogenetics of cytochrome P450 and its applications in drug therapy: The past, present and future. *Trends Pharmacol. Sci.* **2004**, *25*, 193–200. [CrossRef]
42. Gaedigk, A.; Ingelman-Sundberg, M.; Miller, N.A.; Leeder, J.S.; Whirl-Carrillo, M.; Klein, T.E. The Pharmacogene Variation (PharmVar) Consortium: Incorporation of the Human Cytochrome P450 (CYP) Allele Nomenclature Database. *Clin. Pharmacol. Ther.* **2018**, *103*, 399–401. [CrossRef]
43. Broadinstitute. GnomAD. Available online: https://gnomad.broadinstitute.org/ (accessed on 26 October 2020).
44. Mardis, E.R. Next-generation sequencing platforms. *Annu. Rev. Anal. Chem.* **2013**, *6*, 287–303. [CrossRef]
45. Slatko, B.E.; Gardner, A.F.; Ausubel, F.M. Overview of Next-Generation Sequencing Technologies. *Curr. Protoc. Mol. Biol.* **2018**, *122*, e59. [CrossRef] [PubMed]
46. Levy, S.E.; Myers, R.M. Advancements in Next-Generation Sequencing. *Annu. Rev. Genom. Hum. Genet.* **2016**, *17*, 95–115. [CrossRef] [PubMed]
47. Yang, W.; Wu, G.; Broeckel, U.; Smith, C.A.; Turner, V.; Haidar, C.E.; Wang, S.; Carter, R.; Karol, S.E.; Neale, G.; et al. Comparison of genome sequencing and clinical genotyping for pharmacogenes. *Clin. Pharmacol. Ther.* **2016**, *100*, 380–388. [CrossRef] [PubMed]
48. Londin, E.R.; Clark, P.; Sponziello, M.; Kricka, L.J.; Fortina, P.; Park, J.Y. Performance of exome sequencing for pharmacogenomics. *Pers. Med.* **2014**, *12*, 109–115. [CrossRef]
49. Rasmussen-Torvik, L.J.; Almoguera, B.; Doheny, K.F.; Freimuth, R.R.; Gordon, A.S.; Hakonarson, H.; Hawkins, J.B.; Husami, A.; Ivacic, L.C.; Kullo, I.J.; et al. Concordance between Research Sequencing and Clinical Pharmacogenetic Genotyping in the eMERGE-PGx Study. *J. Mol. Diagn.* **2017**, *19*, 561–566. [CrossRef]
50. Ng, D.; Hong, C.S.; Singh, L.N.; Johnston, J.J.; Mullikin, J.C.; Biesecker, L.G. Assessing the capability of massively parallel sequencing for opportunistic pharmacogenetic screening. *Genet. Med.* **2017**, *19*, 357–361. [CrossRef]
51. Cohn, I.; Paton, T.A.; Marshall, C.R.; Basran, R.; Stavropoulos, D.J.; Ray, P.N.; Monfared, N.; Hayeems, R.Z.; Meyn, M.S.; Bowdin, S.; et al. Genome sequencing as a platform for pharmacogenetic genotyping: A pediatric cohort study. *NPJ Genom. Med.* **2017**, *2*, 19. [CrossRef]
52. Gordon, A.S.; Fulton, R.S.; Qin, X.; Mardis, E.R.; Nickerson, D.A.; Scherer, S. PGRNseq: A targeted capture sequencing panel for pharmacogenetic research and implementation. *Pharm. Genom.* **2016**, *26*, 161–168. [CrossRef]
53. Chua, E.W.; Cree, S.L.; Ton, K.N.; Lehnert, K.; Shepherd, P.; Helsby, N.; Kennedy, M.A. Cross-Comparison of Exome Analysis, Next-Generation Sequencing of Amplicons, and the iPLEX((R)) ADME PGx Panel for Pharmacogenomic Profiling. *Front. Pharmacol.* **2016**, *7*, 1. [CrossRef]
54. Ingelman-Sundberg, M.; Sim, S.C. Intronic polymorphisms of cytochromes P450. *Hum. Genom.* **2010**, *4*, 402–405. [CrossRef]
55. Bush, W.S.; Crosslin, D.R.; Owusu-Obeng, A.; Wallace, J.; Almoguera, B.; Basford, M.A.; Bielinski, S.J.; Carrell, D.S.; Connolly, J.J.; Crawford, D.; et al. Genetic variation among 82 pharmacogenes: The PGRNseq data from the eMERGE network. *Pharmacol. Ther.* **2016**, *100*, 160–169. [CrossRef] [PubMed]

56. Gulilat, M.; Lamb, T.; Teft, W.A.; Wang, J.; Dron, J.S.; Robinson, J.F.; Tirona, R.G.; Hegele, R.A.; Kim, R.B.; Schwarz, U.I. Targeted next generation sequencing as a tool for precision medicine. *BMC Med. Genom.* **2019**, *12*, 81. [CrossRef] [PubMed]
57. Aquilante, C.L.; Kao, D.P.; Trinkley, K.E.; Lin, C.T.; Crooks, K.R.; Hearst, E.C.; Hess, S.J.; Kudron, E.L.; Lee, Y.M.; Liko, I.; et al. Clinical implementation of pharmacogenomics via a health system-wide research biobank: The University of Colorado experience. *Pharmacogenomics* **2020**, *21*, 375–386. [CrossRef] [PubMed]
58. National Institute of Health. AllofUs Research Program. Available online: https://allofus.nih.gov/ (accessed on 23 October 2020).
59. Precision Medicine Initiative Work Group. The Precision Medicine Initiative Cohort Program—Building a Research Foundation for 21st Century Medicine; National Institutes of Health. 2015. Available online: https://www.nih.gov/sites/default/files/research-training/initiatives/pmi/pmi-working-group-report-20150917-2.pdf (accessed on 23 October 2020).
60. Caspar, S.M.; Schneider, T.; Meienberg, J.; Matyas, G. Added Value of Clinical Sequencing: WGS-Based Profiling of Pharmacogenes. *Int. J. Mol. Sci.* **2020**, *21*, 2308. [CrossRef] [PubMed]
61. Mantere, T.; Kersten, S.; Hoischen, A. Long-Read Sequencing Emerging in Medical Genetics. *Front. Genet.* **2019**, *10*, 426. [CrossRef] [PubMed]
62. Rhoads, A.; Au, K.F. PacBio Sequencing and Its Applications. *Genom. Proteom. Bioinform.* **2015**, *13*, 278–289. [CrossRef]
63. Bowden, R.; Davies, R.W.; Heger, A.; Pagnamenta, A.T.; de Cesare, M.; Oikkonen, L.E.; Parkes, D.; Freeman, C.; Dhalla, F.; Patel, S.Y.; et al. Sequencing of human genomes with nanopore technology. *Nat. Commun.* **2019**, *10*, 1869. [CrossRef]
64. Wenger, A.M.; Peluso, P.; Rowell, W.J.; Chang, P.C.; Hall, R.J.; Concepcion, G.T.; Ebler, J.; Fungtammasan, A.; Kolesnikov, A.; Olson, N.D.; et al. Accurate circular consensus long-read sequencing improves variant detection and assembly of a human genome. *Nat. Biotechnol.* **2019**, *37*, 1155–1162. [CrossRef]
65. Schüle, B.; McFarland, K.N.; Lee, K.; Tsai, Y.C.; Nguyen, K.D.; Sun, C.; Liu, M.; Byrne, C.; Gopi, R.; Huang, N.; et al. Parkinson's disease associated with pure ATXN10 repeat expansion. *NPJ Park. Dis.* **2017**, *3*, 27. [CrossRef]
66. Ardui, S.; Race, V.; Zablotskaya, A.; Hestand, M.S.; Van Esch, H.; Devriendt, K.; Matthijs, G.; Vermeesch, J.R. Detecting AGG Interruptions in Male and Female FMR1 Premutation Carriers by Single-Molecule Sequencing. *Hum. Mutat.* **2017**, *38*, 324–331. [CrossRef]
67. Qiao, W.; Yang, Y.; Sebra, R.; Mendiratta, G.; Gaedigk, A.; Desnick, R.J.; Scott, S.A. Long-Read Single Molecule Real-Time Full Gene Sequencing of Cytochrome P450-2D6. *Hum. Mutat.* **2016**, *37*, 315–323. [CrossRef] [PubMed]
68. Buermans, H.P.; Vossen, R.H.; Anvar, S.Y.; Allard, W.G.; Guchelaar, H.J.; White, S.J.; den Dunnen, J.T.; Swen, J.J.; van der Straaten, T. Flexible and Scalable Full-Length CYP2D6 Long Amplicon PacBio Sequencing. *Hum. Mutat.* **2017**, *38*, 310–316. [CrossRef] [PubMed]
69. Robarge, J.D.; Li, L.; Desta, Z.; Nguyen, A.; Flockhart, D.A. The star-allele nomenclature: Retooling for translational genomics. *Clin. Pharmacol. Ther.* **2007**, *82*, 244–248. [CrossRef] [PubMed]
70. Numanagic, I.; Malikic, S.; Ford, M.; Qin, X.; Toji, L.; Radovich, M.; Skaar, T.C.; Pratt, V.M.; Berger, B.; Scherer, S.; et al. Allelic decomposition and exact genotyping of highly polymorphic and structurally variant genes. *Nat. Commun.* **2018**, *9*, 828. [CrossRef] [PubMed]
71. Twist, G.P.; Gaedigk, A.; Miller, N.A.; Farrow, E.G.; Willig, L.K.; Dinwiddie, D.L.; Petrikin, J.E.; Soden, S.E.; Herd, S.; Gibson, M.; et al. Constellation: A tool for rapid, automated phenotype assignment of a highly polymorphic pharmacogene, CYP2D6, from whole-genome sequences. *NPJ Genom. Med.* **2016**, *1*, 15007. [CrossRef] [PubMed]
72. Lee, S.B.; Wheeler, M.M.; Thummel, K.E.; Nickerson, D.A. Calling Star Alleles with Stargazer in 28 Pharmacogenes With Whole Genome Sequences. *Clin. Pharmacol. Ther.* **2019**, *106*, 1328–1337. [CrossRef] [PubMed]
73. Twesigomwe, D.; Wright, G.E.B.; Drögemöller, B.I.; da Rocha, J.; Lombard, Z.; Hazelhurst, S. A systematic comparison of pharmacogene star allele calling bioinformatics algorithms: A focus on CYP2D6 genotyping. *NPJ Genom. Med.* **2020**, *5*, 30. [CrossRef]
74. Pratt, V.M.; Everts, R.E.; Aggarwal, P.; Beyer, B.N.; Broeckel, U.; Epstein-Baak, R.; Hujsak, P.; Kornreich, R.; Liao, J.; Lorier, R.; et al. Characterization of 137 Genomic DNA Reference Materials for 28 Pharmacogenetic Genes: A GeT-RM Collaborative Project. *J. Mol. Diagn.* **2016**, *18*, 109–123. [CrossRef]

75. Browning, S.R.; Browning, B.L. Haplotype phasing: Existing methods and new developments. *Nat. Rev. Genet.* **2011**, *12*, 703–714. [CrossRef]
76. McCormack, M.; Alfirevic, A.; Bourgeois, S.; Farrell, J.J.; Kasperavičiūtė, D.; Carrington, M.; Sills, G.J.; Marson, T.; Jia, X.; de Bakker, P.I.; et al. HLA-A*3101 and carbamazepine-induced hypersensitivity reactions in Europeans. *N. Engl. J. Med.* **2011**, *364*, 1134–1143. [CrossRef]
77. Ozeki, T.; Mushiroda, T.; Yowang, A.; Takahashi, A.; Kubo, M.; Shirakata, Y.; Ikezawa, Z.; Iijima, M.; Shiohara, T.; Hashimoto, K.; et al. Genome-wide association study identifies HLA-A*3101 allele as a genetic risk factor for carbamazepine-induced cutaneous adverse drug reactions in Japanese population. *Hum. Mol. Genet.* **2011**, *20*, 1034–1041. [CrossRef] [PubMed]
78. Browning, S.R.; Browning, B.L. Rapid and accurate haplotype phasing and missing-data inference for whole-genome association studies by use of localized haplotype clustering. *Am. J. Hum. Genet.* **2007**, *81*, 1084–1097. [CrossRef] [PubMed]
79. Jin, Y.; Wang, J.; Bachtiar, M.; Chong, S.S.; Lee, C.G.L. Architecture of polymorphisms in the human genome reveals functionally important and positively selected variants in immune response and drug transporter genes. *Hum. Genom.* **2018**, *12*, 43. [CrossRef] [PubMed]
80. Zanger, U.M.; Klein, K.; Saussele, T.; Blievernicht, J.; Hofmann, M.H.; Schwab, M. Polymorphic CYP2B6: Molecular mechanisms and emerging clinical significance. *Pharmacogenomics* **2007**, *8*, 743–759. [CrossRef] [PubMed]
81. Zhou, X.; Batzoglou, S.; Sidow, A.; Zhang, L. HAPDeNovo: A haplotype-based approach for filtering and phasing de novo mutations in linked read sequencing data. *BMC Genom.* **2018**, *19*, 467. [CrossRef] [PubMed]
82. Ingelman-Sundberg, M.; Sim, S.C. Pharmacogenetic biomarkers as tools for improved drug therapy; emphasis on the cytochrome P450 system. *Biochem. Biophys. Res. Commun.* **2010**, *396*, 90–94. [CrossRef] [PubMed]
83. Zhou, Y.; Ingelman-Sundberg, M.; Lauschke, V.M. Worldwide distribution of cytochrome P450 alleles: A meta-analysis of population-scale sequencing projects. *Clin. Pharmacol. Ther.* **2017**, *102*, 688–700. [CrossRef]
84. Wang, K.; Li, M.; Hadley, D.; Liu, R.; Glessner, J.; Grant, S.F.; Hakonarson, H.; Bucan, M. PennCNV: An integrated hidden Markov model designed for high-resolution copy number variation detection in whole-genome SNP genotyping data. *Genome Res.* **2007**, *17*, 1665–1674. [CrossRef]
85. Colella, S.; Yau, C.; Taylor, J.M.; Mirza, G.; Butler, H.; Clouston, P.; Bassett, A.S.; Seller, A.; Holmes, C.C.; Ragoussis, J. QuantiSNP: An Objective Bayes Hidden-Markov Model to detect and accurately map copy number variation using SNP genotyping data. *Nucleic Acids Res.* **2007**, *35*, 2013–2025. [CrossRef]
86. Sun, W.; Wright, F.A.; Tang, Z.; Nordgard, S.H.; Van Loo, P.; Yu, T.; Kristensen, V.N.; Perou, C.M. Integrated study of copy number states and genotype calls using high-density SNP arrays. *Nucleic Acids Res.* **2009**, *37*, 5365–5377. [CrossRef]
87. Darvishi, K. Application of Nexus copy number software for CNV detection and analysis. *Curr. Protoc. Hum. Genet.* **2010**. [CrossRef] [PubMed]
88. Seiser, E.L.; Innocenti, F. Hidden Markov Model-Based CNV Detection Algorithms for Illumina Genotyping Microarrays. *Cancer Inform.* **2014**, *13*, 77–83. [CrossRef] [PubMed]
89. Dellinger, A.E.; Saw, S.M.; Goh, L.K.; Seielstad, M.; Young, T.L.; Li, Y.J. Comparative analyses of seven algorithms for copy number variant identification from single nucleotide polymorphism arrays. *Nucleic Acids Res.* **2010**, *38*, e105. [CrossRef]
90. Fromer, M.; Moran, J.L.; Chambert, K.; Banks, E.; Bergen, S.E.; Ruderfer, D.M.; Handsaker, R.E.; McCarroll, S.A.; O'Donovan, M.C.; Owen, M.J.; et al. Discovery and statistical genotyping of copy-number variation from whole-exome sequencing depth. *Am. J. Hum. Genet.* **2012**, *91*, 597–607. [CrossRef] [PubMed]
91. Krumm, N.; Sudmant, P.H.; Ko, A.; O'Roak, B.J.; Malig, M.; Coe, B.P.; Quinlan, A.R.; Nickerson, D.A.; Eichler, E.E. Copy number variation detection and genotyping from exome sequence data. *Genome Res.* **2012**, *22*, 1525–1532. [CrossRef] [PubMed]
92. GoldenHelix VarSeq. Available online: https://www.goldenhelix.com/products/VarSeq/ (accessed on 25 November 2020).
93. Abyzov, A.; Urban, A.E.; Snyder, M.; Gerstein, M. CNVnator: An approach to discover, genotype, and characterize typical and atypical CNVs from family and population genome sequencing. *Genome Res.* **2011**, *21*, 974–984. [CrossRef]
94. Yao, R.; Zhang, C.; Yu, T.; Li, N.; Hu, X.; Wang, X.; Wang, J.; Shen, Y. Evaluation of three read-depth based CNV detection tools using whole-exome sequencing data. *Mol. Cytogenet.* **2017**, *10*, 30. [CrossRef]

95. Tremmel, R.; Klein, K.; Battke, F.; Fehr, S.; Winter, S.; Scheurenbrand, T.; Schaeffeler, E.; Biskup, S.; Schwab, M.; Zanger, U.M. Copy number variation profiling in pharmacogenes using panel-based exome resequencing and correlation to human liver expression. *Hum. Genet.* **2019**, *139*, 137–149. [CrossRef]
96. Gaedigk, A. Complexities of CYP2D6 gene analysis and interpretation. *Int. Rev. Psychiatry* **2013**, *25*, 534–553. [CrossRef]
97. Gaedigk, A.; Jaime, L.K.; Bertino, J.S., Jr.; Berard, A.; Pratt, V.M.; Bradfordand, L.D.; Leeder, J.S. Identification of Novel CYP2D7-2D6 Hybrids: Non-Functional and Functional Variants. *Front. Pharmacol.* **2010**, *1*, 121. [CrossRef]
98. Lauschke, V.M.; Milani, L.; Ingelman-Sundberg, M. Pharmacogenomic Biomarkers for Improved Drug Therapy-Recent Progress and Future Developments. *AAPS J.* **2017**, *20*, 4. [CrossRef] [PubMed]
99. Kozyra, M.; Ingelman-Sundberg, M.; Lauschke, V.M. Rare genetic variants in cellular transporters, metabolic enzymes, and nuclear receptors can be important determinants of interindividual differences in drug response. *Genet. Med.* **2017**, *19*, 20–29. [CrossRef] [PubMed]
100. Gordon, A.S.; Tabor, H.K.; Johnson, A.D.; Snively, B.M.; Assimes, T.L.; Auer, P.L.; Ioannidis, J.P.; Peters, U.; Robinson, J.G.; Sucheston, L.E.; et al. Quantifying rare, deleterious variation in 12 human cytochrome P450 drug-metabolism genes in a large-scale exome dataset. *Hum. Mol. Genet.* **2014**, *23*, 1957–1963. [CrossRef] [PubMed]
101. Fujikura, K.; Ingelman-Sundberg, M.; Lauschke, V.M. Genetic variation in the human cytochrome P450 supergene family. *Pharm. Genom.* **2015**, *25*, 584–594. [CrossRef]
102. Drogemoller, B.I.; Wright, G.E.; Warnich, L. Considerations for rare variants in drug metabolism genes and the clinical implications. *Expert Opin. Drug Metab. Toxicol.* **2014**, *10*, 873–884. [CrossRef]
103. Ingelman-Sundberg, M.; Mkrtchian, S.; Zhou, Y.; Lauschke, V.M. Integrating rare genetic variants into pharmacogenetic drug response predictions. *Hum. Genom.* **2018**, *12*, 26. [CrossRef]
104. Lauschke, V.M.; Ingelman-Sundberg, M. Requirements for comprehensive pharmacogenetic genotyping platforms. *Pharmacogenomics* **2016**, *17*, 917–924. [CrossRef]
105. Lauschke, V.M.; Ingelman-Sundberg, M. How to Consider Rare Genetic Variants in Personalized Drug Therapy. *Clin. Pharmacol. Ther.* **2018**, *103*, 745–748. [CrossRef]
106. Li, B.; Seligman, C.; Thusberg, J.; Miller, J.L.; Auer, J.; Whirl-Carrillo, M.; Capriotti, E.; Klein, T.E.; Mooney, S.D. In silico comparative characterization of pharmacogenomic missense variants. *BMC Genom.* **2014**, *15* (Suppl. S4), S4. [CrossRef]
107. Han, S.M.; Park, J.; Lee, J.H.; Lee, S.S.; Kim, H.; Han, H.; Kim, Y.; Yi, S.; Cho, J.Y.; Jang, I.J.; et al. Targeted Next-Generation Sequencing for Comprehensive Genetic Profiling of Pharmacogenes. *Clin. Pharmacol. Ther.* **2017**, *101*, 396–405. [CrossRef]
108. Hao, D.; Xiao, P.; Chen, S. Phenotype prediction of nonsynonymous single nucleotide polymorphisms in human phase II drug/xenobiotic metabolizing enzymes: Perspectives on molecular evolution. *Sci. China Life Sci.* **2010**, *53*, 1252–1262. [CrossRef] [PubMed]
109. Kalia, S.S.; Adelman, K.; Bale, S.J.; Chung, W.K.; Eng, C.; Evans, J.P.; Herman, G.E.; Hufnagel, S.B.; Klein, T.E.; Korf, B.R.; et al. Recommendations for reporting of secondary findings in clinical exome and genome sequencing, 2016 update (ACMG SF v2.0): A policy statement of the American College of Medical Genetics and Genomics. *Genet. Med.* **2017**, *19*, 249–255. [CrossRef] [PubMed]
110. Gonsalves, S.G.; Dirksen, R.T.; Sangkuhl, K.; Pulk, R.; Alvarellos, M.; Vo, T.; Hikino, K.; Roden, D.; Klein, T.E.; Poler, S.M.; et al. Clinical Pharmacogenetics Implementation Consortium (CPIC) Guideline for the Use of Potent Volatile Anesthetic Agents and Succinylcholine in the Context of RYR1 or CACNA1S Genotypes. *Clin. Pharmacol. Ther.* **2019**, *105*, 1338–1344. [CrossRef] [PubMed]

2

Pharmacogenomics for Primary Care

Victoria Rollinson *,†, Richard Turner † and Munir Pirmohamed

Wolfson Centre for Personalised Medicine, Institute of Systems, Molecular and Integrative Biology, University of Liverpool, Liverpool L69 3GL, UK; rt34@liverpool.ac.uk (R.T.); munirp@liverpool.ac.uk (M.P.)

* Correspondence: vrollins@liverpool.ac.uk

† These authors contributed equally to this work.

Abstract: Most of the prescribing and dispensing of medicines happens in primary care. Pharmacogenomics (PGx) is the study and clinical application of the role of genetic variation on drug response. Mounting evidence suggests PGx can improve the safety and/or efficacy of several medications commonly prescribed in primary care. However, implementation of PGx has generally been limited to a relatively few academic hospital centres, with little adoption in primary care. Despite this, many primary healthcare providers are optimistic about the role of PGx in their future practice. The increasing prevalence of direct-to-consumer genetic testing and primary care PGx studies herald the plausible gradual introduction of PGx into primary care and highlight the changes needed for optimal translation. In this article, the potential utility of PGx in primary care will be explored and on-going barriers to implementation discussed. The evidence base of several drug-gene pairs relevant to primary care will be outlined with a focus on antidepressants, codeine and tramadol, statins, clopidogrel, warfarin, metoprolol and allopurinol. This review is intended to provide both a general introduction to PGx with a more in-depth overview of elements relevant to primary care.

Keywords: pharmacogenomics; primary care; adverse drug reaction; implementation; antidepressants; warfarin; statins; clopidogrel; drug hypersensitivity

---

1. Introduction

It is increasingly recognised that individuals respond differently to medications. In some cases, these differences in response can be clinically significant leading to failure of therapy or adverse drug reactions (ADRs). The aetiology of this inter-individual variability is complex with multiple contributors including individual characteristics (e.g., age, sex, body mass index), clinical factors (e.g., renal or hepatic impairment; co-medications), environmental exposures (e.g., smoking) and genetics.

Pharmacogenomics (PGx) is the study of the influence of genetic variation on drug response [1] with the aim of increasing the efficacy and safety of current and future treatments. Specifically, it aims to facilitate a move away from the standard empirical trial and error prescribing approach that currently exists and transition towards a more stratified and precise prescribing paradigm.

It is estimated that there are between 19,000 to 21,000 protein-coding genes present in the human genome [2]. Within these genes, multiple types of genetic variations can occur including single nucleotide polymorphisms (SNPs), indels (small insertion/deletions) and larger structural rearrangements; of these, SNPs are the most common. Pharmacokinetics (PK) describes "what the body does to a drug" and pharmacodynamics (PD) "what a drug does to the body". Genomic variation in genes involved in a drug's absorption, distribution, metabolism and elimination (e.g., drug-metabolising enzymes or transporters) can alter a drug's PK profile, influencing systemic exposure and resulting in altered drug response (i.e., influencing its downstream PD). Alternatively, genomic variation in genes that modulate a drug's PD (e.g., its therapeutic on-target and off-target sites) can directly influence drug response. Importantly, in both cases, the altered drug response can attenuate a drug's efficacy or worsen tolerability/safety (Figure 1).

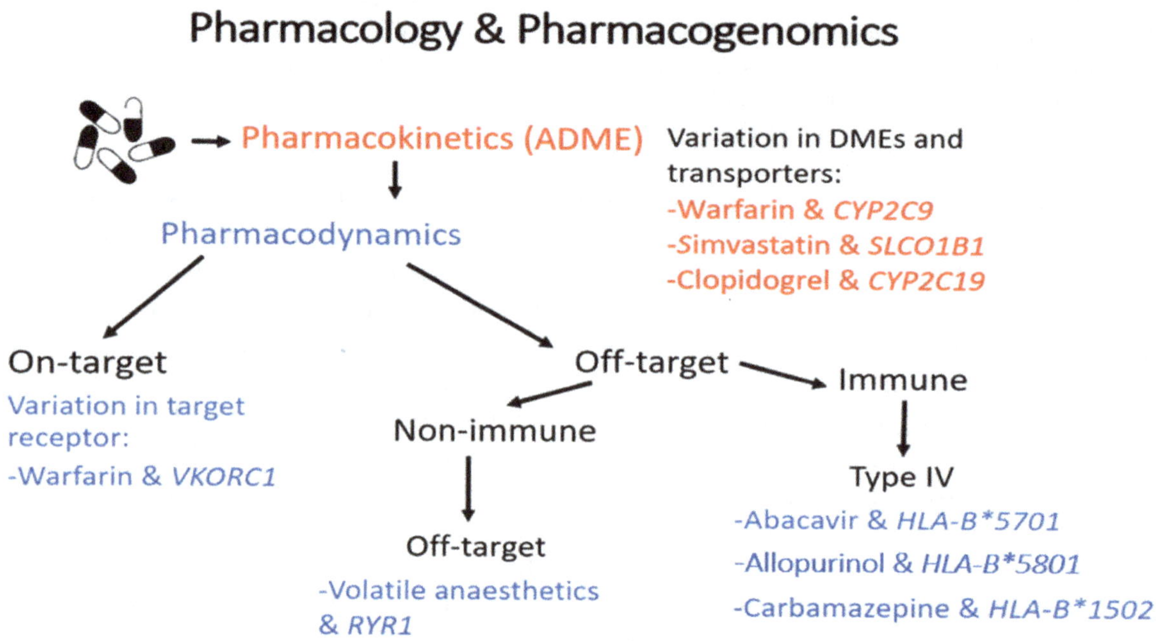

Figure 1. A summary of the mechanisms by which genomic variation can influence the pharmacokinetics and/or pharmacodynamics of a drug, with examples of clinically relevant drug-gene pairs. Genetic changes in drug-metabolising enzymes and transporters can alter a drug's pharmacokinetics, influencing its tissue exposure and so affecting its downstream pharmacodynamics. These changes can lead to underexposure and potentially reduced effectiveness, or increase exposure predisposing often to type A (augmented) adverse drug reactions (ADRs), which are ADRs mediated through excessive action on the drug's therapeutic target and so are predictable (e.g., bleeding after excessive warfarinisation). Secondly, genetic polymorphisms in a drug's therapeutic target can directly modulate drug response, leading to reduced effectiveness or type A ADRs. Lastly, many small molecule drugs bind with varying affinities to unintended off-target molecules, both within and separate to the immune system. Genetic changes in these off-target sites can predispose to less predictable and less common type B (bizarre) ADRs. Of particular note, many rare but serious type B ADRs, such as drug-induced skin injury and drug-induced liver injury, are type IV T-cell mediated delayed type hypersensitivity reactions, and have been very strongly associated with specific human leukocyte antigen (HLA) alleles. It should also be noted that changes in a drug's pharmacokinetics leading to increased exposure can, on occasion, predispose to off-target (type B) ADRs, as is the case, for example, with simvastatin myotoxicity.

The clinical and financial consequences of adverse drug reactions (ADRs) are high, accounting for an estimated 6.5% of hospital admissions [3]. Interestingly, for several of the drugs often implicated in causing hospitalisation, PGx guideline recommendations are now available, such as for warfarin, antiplatelet agents and opioid analgesics [4]. In addition to serious ADRs leading to hospitalisation, it is also known that poor drug tolerability (for example due to mild adverse events) is associated with lower compliance [5], which increases the chances of reduced efficacy and increased medicines wastage.

It is estimated that over 98% of individuals carry at least one pharmacogenetic variant [6]. Importantly, the majority of prescribing and dispensing of medicines happens in primary care, and recent studies in both the US and UK suggest that over 60% of patients within the primary care setting are prescribed a medication with a PGx recommendation [7,8]

The Dutch Pharmacogenomics Working Group (DPWG) and Clinical Pharmacogenetics Implementation Consortium (CPIC) are the two most widely recognised expert groups involved in the development of PGx clinical guidelines. Therapeutic recommendations from CPIC and DPWG, as well as guidelines written by other groups such as the Canadian Pharmacogenomics Network for Drug Safety (CPNDS), are curated and housed by the Pharmacogenomics Knowledge Base (https://www.pharmgkb.org/), and can be accessed online for free by healthcare professionals and other individuals with an interest. To date, PGx associations with actionable PGx recommendations for clinical practice have been developed for just over 80 drugs [9]. Almost two-thirds of these actionable drug-gene associations involve drug metabolizing enzyme genes, with ~80% of these being genes encoding cytochrome P450 (CYP) enzymes. A small number of actionable drug-gene associations involve transporter genes, and just under a third involve genes that influence drug PD (~5% on-target, ~26% off-target, with almost a third of the latter involving human leukocyte antigen (*HLA*) genes). The US Food & Drug Administration (FDA) has also evaluated drug-gene associations, deeming 47 drugs to have sufficient evidence for PGx therapeutic recommendations and another 16 drugs to have PGx associations that potentially impact clinical safety or response [10]; there is notably overlap between the drug-gene associations considered actionable by the guideline committees and the FDA.

A list of drugs (though not exhaustive) commonly prescribed in primary care with PGx guidelines currently available is outlined in Table 1.

Despite the growing availability of guidelines, adoption of PGx in primary care has been slow. Nevertheless, a nationwide study from the Netherlands inferred that 1 out of every 19 new prescriptions in primary care could have undergone an adjustment had PGx data been available [11]. Within the UK and in many other countries, PGx testing largely remains within the remit of specialist secondary and tertiary care settings (e.g., with abacavir-*HLA B*57:01* testing). Table 2 provides a summary, albeit non-exhaustive, of recent and large interventional studies that have assessed PGx and are relevant to primary care.

A recent analysis identified the following pharmacogenes to be most commonly linked to primary care prescriptions in England: *CYP2D6*, *CYP2C19* and *SLCO1B1* (solute carrier organic anion transporter family member 1B1), followed by *CYP2C9*, *VKORC1* (vitamin K epoxide reductase complex 1), *CYP4F2* and *HLA-B* (8).Therefore, the subsequent sections in this review provide an overview of the role PGx can play in primary care in the prescribing and monitoring of specific medications related to these genes. Drug-specific literature searches were conducted between June and October 2020.

Table 1. Commonly used drugs in primary care with available pharmacogenomics guidelines.

Class	Drug	Gene	Actionable Result	Guideline Availability		Therapeutic Recommendations [1]
				DPWG	CPIC	
Lipid lowering agents	Atorvastatin	*SLCO1B1*	rs4145096 (521T > C) carriers	√	-	AD
	Simvastatin	*SLCO1B1*		√	√	LD, AD, M
Antidepressants	Citalopram	*CYP2C19*	PM, UM	√	√	LD (PM), AD (PM, UM)
	Sertraline	*CYP2C19*	PM, UM	√	√	LD (PM), AD (PM, UM)
	Amitriptyline	*CYP2C19*	PM, RM, UM	-	√	LD (PM), AD (PM, RM, UM)
		CYP2D6	IM, PM, UM	√	√	LD (IM, PM), AD (PM, UM)
Analgesics	Codeine	*CYP2D6*	IM, PM, UM	√	√	AD (UM, PM), M (IM)
	Tramadol	*CYP2D6*	IM, PM, UM	√	-	AD (IM, PM, UM), ID (IM, PM), LD (UM)
Anti-platelet	Clopidogrel	*CYP2C19*	IM, PM	√	√	AD
Anticoagulant	Warfarin	*VKORC1*	*VKORC1 c.-1639G > A*	√	√	LD [2]
		CYP2C9	**2, *3, *5, *6, *8, *11*	√	√	LD [2]
		CYP2C region	rs12777823		√	LD
Anticonvulsant	Carbamazepine	*HLA-B*	*HLA-B*15:02* detected	-	√	AD, M
		HLA-A	*HLA-A*31:01* detected	-	√	AD, M
Antibiotic	Flucloxacillin	*HLA-B*	*HLA-B*57:01* detected	√	-	AD, M
Contraception	Oestrogen-containing contraceptives	*F5*	rs6025 (p.R534Q) carriers	√	-	AD
Xanthine oxidase inhibitor	Allopurinol	*HLA-B*	*HLA-B*58:01* detected	-	√	AD

[1] = Where a drug-gene pair has guidance available from both CPIC and DPWG, the CPIC recommendations are detailed here. [2] = VKORC1 -1639G > A and CYP2C9 alleles are often combined together into an algorithm, alongside clinical variables, to guide initial warfarin dosing. Please note that CYP2C9 *1/*2 does not lead to recommended warfarin dose changes unless the VKORC1 -1639A allele is also present, and VKORC1 -1639GA does not lead to a dose change unless a CYP2C9 reduction-of-function allele is also present [9]. AD = alternative drug; CPIC = Clinical Pharmacogenetics Implementation Consortium; DPWG = Dutch Pharmacogenetics Working Group; LD = lower dose; ID = increase dose; M = consider additional monitoring (e.g., routine CK surveillance for simvastatin); PM = poor metaboliser; UM = ultra-rapid metaboliser; √ = guideline available; - = no guideline available.

Table 2. A non-exhaustive summary of recent interventional studies investigating pharmacogenomics of relevance to primary care. 1° = primary endpoint, 2° = secondary endpoints, RCT = randomised controlled trial, SoC = standard of care treatment.

Study	N	Genes	Treatment	Design	Duration	Intervention	Comparator	Endpoint	Outcome
Greden et al. 2019 (GUIDED) [12]	1167	Panel of 8 genes (including *CYP2C19* and *CYP2D6*)	SSRI, SNRI, TCA, other antidepressants, typical and atypical antipsychotics	RCT	24 weeks	PGx guided treatment	Standard of care treatment	1°–Symptoms (8 weeks) 2°–Response rate and remission (8 weeks)	1°–Symptom ↓ of 27.2% PGx vs. 24.4% SoC ($p = 0.107$) 2°–Response: 26.0% vs. 19.9% ($p = 0.013$) Remission: 15.3% vs. 10.1% ($p = 0.007$)
Perez et al. 2017 [13]	316	Panel of 30 genes (including *CYP2C19* and *CYP2D6*)	SSRI, SNRI, TCA, MAOI, other antidepressants	RCT	12 weeks	PGx guided treatment	Standard of care treatment	1°–% of patients with sustained response (12 weeks) 2°–Responder rate and side effect burden (12 weeks)	1°–38.5% PGx vs. 34.4% SoC ($p = 0.4735$) 2°–Responder rate: 47.8% vs. 36.1% ($p = 0.0476$) 2°–Side effect burden: 68.5% vs. 51.4% ($p = 0.0260$)
Bradley et al. 2018 [14]	685	Panel of 10 genes (including *CYP2C19* and *CYP2D6*)	SSRI, SNRI, TCA, other antidepressants, benzodiazepines, buspirone	RCT	12 weeks	PGx guided treatment	Standard of care treatment	Remission & response depression (12 weeks) Symptom severity & response anxiety (12 weeks)	Depression: Remission: 35% PGx vs. 13% SoC ($p = 0.02$) Response: 73% vs. 36% ($p = 0.001$) Anxiety: Symptom ↓ of 54% vs. 42% ($p = 0.02$) Response: 63% vs. 50% ($p = 0.04$)
Pirmohamed et al. 2013 (EU-PACT) [15]	455	*CYP2C9* and *VKORC1*	Warfarin	RCT	12 weeks	PGx guided treatment	Standard of care treatment	1°–% of time in INR range 2.0 to 3.0	1°–67.4% PGx vs. 60.3% SoC ($p < 0.001$)
Kimmel et al. 2013 (COAG) [16]	1015	*CYP2C9* and *VKORC1*	Warfarin	RCT	28 days	PGx guided treatment	Clinical dosing algorithm	1°–% of time in INR range 2.0 to 3.0	1°–45.2% PGx vs. 45.4% SoC ($p = 0.91$)
Gage et al., 2017 (GIFT) [17]	1650	*CYP2C9*, *VKORC1* and *CYP4F2*	Warfarin	RCT		PGx guided treatment	Clinical dosing algorithm	1°–composite of major bleeding, INR ≥ 4, death (all in 30 days) or VTE (in 60 days)	1°–10.8% PGx vs. 14.7% SoC ($p = 0.02$)

Table 2. *Cont.*

Study	N	Genes	Treatment	Design	Duration	Intervention	Comparator	Endpoint	Outcome
Pereira et al. 2020 (TAILOR-PCI) [18]	5302	*CYP2C19*	Clopidogrel	RCT	12 months	PGx guided oral P2Y12 inhibitor treatment	Standard of care (Clopidogrel)	1°–composite of cardiovascular death, myocardial infarction, stroke, stent thrombosis, and severe recurrent ischemia (12 months)	1°–in 4.0% PGx LOF carriers vs. 5.9% SoC LOF carriers ($p = 0.06$)
Claassens et al. 2019 (POPular) [19]	2488	*CYP2C19*	Clopidogrel	RCT	12 months	PGx guided oral P2Y12 inhibitor Tx	Standard of care (Ticagrelor or prasugrel)	1°–Net adverse clinical events (12 months) 1°–Major or minor bleeding (12 months)	Net events: 5.1% PGx vs. 5.9% SoC ($p < 0.001$ for noninferiority) Bleeding: 9.8% vs. 12.5% ($p = 0.04$)
Ko et al. 2015 [20]	2926	*HLA-B*58:01*	Allopurinol	Cohort	9 months	Allopurinol avoided in *HLA-B*58:01* +ve patients	Allopurinol given in *HLA-B*58:01*-ve patients	1°–Incidence of SCARs in cohort compared to historical national average	1°–No cases of SCARs in prospective cohort (within 9 month follow up) vs. 7 cases to be expected based on historical average (0.3% per year), $p = 0.0026$

2. Antidepressants

Prescribed for a variety of indications, the number of prescriptions for antidepressants in the UK primary care sector is increasing annually [21]. Whilst they are effective therapies, these drugs have variable success rates [22], with up to 50% of patients nonresponsive to treatment. Some of this heterogeneity in response may be accounted for by PGx variation.

In the UK, selective serotonin re-uptake inhibitors (SSRIs) account for over 50% of primary care antidepressant prescriptions [23]; tricyclic antidepressants (TCAs), serotonin-norepinephrine reuptake inhibitors (SNRIs) and atypical antidepressants (e.g., mirtazapine) are also utilised.

There are 57 putatively functional CYP genes within the human genome, of which around 12 are involved in the biotransformation of 70–80% of all therapeutics used in clinical practice [24]. Most antidepressants are, in some part, metabolized via the CYP enzyme system, with CYP2D6 and CYP2C19 [25] widely regarded as the most influential enzymes for antidepressant biotransformation.

CYP2D6 is highly polymorphic with over 100 allelic variants recorded [26]. Due to the number of possible diplotypes within a population the translation of genotype to phenotype for *CYP2D6* is often performed using an "activity score" wherein alleles are given a numeric value based on their functionality and the sum of the values present in an individual is subsequently categorised into one of the following "metaboliser phenotypes": ultra-rapid metabolizer (UM), extensive (normal) metabolizer (EM), intermediate metabolizer (IM), and poor metabolizer (PM) [27].

Allelic frequencies in *CYP2D6* vary substantially across populations. The most common non-functioning variant, *CYP2D6*4* (rs3892097, 1846G > A), which is a splicing defect, is found at the highest frequency within Caucasian populations [28]; related to this observation Caucasian populations have a higher frequency of PMs (around 5–10%) compared to Asian and African-American populations. CYP2D6 is also subject to copy number variation (CNV) that can lead to deletion of a CYP2D6 allele (*5) or CYP2D6 duplication or multiplication; whilst the former decreases CYP2D6 function, an increased number of functional CYP2D6 alleles results in the UM phenotype (*xN). UMs are less frequent in Caucasian populations at approximately 2%, but the frequency of UMs has been noted to be much higher in other specific populations, such as those with North African ancestry (c.25%) [29].

Studies have demonstrated that the presence of the *CYP2D6*4* allele in PMs correlated to increased side effect frequency with some antidepressants including venlafaxine [30] and lower dose requirements of SSRIs and TCAs (e.g., amitriptyline, nortriptyline; see below) [31]. Additionally, studies have indicated that *CYP2D6* UMs taking paroxetine have low plasma concentrations in comparison to EMs [32] and this may be a risk factor for therapeutic failure. In the case of both fluvoxamine and paroxetine, the CPIC guideline highlights the possibility of ADRs potentiated by higher plasma concentrations in *CYP2D6* PMs [33]. Some evidence exists to correlate increased ADRs with mirtazapine in *CYP2D6* IM and PM patients [34,35]. However, at this time, no clinically actionable PGx recommendation exists for mirtazapine.

CYP2C19 is similarly highly polymorphic: 34 conventional star alleles are currently recognised [36] and over 2000 *CYP2C19* variants have been identified, although the majority are intronic [37]. The most prevalent reduction-of-function (ROF) allele is *2 (rs4244285, c.681G > A), a splice defect, followed by **3* (rs4986893, c.636G > A) which results in a premature stop codon. *CYP2C19*2* is most common in individuals of Asian ancestry with minor allele frequencies (MAFs) of 31–36% [38], whilst occurring in ~16% of African and European individuals. *CYP2C19*3* occurs in ~6% of East Asian individuals, but is rare in African and European populations. Conversely, *CYP2C19*17* (rs12248560), which is a common variant in the promotor region of the gene, is associated with increased transcription and enzymatic function [39].

Similar to *CYP2D6*, individuals can be categorised according to genotype into anticipated CYP2C19 EMs (*1/*1 wild-type), IMs (one ROF allele), PMs (two ROF alleles), and UMs (*17/*17). Unlike conventional *CYP2D6* phenotype categorisation, a *CYP2C19* rapid metaboliser (RM, *1/*17) phenotype category is also recognised with functionality between EMs and UMs.

Sertraline, citalopram and escitalopram are all extensively metabolised by CYP2C19 and, in PMs, elevated plasma concentrations may lead to potential ADRs [40,41]. Presently, however, a formal drug label warning only exists for escitalopram, which recommends a reduced starting dose for *CYP2C19* PMs due to the risk of QT interval prolongation [42].

Amitriptyline undergoes CYP2C19-mediated demethylation to its active metabolite, nortriptyline, which is also available on prescription. Whilst both are classed as TCAs, amitriptyline blocks serotonin and noradrenaline reuptake equally, whereas nortriptyline inhibits noradrenaline uptake more potently [43]. As a result, *CYP2C19* PMs are expected to show reduced conversion to nortriptyline, increased systemic exposure to amitriptyline and an increased risk of amitriptyline-related side effects [44]. Although TCAs are now more commonly used at lower doses for the treatment of neuropathic pain, rather than for major depressive disorder, the CPIC guidelines for amitriptyline still recommend consideration of alternative therapy in *CYP2C19* UMs due to an increased risk of treatment failure irrespective of indication [45]. Additionally, amitriptyline and nortriptyline also undergo *CYP2D6* metabolism to a less active metabolite. Whereas *CYP2C19* influences the ratio of metabolites, *CYP2D6* plays a greater role in drug clearance. This may lead to raised plasma concentrations of amitriptyline and nortriptyline in CYP2D6 PMs or in patients co-administered a CYP2D6 inhibitor [46]. CPIC guidelines therefore recommend a lower starting dose when used at dosing ranges for depression [47].

A recent meta-analysis of five randomised clinical trials (RCTs) reported that patients receiving PGx guided dosing were 1.71 (95% CI: 1.17–2.48, $p = 0.005$) times more likely to achieve symptom remission for major depressive disorder (MDD) than those on standard care [48]. Details of some of the most recent RCTs are in Table 2.

While there is still work to be done on the utilisation of PGx in antidepressant prescribing, there are multiple potential benefits to having PGx information at hand when selecting treatments. An analysis of UK healthcare data from 2016 identified that the age categories with highest antidepressant use were ages 55–64 and 75–84 [49]. Additionally, the same data set demonstrated an increasing trend for polypharmacy with increasing age, particularly in the over 75-years-old age bracket. PGx testing has the potential to circumvent some of the risks associated with polypharmacy by guiding the prescribing of suitable medications [50].

In addition to patient benefits, analyses have shown that utilising PGx information in mental health prescribing may offer significant financial savings via a reduction in the number of failed treatments and subsequent medicines wastage [51].

3. Opioid Analgesics

Codeine and tramadol are commonly prescribed weak opioid analgesics indicated for mild to moderate (non-neuropathic) pain; they are positioned on the second rung of the World Health Organisation's three step pain ladder. Codeine is an inactive prodrug; 0–15% undergoes O-demethylation catalysed by CYP2D6 to form active morphine, which has an affinity for the μ-opioid receptor 200-fold more than that of parent codeine [52]. Similarly, tramadol undergoes CYP2D6-mediated O-demethylation to O-desmethyltramadol [53], which has an affinity for the μ-opioid receptor that is also significantly higher than that of tramadol [54]. Whereas the majority of codeine's analgesic effect stems from morphine agonism on opioid receptors, for tramadol, the analgesia conferred by O-desmethyltramadol agonism of the μ-opioid receptor is complemented by inhibition of serotonin and noradrenaline reuptake by parent tramadol.

In *CYP2D6* EM individuals, at least 80% of codeine metabolism results in inactive metabolites, with around 5–10% undergoing biotransformation into morphine [55]. This percentage increases in UMs [56] whilst, in PMs, there may be very little if any conversion (52). PK and PD studies have demonstrated that the increased codeine biotransformation in *CYP2D6* UMs can result in opiate toxicity even with low doses of codeine [57]. Conversely, *CYP2D6* PMs are likely to obtain little to no therapeutic benefit [58]. In addition, due to the heterogeneity in *CYP2D6* allele functionality, some patients within the broad EM category may also experience an increased number of adverse events compared with others. These "ultra-rapid EMs" have alleles leading to a greater activity score, but which still fall within the EM activity score reference range, and thus ideally require lower doses to circumvent possible ADRs [59].

The PGx of codeine received international attention following reports of infant opiate toxicity from higher levels of morphine in the breast milk of UM mothers. Reviews of this phenomenon resulted in amended FDA and European Medicines Agency (EMA) guidance to avoid the use of codeine when breastfeeding [60].

Similarly, regulatory changes followed case reports of children with obstructive sleep apnoea receiving codeine post-tonsillectomy and/or adenoidectomy leading to codeine toxicity and fatalities, with these children having evidence of being *CYP2D6* UMs [61,62]. This led to blanket regulation from authorities such as the UK Medicines and Healthcare products Regulatory Agency (MHRA) [63] restricting the use of codeine in children under 12 irrespective of *CYP2D6* metaboliser status. This same MHRA guidance extends to cover all patients (i.e., 12 years and older) with a documented *CYP2D6* UM status, although in practice this is seldom known. Both CPIC and the DPWG have developed PGx guidelines for codeine that advocate avoiding codeine in UM and PM patients. However, there are nuanced differences between these recommendations. Most pertinently, in UMs, CPIC recommends simply avoiding codeine, whereas the DPWG guidance suggests no additional action is required in UM patients that receive lower doses of codeine and have no additional risk factors (e.g., concomitant CYP3A4-inhibiting drugs) that would predispose to exaggerated biotransformation to morphine.

In addition to the influence of *CYP2D6*, there is emerging evidence for the influence of polymorphisms within other genes including the μ-opioid receptor gene, *OPRM1*, and the phase 2 metabolising enzyme *UGT2B7* [64]. While associations with variation in these genes remain inconclusive, they are important areas for future research.

Within the UK, the use of the weak opioid tramadol has increased over the past two decades [65]. In keeping with codeine, studies have demonstrated a probable reduced efficacy with tramadol in *CYP2D6* PMs patients and, additionally, a lower risk of ADRs [66]. Again, the risk of ADRs including potentially severe reactions appears greater in UMs [67,68]. A systematic review of the CYP2D6*10 C188T polymorphism which included 9 studies and 809 subjects showed a relationship between this polymorphism and pharmacokinetics of tramadol (half-life, AUC and clearance) and analgesic effect, but not with the adverse effects of nausea and vomiting [69].

Although CPIC has yet to develop guidance for tramadol, the DPWG guidelines recommend avoiding tramadol in UMs or, if not possible, using just 40% of the standard dose, to minimise the risk of opioid receptor-mediated ADRs. For PMs, an increased alertness to reduced effectiveness is primarily recommended. This is because it is difficult to predict the influence of decreased CYP2D6 metabolism on the overall analgesic effects experienced by an individual, because the resulting increased proportion of parent tramadol to O-desmethyltramadol may enable the potentiated SNRI properties of parent tramadol to mitigate some of the lost O-desmethyltramadol opioid receptor-mediated analgesic effects.

4. Statins

Statins are first line lipid-lowering agents for both primary and secondary prevention of cardiovascular disease, are widely prescribed, and are generally safe and well tolerated. Statins are, however, associated with an increased risk of type 2 diabetes mellitus and muscle toxicity, which is phenotypically heterogeneous ranging from myalgias with normal plasma creatine kinase (CK, ~5% of individuals [70]) to infrequent myopathies to rare rhabdomyolysis, and finally extremely rare immune-mediated necrotizing myopathy (IMNM) [71]. A recent study [72] showed that the risk of myopathy (CK > 10 × the upper limit of normal) with simvastatin was 9 per 10,000 person-years of therapy. Independent risk factors for myopathy included simvastatin dose, ethnicity, sex, age, body mass index, medically treated diabetes, and concomitant use of certain drugs (niacin-laropiprant, verapamil, β-blockers, diltiazem and diuretics), which collectively predicted more than a 30-fold risk difference between the top and bottom thirds of a clinical myopathy score. This risk score was less strongly associated with milder myopathy, and not associated with reports of any muscle symptoms, and so the authors concluded that muscle presentations other than myopathy were unlikely to be related to statins [73].

Statins competitively inhibit 3-hydroxy-3-methylglutaryl-Coenzyme A reductase (HMGCR) in the liver, resulting in decreased circulating low-density lipoprotein cholesterol (LDL-C). Organic anion-transporting polypeptide 1B1 (OATP1B1) is a liver-specific transporter expressed on the basolateral (sinusoidal) side of hepatocytes [74], is encoded by *SLCO1B1* and is involved in hepatic uptake of statins and other drugs (e.g., letermovir [73]). A common ROF *SLCO1B1* missense variant, rs4149056 (c.521T > C, p.V174A, present in SLCO1B1*5, *15 and *17), is associated with a 221% increased systemic exposure to simvastatin acid in 521CC compared to wild-type 521TT individuals. Moreover, the C allele is associated with elevated exposures to all statins, except fluvastatin, albeit to lesser extents [75]. For example, the corresponding increase with atorvastatin is 145%. The MAF of rs4149056 in African, East Asian and European populations is 1%, 12% and 16%, respectively.

Importantly, it was shown in a genome-wide association study (GWAS) that 521TC and 521CC patients taking simvastatin 80mg daily had an odds ratio (OR) for myopathy of 4.5 (95% confidence interval (CI) 2.6–7.7) and 16.9 (95% CI 4.7–61.1) compared to wild-type patients, respectively [76]. In 521TC patients on simvastatin 40mg, the relative risk was 2.6 (95% CI 1.3–5.0). Furthermore, the 521C allele is associated with a two-fold increase in statin intolerance in patients predominantly taking simvastatin, and this intolerance can reduce lipid-lowering efficacy [77]. Thus, the strength of *SLCO1B1*-myotoxicity association increases with 521C allele dose, simvastatin dose and myopathy severity.

Several other studies [78] including a recent large-scale GWAS [79] have replicated the simvastatin-521T > C association. The consistent association with simvastatin mirrors the PK observations that 521T > C has the largest impact on simvastatin exposure, reflects the high prevalence of simvastatin use in clinical practice leading to reliance on simvastatin myotoxicity cases in research studies, and the in vitro observations that simvastatin (lactone) is particularly myotoxic [80]. Elevated simvastatin systemic exposure presumably increases skeletal muscle exposure, predisposing to myotoxicity by mechanisms that are incompletely understood but likely to include mitochondrial dysfunction, calcium signalling disruption and reduced prenylation.

The evidence for an association between SLCO1B1 521T > C and other statins is less clear. Some studies have suggestively associated 521C with atorvastatin myotoxicity [81–83], but others found no association [84–86]. Interestingly, a recent study in patients on high dose atorvastatin for secondary prevention found 521C was associated with both muscular symptoms and atorvastatin intolerance, suggesting that 521T > C may be more relevant in patients on high dose (e.g., 80 mg) atorvastatin [87]. For rosuvastatin, 521C was not associated with myalgias in patients of European descent [88], but recently has been associated with myotoxicity (myalgias to rhabdomyolysis) in Chinese ancestry patients [89]. *SLCO1B1* 521T > C has not been associated with pravastatin myotoxicity.

A recent international whole-exome sequencing endeavour of patients with statin (most commonly simvastatin) myopathy identified no novel variants [90]. Nevertheless, a candidate missense variant (rs12975366, p.D247G) within leukocyte immunoglobulin-like receptor subfamily B member 5 (*LILRB5*) was recently associated with statin myotoxicity, including intolerance and myalgia, implicating the immune system in these more mild phenotypes [91]; an intervention study is underway [92]. Moreover, *CYP3A4*22* and *CYP3A5* non-expressors have been associated with modestly elevated simvastatin exposure [93], *CYP3A7*1C* with increased atorvastatin hydroxylation [89], and *ABCG2* rs2231142 (c.421C > A) with elevations in exposure to simvastatin, atorvastatin, fluvastatin and especially rosuvastatin [75,94]. Nevertheless, despite signals, these candidate genes and others (e.g., *ABCB1*) have not been consistently associated with statin myotoxicity across studies. Similarly, *CYP3A4* [95], *CYP3A5* [96] and *CYP2D6* [97] have been investigated as potential biomarkers of statin efficacy, but results have varied and, of note, none were identified in a GWAS meta-analysis of statin lipid-lowering efficacy [98]. Nevertheless, the influence of more complex interactions, such as those involving combined genetic variation in both *SLCO1B1* and *CYP* and/or other transporter genes, on statin pharmacokinetics and clinical effects, warrants further study. In addition, *CYP2C9* ROF variants have been associated with increased adverse events (primarily myotoxicity [99]) and potentially increased lipid-lowering efficacy [100]. Fluvastatin has arguably received less research attention than simvastatin and atorvastatin, yet *CYP2C9* is important in fluvastatin's metabolism, and so follow up studies are warranted to further investigate these findings.

SLCO1B1 521T > C has been associated with the spectrum of myotoxicity, at least for simvastatin, except for IMNM. A subtype of IMNM is anti-HMGCR myopathy [101]; most patients with anti-HMGCR myopathy have a history or statin exposure, develop muscle weakness with highly elevated CK levels that persist despite statin cessation, are identified by the presence of circulating anti-HMGCR autoantibodies that can be directly pathogenic, and normally require treatment with immunosuppressive drugs or intravenous immunoglobulins [102]. Interestingly, *HLA-DRB1*11:01* has been significantly associated with anti-HMGCR myopathy [103,104] with estimated OR of ~25–57 dependent on ethnicity. Whilst this HLA association may catalyse research into underlying mechanisms and aid diagnosis, the rarity of anti-HMGCR myopathy suggests this PGx association will not have utility in guiding statin initiation.

Both CPIC and the DPWG have developed clinical guidelines for simvastatin-SLCO1B1 [105,106], and the DPWG have also developed atorvastatin-SLCO1B1 guidance. In patients that carry 521C, they recommend starting an alternate statin or using a lower simvastatin dose. For atorvastatin, the DPWG guideline recommends an alternative statin in 521C carriers that have additional clinical myotoxicity risk factors. Nevertheless, few patients are now started on simvastatin 80 mg following an FDA warning about its increased myopathy risk [107]. Interestingly, a recent randomized trial in 159 patients with previous statin myalgia has demonstrated that providing *SLCO1B1* 521T > C genotype with recommendations increases statin re-initiation in primary care [108]. As muscle symptoms are associated with statin discontinuation and non-adherence [5], which in turn increase the risk of cardiovascular events [109], 521T > C genotyping may help reduce cardiovascular events as well as myotoxicity in clinical practice, although this remains to be substantiated.

5. Clopidogrel

Clopidogrel is an antiplatelet drug indicated in acute coronary syndrome (ACS), percutaneous coronary intervention (PCI), stroke, transient ischaemic attack (TIA), peripheral artery disease (PAD) and atrial fibrillation (AF). Clopidogrel is a prodrug: of the ~50% absorbed, ~85% is rapidly hydrolysed to inactive clopidogrel carboxylic acid via carboxylesterase 1 (CES1) and ~15% undergoes a two-step oxidative biotransformation to produce the active thiol metabolite that irreversibly inhibits platelet P2Y12 receptors [110].

CYP2C19 is the only CYP substantially involved in both oxidative steps, contributing 45% and 21% to the first and second steps, respectively [111]. *CYP2C19* ROF alleles are associated with decreased levels of circulating clopidogrel active metabolite [112] and increased ex vivo high on-treatment platelet reactivity (HTPR) [113]. A meta-analysis of 9685 patients, of whom 91% had undergone PCI (55% ACS), demonstrated that *CYP2C19* ROF alleles were associated with an increased risk of major adverse cardiovascular events (MACE) and stent thrombosis, with a gene-dose trend evident [114]. However, a second meta-analysis assessing *CYP2C19* genotype and cardiovascular outcomes in 26, 251 individuals found no overall association with cardiovascular outcomes after exclusion of small studies, although an increased risk of stent thrombosis remained evident [115]. This meta-analysis included a wider spectrum of indications for clopidogrel, including atrial fibrillation. To resolve these discrepant observations, clopidogrel indication-specific PGx has been posited. Thus, these (mostly) observational data have been considered to support an association between *CYP2C19* ROF variants and cardiovascular events in post-PCI patients, because this patient population's high baseline risk for cardiovascular events makes them more susceptible to suboptimal treatment, but does not support an association in other (mainly cardiac) settings where the overall benefit of clopidogrel is modest anyway [116].

To investigate whether interventions based on *CYP2C19* ROF alleles improve clinical outcomes, two large randomized clinical trials (RCTs) have been undertaken and recently reported (Table 2) [18,19]. The Patient Outcome after primary PCI (POPular) Genetics trial included 2488 patients with an ST-elevation myocardial infarction (STEMI) that underwent primary PCI with stent insertion and compared standard-treatment (ticagrelor or prasugrel) to a genotype-informed antiplatelet strategy that allocated ticagrelor/prasugrel to *CYP2C19**2 or *3 carriers and clopidogrel to noncarriers. POPular Genetics reported the genotype strategy was non-inferior to standard-treatment for net adverse clinical events (MACE plus major bleeding, $p < 0.001$ for noninferiority), but reduced (mostly minor) bleeding (hazard ratio (HR) 0.78, 95% CI 0.61–0.98, $p = 0.04$). The Tailored Antiplatelet Initiation to Lessen Outcomes Due to Decreased Clopidogrel Response after PCI (TAILOR-PCI) RCT [18] recruited 5302 patients undergoing PCI with stent insertion (for ACS or stable coronary artery disease) and compared standard-treatment clopidogrel to an equivalent CYP2C19-informed antiplatelet strategy to that used in POPular Genetics. The primary result of TAILOR-PCI was a reduction in first MACE in the genotype strategy arm compared to the standard (clopidogrel) arm, although it narrowly missed statistical significance (HR 0.66, 95% CI 0.43–1.02, $p = 0.06$). A pre-specified sensitivity analysis showed a significant reduction in all cumulative MACE events (HR 0.60, 95% CI 0.41–0.89, $p = 0.01$) with genotyping. There was no difference in bleeding risk between arms. Of note, the power to detect a difference in TAILOR-PCI was lower than originally planned because the event rate was lower than anticipated, in keeping with use of newer generation drug-eluting stents [18].

*CYP2C 19**17 has been associated with decreased HTPR, and inconsistently with increased bleeding risk and reduced MACE [117]. Given the inconsistent findings, less observational research has focused on *17 compared to *CYP2C19* ROF alleles, and that *17 was not included in the POPular Genetics or TAILOR-PCI primary analyses, the clinical relevance of *17 remains undetermined.

There has been an increased focus recently on the impact of *CYP2C19* ROF alleles in patients following a stroke. A recent meta-analysis of studies of patients prescribed clopidogrel for ischaemic stroke/TIA found *CYP2C19* ROF carriers had an increased risk of recurrent stroke and MACE [118]. *CYP2C19* ROF alleles have also been associated with increased in-stent restenosis in patients with PAD [119]. On the other hand, a genetic analysis of the large EUCLID trial (n = 13,885) that recruited patients with symptomatic PAD reported no difference in cardiovascular outcomes between patient subgroups with different *CYP2C19* genotypes [120]. However, EUCLID excluded *CYP2C19* PM patients from entry into the trial, limiting interpretation of these findings.

Beyond *CYP2C19*, there is growing evidence for a role of *CES1* in clopidogrel PGx. *CES1* catalyses clopidogrel to its inactive metabolite; the variant allele of rs71647871 (p.G143E, MAF ~1%) in *CES1* has been associated with increased circulating clopidogrel active metabolite, reduced ex vivo platelet reactivity, and a nonsignificant trend towards decreased MACE [121]. Moreover, the variant allele of CES1 rs2307240 (p.S75N, MAF ~5%) was recently associated with reduced subsequent MACE in clopidogrel-treated ACS patients [106].

Both CPIC [121] and DPWG (106) have produced clinical guidelines for clopidogrel-CYP2C19: CPIC focuses on ACS patients undergoing PCI, and DPWG on PCI for any indication, as well as stroke and TIA. The main recommendation is alternative antiplatelet therapy in those with *CYP2C19* ROF alleles, although the DPWG guidance also permits doubling the dose of clopidogrel in *CYP2C19* IMs. A multi-site real world implementation of *CYP2C19* genotyping to guide antiplatelet stratification after PCI (n = 1815) has been reported, and importantly demonstrated clinical benefit [122]. On balance, taking all evidence together, we contend that clinical implementation of clopidogrel-CYP2C19 genotyping is justifiable and beneficial.

6. Warfarin

The oral vitamin K antagonist, warfarin, is indicated to prevent and treat venous thromboembolism (VTE) and to prevent thromboembolism in atrial fibrillation (AF) and following mechanical heart valve transplantation. Warfarin is a racemate that competitively inhibits VKORC1 within the vitamin K cycle, leading to hypofunctional clotting factors II, VII, IX and X. The extent of anticoagulation is measured by the international normalised ratio (INR) and, for most indications, the target therapeutic INR is 2.0–3.0 [123]. Warfarin stable dose (WSD) requirements vary ~30-fold between patients [124], and its narrow therapeutic index underlies warfarin being the third most common drug to lead to hospitalisation due to ADRs(3). A 10% increase in time outside the therapeutic INR range (TTR) is associated with increased thromboembolic events and mortality [125], and supratherapeutic INRs increase the risk of major bleeding [126].

Overall, ~60% of the observed variation in warfarin stable dose requirements can be explained, and several clinical factors including age, smoking and interacting drugs contribute [127]. However, genetic factors explain the majority of this observed variation. Specifically, rs9923231 (-1639G > A) in *VKORC1* accounts for 6–25% of observed variation, variation in *CYP2C9* another ~15%, and *CYP4F2*3* (rs2108622, p.V433M) 1–7% [128–130].

-1639G > A lies within *VKORC1's* promoter region; -1639A alters a transcription factor binding site reducing *VKORC1* transcription [131], increasing sensitivity to warfarin and reducing WSD requirements [132]. The MAF of -1639A in African, East Asian, South Asian and European populations is ~5%, ~90%, ~15% and ~40%, demonstrating allele reversal in East Asians. The variation in -1639A MAF perhaps underlies why -1639G > A explains only 6% of WSD variation in African-Americans but ~20–25% in Asian and Caucasian populations [133].

CYP2C9 metabolises the more potent S-warfarin enantiomer and *CYP2C9* ROF variants reduce WSD requirements. *CYP2C9*2* (rs1799853, p.R144C) and **3* (rs1057910, p.I359L) are common ROF alleles in European populations with MAFs of ~12% and ~7%, respectively, and *CYP2C9*3* is common in Asian populations (MAF 3–11%). However, *CYP2C9*2* is infrequent in Asians (0–3%) and both are rare or infrequent in African populations (0–3.6% for *2, and 0.3–2% for *3) [134]. Interestingly, distinct warfarin-associated variants have been described in African ancestry patients (primarily Africa-Americans). *CYP2C9*5, *6, *8* and **11* are ROF alleles with a collective frequency of ~20% in African ancestry individuals [135], but are rare in other ethnicities. All of these variants, except *CYP2C9*8*, have been confirmed by meta-analysis to reduce warfarin dose requirements in black African patients [136]. The non-coding variant, rs12777823, within the *CYP2C* cluster upstream of *CYP2C18*, has also been associated with reduced WSD requirements, independent of *CYP2C9* [137].

CYP4F2 mediates removal of active (reduced) vitamin K from the vitamin K cycle. *CYP4F2*3* is associated with lower hepatic CYP4F2 [138] and increased WSD requirements in Asian [139] and European ancestry patients, but not in those of African ancestry [140,141].

Beyond *VKORC1/CYP2C9/CYP4F2*, many other candidate genes have been investigated for their role in variable warfarin dose requirements, although findings have been mostly contradictory, and not supported by GWAS. Interestingly however, rs7856096 in the folate homeostasis gene, folylpolyglutamate synthase (*FPGS*), was identified in African-Americans by exome sequencing and replicated [142]. It decreases *FPGS* transcription and is associated with reduced WSD requirements, although the causative mechanism remains unknown.

Several RCTs have investigated the utility of genetic-guided warfarin dosing algorithms (Table 2). The largest trial to date, the Genetic Informatics Trial (GIFT), recruited patients initiating warfarin for elective hip or knee surgery [17]. GIFT compared 808 patients that received genotype-guided dosing (considering *VKORC1* -1639G > A, *CYP2C9*2, CYP2C9*3, CYP4F2*3*) to 789 that received clinically-guided dosing. The primary clinical composite endpoint of major bleeding, INR ≥ 4, VTE or death occurred in 10.8% of patients in the genotyped arm versus 14.7% in the clinically-guided arm ($p = 0.02$). The high-risk subgroup of patients (those with a difference of at least 1.0mg/day between clinically guided and genotype-predicted warfarin doses), which plausibly had a higher number of warfarin sensitive alleles, particularly benefitted from genotyping with a larger (7%) increase in TTR. The findings in GIFT were consistent with the EU-PACT RCT, but not with COAG (Table 2) [15,16,131]

Both CPIC [143] and DPWG have developed warfarin PGx guidelines for commencing warfarin that recommend validated genetic algorithms (e.g., the EU-PACT loading algorithm [15] or International Warfarin Pharmacogenetics Consortium (IWPC) algorithm [144]) or percent dose alterations. Importantly, point-of-care genotype-guided warfarin dosing has been shown to significantly improve TTR following implementation in real world anticoagulation clinics [145], and appears cost-effective [16].

The majority of patients investigated have been of European ancestry.As described above, ethnicity influences the prevalence of warfarin risk alleles, particularly in those of Sub-Saharan African origin. Thus, ethnicity-specific algorithms have been developed, although prospective testing of these algorithms is currently limited [146,147]. Moreover, self-reported ethnicity may not represent genetic ancestry well, especially for admixed individuals [148]. Nonetheless, it has been recently shown that an individual's genetic ancestry can be reasonably determined from clinically focused PGx SNP panels (122 and 243 SNPs) compared with genome-wide genotyping [149]. This approach could stratify individual's by genetic ancestry to facilitate implementation of ethnicity-specific warfarin algorithms.

Although warfarin remains commonly prescribed, it is clear that the use of direct oral anticoagulants (DOACs) is increasing [150]. DOACs are at least as safe and effective as warfarin in the prevention of stroke in non-valvular AF [151] and monitoring is not required. However, their current high price restricts access to them in many healthcare systems, and concerns over long term adherence [152], as well as patient choice, mean they are not suitable for all patients. Interestingly, bleeding risk appears equivalent between DOACs and warfarin in patients who have no *VKORC1/CYP2C9* warfarin risk alleles [153] or their anticoagulation centre-based TTR is ≥66% [154], and thus anticoagulant stratification based on *VKORC1/CYP2C9* genotypes has been posited [155]. Moreover, no DOAC is indicated following mechanical heart valve surgery or in those with a creatinine clearance <15mL/min; thus, further research into the utility of warfarin PGx in these specific settings is warranted.

7. Metoprolol

Metoprolol is a racemate cardioselective β1-adrenoreceptor blocking agent used for indications including hypertension, heart failure, angina pectoris, arrhythmias and migraine prophylaxis. Around 70% of an oral dose undergoes metabolism by CYP2D6 to inactive metabolites [156]. Plasma levels of metoprolol have been found to be significantly higher (around 4–5 ×) in *CYP2D6* PMs compared with EMs [157].

Metoprolol decreases cardiac output via negative chronotropic, as well as inotropic effects, thus reducing heart rate [158]. Retrospective and prospective studies have demonstrated significantly greater reductions in heart rate in PMs vs. non-PMs [159,160] and an increased risk of bradycardia [161]. Although, there is observed heterogeneity in the incidence of bradycardia between studies, a recent meta-analysis identified that overall the prevalence of bradycardia is statistically significantly higher in PMs [162]. Nevertheless, the clinical relevance of this finding is presently unclear, given that many of the instances of bradycardia have been asymptomatic (e.g., detected on an electrocardiogram performed as part of a study protocol) with comparatively little reported around symptomatic bradyarrhythmias.

The DPWG guideline for metoprolol in CYP2D6 PM and IM patients suggest a dose reduction (to 25% and 50% of the standard dose, respectively) where a gradual reduction in heart rate is required (for example, in chronic heart failure) or symptomatic bradycardia occurs. As there may be increased conversion to inactive metabolites in UM patients blunting the efficacy of metoprolol, dose increases beyond the usual maximum dose or selection of an alternative β-blocker (indication dependent) may be required [106]. While other β-blockers including carvedilol, nebivolol and propranolol are also metabolized by CYP2D6, the extent of their CYP2D6-dependent metabolism is less than for metoprolol [163]. Moreover, atenolol is not metabolised, and bisoprolol undergoes balanced elimination with half excreted via the kidneys and the other half undergoing metabolism by CYP3A4 and CYP2D6; CYP2D6 does not appear to be an important predictor of bisoprolol exposure or function [164,165].

8. Allopurinol

The xanthine oxidase inhibitor, allopurinol, is commonly prescribed in primary care for the prophylaxis of gout; it is also indicated in other hyperuricaemic conditions including tumour lysis syndrome. Although allopurinol is generally well tolerated, severe cutaneous adverse reactions (SCARs) represent a rare (0.1–0.4% of patients) but serious allopurinol ADR. The SCARs, Stevens–Johnson syndrome (SJS), toxic epidermal necrolysis (TEN), and drug reaction with eosinophilia and systemic symptoms (DRESS), have all been reported following allopurinol exposure [166].

SCARs have overlapping clinical features including eosinophilia, hepatic/renal dysfunction and rash or skin detachment. SJS and TEN are considered to represent different severities along a continuum of the same disease process; SJS is diagnosed when ≤10% body surface area is affected, TEN when >30% is affected, and an overlap syndrome occurs with 10–30% body surface area involvement [167]. Allopurinol is the most common cause of SCARs in Europe [168]. Furthermore, SCARs have high morbidity and mortality rates [167,169] and the mortality specifically from allopurinol-associated SCARs has been reported to approach 25% [168,170].

Studies have shown strong associations between allopurinol-related SCARs and carrying *HLA-B*58:01* [171,172]. In an interventional cohort study in Taiwan, genotyping *HLA-B*58:01* and giving alternate treatment to *HLA-B*58:01* positive patients, whilst *HLA-B*58:01* negative patients received allopurinol, resulted in no SCAR cases, compared to an estimated seven cases based on the historical average ($p = 0.0026$) [20].

The allopurinol SCAR-*HLA-B* association is considered to be a type IV hypersensitivity reaction and is T-cell mediated [173]; typically, such reactions occur up to 3 months after drug initiation (most cases occurring within 8–9 weeks [174] and are delayed in onset (as opposed to anaphylactic reactions with other drugs which are immediate) [175]. Other identified clinical factors that increase the risk of allopurinol SCAR include older age, female sex, chronic kidney disease and higher starting doses, which all plausibly increase systemic exposure [176]. Following oral administration, allopurinol is almost completely metabolised into its active metabolite, oxypurinol, which has an elimination half-life of 15 h, compared to 1–2 h for allopurinol [177]. Regarding immunopathogenesis, both allopurinol and oxypurinol have been shown to directly bind *HLA-B*58:01* and Arg97 of *HLA-B*58:01* is a plausible binding site for oxypurinol via hydrogen bond formation [178]. Oxypurinol-sensitive T-cell lines can have mixed populations of CD4+ and CD8+ T-cells. Moreover, in vitro T-cell activation assays after culturing peripheral blood mononuclear cells from patients with previous allopurinol-associated SCARs demonstrated that oxypurinol increased granulysin in a concentration- and time-dependent manner, but allopurinol and febuxostat did not, indicative of oxypurinol-induced T-cell activation [179]. Sequencing the T-cell receptors demonstrated that clonotype-specific T-cells that secrete granulysin in response to oxypurinol likely participate in the pathogenesis [179]. Overall, these observations are consistent with the p-i hypothesis (direct pharmacological interaction between a drug/metabolite and HLA molecules) whereby allopurinol-associated SCARs are the result of MHC Class I-driven activation of oxypurinol-specific T-cell clones through an antigen-processing independent route.

The frequency of *HLA-B*58:01* varies with ethnicity, but occurs at a higher prevalence in East Asian populations [180]. *HLA-B* expression is co-dominant and individuals need only carry one copy of *HLA-B*58:01* to be at increased risk of SCARs. Accordingly, genotyping results are usually reported as *HLA-B*58:01* positive, where one of more copies of the allele are detected, or negative where the allele is not detected. This association is now mentioned within the European drug label and CPIC guidelines for allopurinol advise against its use in known *HLA-B*58:01* carriers [170,181]

More generally, associations between specific *HLA* alleles and serious ADRs due to at least 24 different drugs have now been reported [182], highlighting the importance of the *HLA* locus to immune-mediated type IV hypersensitivity reactions. Like, allopurinol, several of these associations are very strong (e.g., odds ratios in the tens-thousands) and related to drug-induced skin injury, such as between carbamazepine-*HLA-B*15:02* and SJS-TEN, and carbamazepine-*HLA-A*31:01* that is associated with both specific SCARs (DRESS and SJS-TEN) and more mild but common (up to 10% of patients [183]) maculopapular exanthema [184]. *HLA* alleles have also been associated with drug-induced liver injury, such as between flucloxacillin and *HLA-B*57:01* [185]. Of note, *HLA-B*57:01* is also associated with abacavir hypersensitivity syndrome [186]. As previously mentioned, *HLA-DRB1*11:01* has been significantly associated with statin-related anti-HMGCR myopathy [103]. These associations provide mechanistic insight and can aid in preventing or diagnosing a serious ADR.

9. Transitioning to the Future

The current literature demonstrates that many primary healthcare providers including physicians and pharmacists are hopeful about the role of PGx in enhancing the care of their patients [187,188] but often highlight that there are still multiple barriers impeding translation into daily practice [189]. Potential pathways of how GPs may encounter PGx tests are shown in Figure 2. Recent studies have identified that barriers to PGx implementation specifically within primary care include a perceived lack of evidence for clinical utility, unclear cost effectiveness and reimbursement strategies, how to educate the primary care workforce regarding PGx, unclear roles and responsibilities particularly between general practitioners and pharmacists, the need for informatics to support PGx-informed clinical prescribing decisions, and concerns over the principles of data sharing as well as other ethical, legal and social implications (ELSI) surrounding PGx [190,191].

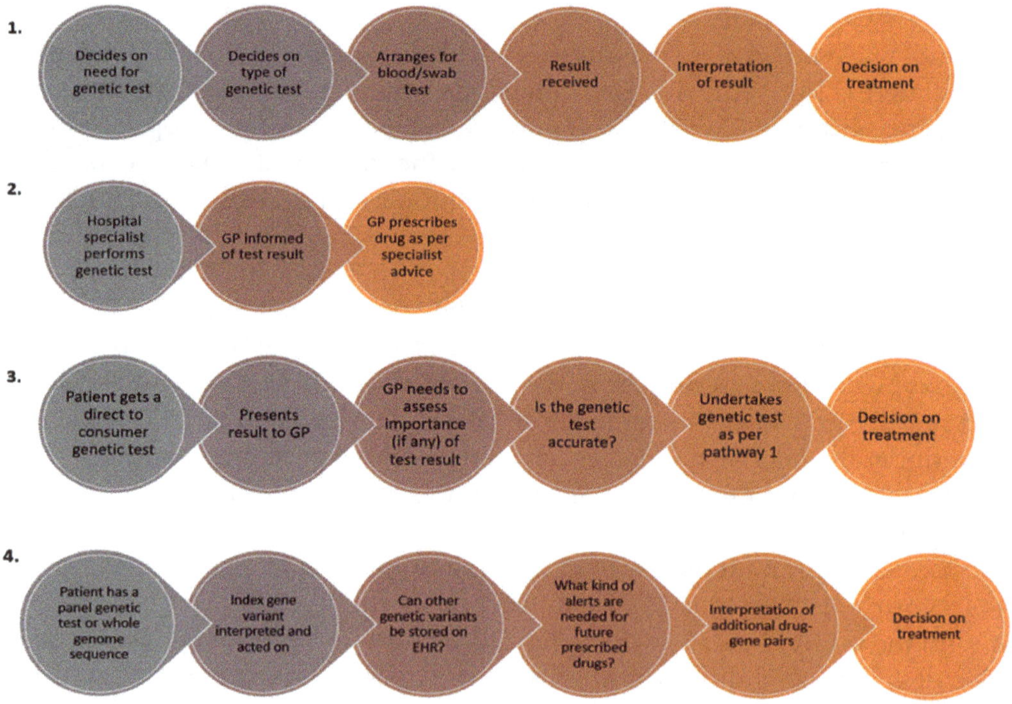

Figure 2. Four hypothetical pathways through which GPs may encounter pharmacogenetic tests within their primary care practice. Pathway 1 is where the GP initiates the test themselves; pathway 2 is where the genetic test is carried out in secondary care and the GP is informed of the test result; and pathway 3 is where the patient presents to the GP having undertaken a test privately or via a direct to consumer genetic testing laboratory. Pathways 1–3 represent situations where a single gene/variant test is undertaken for one gene-drug pair. Pathway 4 represents the situation where the patient has undergone a panel test or exome/whole genome sequencing, where there is the added complexity of storing the rest of the genetic data and having the ability to retrieve it, and use it appropriately in a pre-emptive fashion when a patient is prescribed a new drug(s).

Efforts to overcome these barriers and facilitate PGx translation are ongoing. Within Europe, the Ubiquitous Pharmacogenomics Consortium (U-PGx) is undertaking a large, international implementation project (PREemptive Pharmacogenomic testing for prevention of Adverse drug REactions (PREPARE)) within both primary and secondary care settings [192]. This study aims to recruit around 7000 patients to determine the clinical utility and cost effectiveness of testing a panel of 44 PGx variants in 12 genes relevant to 42 drugs for which a DPWG PGx guideline has been developed; the primary focus of PREPARE is to investigate whether PGx implementation reduces ADRs within the first 12 weeks of starting one of these 42 drugs, compared to standard care. Similar initiatives adopting panel-based testing are ongoing around the world, including the Pharmacogenomic Resource for Enhanced Decisions in Care and Treatment program (PREDICT) in the US, which has pre-emptively tested over 10,000 patients to date [6]. Moreover, in the UK, the NHS Genomic Medicine Service (GMS) outlined its plans to have genomic medicine fully integrated into routine practice by 2025 [193].

Despite the cost of genetic tests decreasing, cost-effectiveness remains a concern for PGx testing. While some drug-gene pairs, such as abacavir-*HLA-B*57:01* and allopurinol-*HLA-B*58:01*, have demonstrated cost-effectiveness compared with no genetic testing, others such as factor V Leiden testing prior to oral contraception, have shown mixed and inconclusive results [194]. Panel testing is the most common form of PGx testing currently being utilised in large scale studies such as PREPARE, and is likely more cost effective than single gene testing [195]. Although panel testing does not offer the same in-depth information for a gene compared to whole genome sequencing, its upfront costs are less, test turnaround times are shorter, and interpretation of gene regions is less complicated, which arguably makes it a better suited technology for larger scale implementation in the near to medium term.

Patient focus groups have shown a preference for a familiar healthcare provider to be involved with delivering PGx services [196]. In addition, the uptake of direct-to-consumer testing is increasing and so there is a need to upskill the primary care workforce at large to improve its genetic literacy [197]. It is clear that wider implementation of PGx into the primary care sector will be soon upon us, and it is essential that all areas are able to access the resources to become more comfortable with PGx and overcome the aforementioned barriers.

One critical area for implementation is the development of appropriate clinical decision support systems (CDSS) that facilitate use of PGx information at the point of prescribing and, ideally, integrate this information with other factors routinely considered in the prescribing decision-making process, such as co-medications and comorbidities. In the UK at least, the widespread and early adoption of electronic medical patient records in primary care, which are provided by only a handful of service providers (e.g., EMIS and SystemOne), provide a pre-existing technological infrastructure to build PGx CDSS into. In contrast, the varying uptake of electronic records in secondary care and the greater heterogeneity in providers poses additional barriers to implementing PGx in hospital settings.

As the implementation infrastructure for PGx is gradually erected, it will be important to transition to healthcare learning systems where clinical and research activities are more clearly linked. Thus, ideally, novel clinically relevant and validated discoveries can then be implemented in a shorter time frame than currently, and the effects in the real-world of new interventions observed, measured and iteratively fed back to the research arm to inform future enquiry. A key component of an effective healthcare learning system will be merging presently disparate data sources together and putting systems in place to efficiently collect future clinical data as it is generated to enable big data analyses, and there is little reason why PGx cannot be at the forefront of such endeavours. For example, combining primary care records with array genetic data at scale within UK Biobank has enabled recent PGx analysis investigating interactions between 200 drugs and nine genes in 200,000 subjects, leading to confirmation of several established drug-gene pairs, as well as providing genetic evidence of more novel associations such as between citalopram and reduced incidence of herpes zoster in *CYP2C19* IMs [198].

It should be noted that, to date, the majority of PGx associations involve common variants, including the drug-gene variant associations highlighted in this review. Rare variants (i.e., those with a minor allele frequency < 1%) are often missed in small clinical studies or GWAS analyses, but some may have large effects on outcomes [199]. Case studies of rare and serious ADRs have highlighted the clinical impact of rare variation in pharmacogenes. For example, a recent case report detailed development of reversible encephalopathy and coma after a paediatric patient received a single dose of ivermectin, attributable to compound heterozygosity from two nonsense mutations in *ABCB1*, which encodes P-glycoprotein [200]. Furthermore, the increasing use of next generation sequencing (NGS) technologies in national and other large genomic medicine projects heralds a new era for investigating rare variation at scale. It is currently estimated that, overall, 10–40% of genetic functional variation in pharmacogenes is attributable to rare ght to account for 9% and 39% of the functional variation in *SLCO1B1* and *ABCC1*, respectively variation, although it varies considerably between genes [201]. For example, rare variation is thou Machine learning and other advanced methodologies will likely be needed to parse this rich sequence data, particularly when combined with other data types (e.g., clinical and other omics datasets), to aid functional interpretation and variant discovery, refine genotype-to-phenotype predictions, stratify patient groups, and predict drug response [202,203].

10. Conclusions

The majority of prescribing happens in primary care. Owing to interindividual variation, some patients experience reduced effectiveness and others ADRs. Extensive research into PGx has identified and replicated multiple drug-gene pairs, mainly associated with ADRs, with several of the associated drugs commonly prescribed in primary care. The ongoing development of PGx guidelines by CPIC, DPWG and others offers a standardised approach to translating drug-gene associations into actionable prescribing recommendations based on the collective evidence available. Nevertheless, several barriers still exist to wider adoption of PGx into primary care, although these are gradually being addressed. Moving forward, a transition towards healthcare learning systems that harness big data and advanced analytical techniques with implementation of clinically relevant findings is anticipated to advance patient care. One area for focus is the surge in multimorbidity and related polypharmacy that multiple primary care and wider healthcare systems are facing. Although further research is required, it is envisaged that PGx will play a meaningful role in optimising medicines and managing polypharmacy [50]. Overall, it is hoped that implementation of PGx in primary care will be a major activity over the next five years, with ongoing PGx discoveries further boosting the case for implementation.

Author Contributions: Conceptualization, V.R. and R.T.; writing—original draft preparation, V.R. and R.T.; writing—review and editing, M.P.; All authors have read and agreed to the published version of the manuscript.

Acknowledgments: Not applicable.

References

1. Evans, W.E.; McLeod, H.L. Pharmacogenomics—Drug disposition, drug targets, and side effects. *N. Engl. J. Med.* **2003**, *348*, 538–549. [CrossRef] [PubMed]

2. Gray, K.A.; Yates, B.; Seal, R.L.; Wright, M.W.; Bruford, E.A. Genenames.org: The HGNC resources in 2015. *Nucleic Acids Res.* **2015**, *43*, 1079–1085. [CrossRef] [PubMed]
3. Pirmohamed, M.; James, S.; Meakin, S.; Green, C.; Scott, A.K.; Walley, T.J.; Farrar, K.; Park, B.K.; Breckenridge, A.M. Adverse drug reactions as cause of admission to hospital: Prospective analysis of 18 820 patients. *BMJ* **2004**, *329*, 15–19. [CrossRef] [PubMed]
4. Howard, R.L.; Avery, A.J.; Slavenburg, S.; Royal, S.; Pipe, G.; Lucassen, P.; Pirmohamed, M. Which drugs cause preventable admissions to hospital? A systematic review. *Br. J. Clin. Pharmacol.* **2007**, *63*, 136–147. [CrossRef] [PubMed]
5. Wei, M.Y.; Ito, M.K.; Cohen, J.D.; Brinton, E.A.; Jacobson, T.A. Predictors of statin adherence, switching, and discontinuation in the USAGE survey: Understanding the use of statins in America and gaps in patient education. *J. Clin. Lipidol.* **2013**, *7*, 472–483. [CrossRef] [PubMed]
6. Van Driest, S.L.; Shi, Y.; Bowton, E.A.; Schildcrout, J.S.; Peterson, J.F.; Pulley, J.; Denny, J.C.; Roden, D.M. Clinically Actionable Genotypes Among 10,000 Patients With Preemptive Pharmacogenomic Testing. *Clin. Pharmacol. Ther.* **2014**, *95*, 423–431. [CrossRef] [PubMed]
7. Schildcrout, J.S.; Denny, J.C.; Bowton, E.; Gregg, W.; Pulley, J.M.; Basford, M.A.; Cowan, J.D.; Xu, H.; Ramirez, A.H.; Crawford, D.C.; et al. Optimizing Drug Outcomes Through Pharmacogenetics: A Case for Preemptive Genotyping. *Clin. Pharmacol. Ther.* **2012**, *92*, 235–242. [CrossRef]
8. Kimpton, J.; Carey, I.M.; Threapleton, C.J.; Robinson, A.; Harris, T.; Cook, D.G.; Dewilde, S.; Baker, E.H. Longitudinal exposure of English primary care patients to pharmacogenomic drugs: An analysis to inform design of pre-emptive pharmacogenomic testing. *Br. J. Clin. Pharmacol.* **2019**, *85*, 2734–2746. [CrossRef]
9. Pharmacogenomics Knowledge Base (PharmGKB). Clinical Guideline Annotations. Available online: https://www.pharmgkb.org/guidelineAnnotations (accessed on 29 October 2020).
10. Food and Drug Administration (FDA). Table of Pharmacogenetic Associations. Available online: https://www.fda.gov/medical-devices/precision-medicine/table-pharmacogenetic-associations (accessed on 27 October 2020).
11. Bank, P.C.D.; Swen, J.J.; Guchelaar, H.J. Estimated nationwide impact of implementing a preemptive pharmacogenetic panel approach to guide drug prescribing in primary care in The Netherlands. *BMC Med.* **2019**, *17*, 1–14. [CrossRef]
12. Greden, J.F.; Parikh, S.V.; Rothschild, A.J.; Thase, M.E.; Dunlop, B.W.; Debattista, C.; Conway, C.R.; Forester, B.P.; Mondimore, F.M.; Shelton, R.C.; et al. Impact of pharmacogenomics on clinical outcomes in major depressive disorder in the GUIDED trial: A large, patient- and rater-blinded, randomized, controlled study. *J. Psychiatr. Res.* **2019**, *111*, 59–67. [CrossRef]
13. Pérez, V.; AB-GEN Collaborative Group; Salavert, A.; Espadaler, J.; Tuson, M.; Saiz-Ruiz, J.; Sáez-Navarro, C.; Bobes, J.; Baca-García, E.; Vieta, E.; et al. Efficacy of prospective pharmacogenetic testing in the treatment of major depressive disorder: Results of a randomized, double-blind clinical trial. *BMC Psychiatry* **2017**, *17*, 250. [CrossRef] [PubMed]
14. Bradley, P.; Shiekh, M.; Mehra, V.; Vrbicky, K.; Layle, S.; Olson, M.C.; Maciel, A.; Cullors, A.; Garces, J.A.; Lukowiak, A.A. Improved efficacy with targeted pharmacogenetic-guided treatment of patients with depression and anxiety: A randomized clinical trial demonstrating clinical utility. *J. Psychiatr. Res.* **2018**, *96*, 100–107. [CrossRef] [PubMed]
15. Pirmohamed, M.; Burnside, G.; Eriksson, N.; Jorgensen, A.L.; Toh, C.-H.; Nicholson, T.; Kesteven, P.; Christersson, C.; Wahlström, B.; Stafberg, C.; et al. A Randomized Trial of Genotype-Guided Dosing of Warfarin. *N. Engl. J. Med.* **2013**, *369*, 2294–2303. [CrossRef] [PubMed]
16. Kimmel, S.E.; French, B.; Kasner, S.E.; Johnson, J.A.; Anderson, J.L.; Gage, B.F.; Rosenberg, Y.D.; Eby, C.S.; Madigan, R.A.; McBane, R.B.; et al. A Pharmacogenetic versus a Clinical Algorithm for Warfarin Dosing. *N. Engl. J. Med.* **2013**, *369*, 2283–2293. [CrossRef]
17. Gage, B.F.; Bass, A.R.; Lin, H.; Woller, S.C.; Stevens, S.M.; Al-Hammadi, N.; Philip, M.J.; Rodríguez, T.; Miller, J.P.; McMillin, G.A.; et al. Effect of Genotype-Guided Warfarin Dosing on Clinical Events and Anticoagulation Control Among Patients Undergoing Hip or Knee Arthroplasty: The GIFT Randomized Clinical TrialEffect of Genotype-Guided Warfarin Dosing on Events and Anticoagulation Control Effect of Genotype-Guided Warfarin Dosing on Events and Anticoagulation Control. *JAMA* **2017**, *318*, 1115–1124. [CrossRef]

18. Pereira, N.L.; Farkouh, M.E.; So, D.; Lennon, R.; Geller, N.; Mathew, V.; Bell, M.; Bae, J.-H.; Jeong, M.H.; Chavez, I.; et al. Effect of Genotype-Guided Oral P2Y12 Inhibitor Selection vs Conventional Clopidogrel Therapy on Ischemic Outcomes After Percutaneous Coronary Intervention: The TAILOR-PCI Randomized Clinical Trial. *JAMA* **2020**, *324*, 761–771. [CrossRef]
19. Claassens, D.M.; Vos, G.J.; Bergmeijer, T.O.; Hermanides, R.S.; van't Hof, A.W.V.; Van Der Harst, P.; Barbato, E.; Morisco, C.; Gin, R.M.T.J.; Asselbergs, F.W.; et al. A Genotype-Guided Strategy for Oral P2Y12 Inhibitors in Primary PCI. *N. Engl. J. Med.* **2019**, *381*, 1621–1631. [CrossRef]
20. Ko, T.M.; Tsai, C.Y.; Chen, S.Y.; Chen, K.-S.; Yu, K.-H.; Chu, C.-S.; Huang, C.-M.; Wang, C.-R.; Weng, C.-T.; Yu, C.-L.; et al. Use of HLA-B*58:01 genotyping to prevent allopurinol induced severe cutaneous adverse reactions in Taiwan: National prospective cohort study. *BMJ* **2015**, 351. [CrossRef]
21. Lacobucci, G. NHS prescribed record number of antidepressants last year. *BMJ* **2019**, *364*, l1508. [CrossRef]
22. Henssler, J.; Kurschus, M.; Franklin, J.; Bschor, T.; Baethge, C. Trajectories of Acute Antidepressant Efficacy: How Long to Wait for Response? A Systematic Review and Meta-Analysis of Long-Term, Placebo-Controlled Acute Treatment Trials. *J. Clin. Psychiatry* **2018**, *79*. [CrossRef]
23. Mars, B.; Heron, J.; Kessler, D.; Davies, N.M.; Martin, R.M.; Thomas, K.H.; Gunnell, D. Influences on antidepressant prescribing trends in the UK: 1995–2011. *Soc. Psychiatry Psychiatr. Epidemiol.* **2016**, *52*, 193–200. [CrossRef] [PubMed]
24. Zanger, U.M.; Turpeinen, M.; Klein, K.; Schwab, M. Functional pharmacogenetics/genomics of human cytochromes P450 involved in drug biotransformation. *Anal. Bioanal. Chem.* **2008**, *392*, 1093–1108. [CrossRef] [PubMed]
25. Licinio, J.; Wong, M.-L. Pharmacogenomics of antidepressant treatment effects. Dialog. *Clin. Neurosci.* **2011**, *13*, 63–71.
26. Pharmvar Pharmacogenomics Variation Consortium. CYP2D6. Available online: https://www.pharmvar.org/gene/CYP2D6 (accessed on 28 June 2020).
27. Gaedigk, A.; Dinh, J.C.; Jeong, H.; Prasad, B.; Leeder, J.S. Ten Years' Experience with the CYP2D6 Activity Score: A Perspective on Future Investigations to Improve Clinical Predictions for Precision Therapeutics. *J. Pers. Med.* **2018**, *8*, 15. [CrossRef] [PubMed]
28. Gaedigk, A.; Sangkuhl, K.; Whirl-Carrillo, M.; Klein, T.E.; Leeder, J.S. Prediction of CYP2D6 phenotype from genotype across world populations. *Genet. Med.* **2017**, *19*, 69–76. [CrossRef] [PubMed]
29. Roke, Y.; Van Harten, P.N.; Franke, B.; Galesloot, T.E.; Boot, A.M.; Buitelaar, J.K. The effect of the Taq1A variant in the dopamine D (2) receptor gene and common CYP2D6 alleles on prolactin levels in risperidone-treated boys. *Pharm. Genom.* **2013**, *23*, 487–493. [CrossRef] [PubMed]
30. Shams, M.E.E.; Arneth, B.; Hiemke, C.; Dragicevic, A.; Muller, M.J.; Kaiser, R.; Lackner, K.; Hartter, S. CYP2D6 polymorphism and clinical effect of the antidepressant venlafaxine. *J. Clin. Pharm. Ther.* **2006**, *31*, 493–502. [CrossRef]
31. Bijl, M.J.; Visser, L.E.; Hofman, A.; Vulto, A.G.; Van Gelder, T.; Stricker, B.H.; Van Schaik, R.H.N. Influence of the CYP2D6*4 polymorphism on dose, switching and discontinuation of antidepressants. *Br. J. Clin. Pharmacol.* **2007**, *65*, 558–564. [CrossRef]
32. Güzey, C.; Spigset, O. Low Serum Concentrations of Paroxetine in CYP2D6 Ultrarapid Metabolizers. *J. Clin. Psychopharmacol.* **2006**, *26*, 211–212. [CrossRef]
33. Hicks, J.K.; Bishop, J.R.; Sangkuhl, K.; Müller, D.J.; Ji, Y.; Leckband, S.G.; Leeder, J.S.; Graham, R.L.; Chiulli, D.L.; LLerena, A.; et al. Clinical Pharmacogenetics Implementation Consortium (CPIC) Guideline for CYP2D6 and CYP2C19 Genotypes and Dosing of Selective Serotonin Reuptake Inhibitors. *Clin. Pharmacol. Ther.* **2015**, *98*, 127–134.
34. Zastrozhin, M.; Skryabin, V.Y.; Smirnov, V.; Grishina, E.; Ryzhikova, K.; Chumakov, E.; Bryun, E.; Sychev, D. Effects of CYP2D6 activity on the efficacy and safety of mirtazapine in patients with depressive disorders and comorbid alcohol use disorder. *Can. J. Physiol. Pharmacol.* **2019**, *97*, 781–785. [CrossRef] [PubMed]
35. Ramaekers, J.G.; Conen, S.; De Kam, P.J.; Braat, S.; Peeters, P.; Theunissen, E.L.; Ivgy-May, N. Residual effects of esmirtazapine on actual driving performance: Overall findings and an exploratory analysis into the role of CYP2D6 phenotype. *Psychopharmacology* **2011**, *215*, 321–332. [CrossRef] [PubMed]
36. Pharmvar. CYP2C19. Available online: https://www.pharmvar.org/gene/CYP2C19 (accessed on 8 June 2020).
37. Pereira, N.L.; Rihal, C.S.; So, D.Y.; Rosenberg, Y.; Lennon, R.J.; Mathew, V.; Goodman, S.G.; Weinshilboum, R.M.; Wang, L.; Baudhuin, L.M.; et al. Clopidogrel Pharmacogenetics: State of the Art Review and the TAILOR-PCI Study. *Circ. Cardiovasc. Interv.* **2019**, *12*, e007811. [CrossRef] [PubMed]

38. Desta, Z.; Zhao, X.; Shin, J.G.; Flockhart, D.A. Clinical significance of the cytochrome P450 2C19 genetic polymorphism. *Clin. Pharmacokinet.* **2002**, *41*, 913–958. [CrossRef] [PubMed]
39. Sim, S.C.; Risinger, C.; Dahl, M.-L.; Aklillu, E.; Christensen, M.; Bertilsson, L.; Ingelman-Sundberg, M. A common novel CYP2C19 gene variant causes ultrarapid drug metabolism relevant for the drug response to proton pump inhibitors and antidepressants. *Clin. Pharmacol. Ther.* **2006**, *79*, 103–113. [CrossRef] [PubMed]
40. Grasmader, K.; Verwohlt, P.L.; Rietschel, M.; Dragicevic, A.; Müller, M.; Hiemke, C.; Freymann, N.; Zobel, A.; Maier, W.; Rao, M.L. Impact of polymorphisms of cytochrome-P450 isoenzymes 2C9, 2C19 and 2D6 on plasma concentrations and clinical effects of antidepressants in a naturalistic clinical setting. *Eur. J. Clin. Pharmacol.* **2004**, *60*, 329–336. [CrossRef] [PubMed]
41. Fudio, S.; Borobia, A.M.; Piñana, E.; Ramírez, E.; Tabarés, B.; Guerra, P.; Carcas, A.; Frias, J. Evaluation of the influence of sex and CYP2C19 and CYP2D6 polymorphisms in the disposition of citalopram. *Eur. J. Pharmacol.* **2010**, *626*, 200–204. [CrossRef]
42. FDA. Lexapro (Escitalopram Oxalate)—Prescribing Information. Available online: https://www.accessdata.fda.gov/drugsatfda_docs/label/2017/021323s047lbl.pdf (accessed on 28 June 2020).
43. Hyttel, J.; Christensen, A.V.; Fjalland, B. Neuropharmacological Properties of Amitriptyline, Nortriptyline and their Metabolites. *Acta Pharmacol. Toxicol.* **2009**, *47*, 53–57. [CrossRef]
44. Shimoda, K.; Someya, T.; Yokono, A.; Morita, S.; Hirokane, G.; Takahashi, S.; Okawa, M. The Impact of CYP2C19 and CYP2D6 Genotypes on Metabolism of Amitriptyline in Japanese Psychiatric Patients. *J. Clin. Psychopharmacol.* **2002**, *22*, 371–378. [CrossRef]
45. Hicks, J.K.; Swen, J.J.; Thorn, C.F.; Sangkuhl, K.; Kharasch, E.D.; Ellingrod, V.L.; Skaar, T.C.; Müller, D.J.; Gaedigk, A.; Stingl, J.C. Clinical Pharmacogenetics Implementation Consortium Guideline for CYP2D6 and CYP2C19 Genotypes and Dosing of Tricyclic Antidepressants. *Clin. Pharmacol. Ther.* **2013**, *93*, 402–408. [CrossRef]
46. Chaudhry, M.; Alessandrini, M.; Rademan, J.; Dodgen, T.M.; Steffens, F.E.; Van Zyl, D.G.; Gaedigk, A.; Pepper, M.S. Impact of CYP2D6 genotype on amitriptyline efficacy for the treatment of diabetic peripheral neuropathy: A pilot study. *Pharmacogenomics* **2017**, *18*, 433–443. [CrossRef] [PubMed]
47. Hicks, J.K.; Sangkuhl, K.; Swen, J.J.; Ellingrod, V.L.; Müller, D.J.; Shimoda, K.; Bishop, J.R.; Kharasch, E.D.; Skaar, T.C.; Gaedigk, A.; et al. Clinical pharmacogenetics implementation consortium guideline (CPIC) for CYP2D6 and CYP2C19 genotypes and dosing of tricyclic antidepressants: 2016 update. *Clin. Pharmacol. Ther.* **2017**, *102*, 37–44. [CrossRef] [PubMed]
48. Bousman, C.A.; Arandjelovic, K.; Mancuso, S.G.; Eyre, H.A.; Dunlop, B.W. Pharmacogenetic tests and depressive symptom remission: A meta-analysis of randomized controlled trials. *Pharmacogenomics* **2019**, *20*, 37–47. [CrossRef] [PubMed]
49. NHS Digital. Health Survey for England 2016: Adult Prescribed Medications—Tables. Available online: https://digital.nhs.uk/data-and-information/publications/statistical/health-survey-for-england/health-survey-for-england-2016 (accessed on 1 August 2020).
50. Sharp, C.N.; Linder, M.W.; Valdes, R. Polypharmacy: A healthcare conundrum with a pharmacogenetic solution. *Crit. Rev. Clin. Lab. Sci.* **2019**, *57*, 161–180. [CrossRef]
51. Brown, L.C.; Lorenz, R.A.; Li, J.; DeChairo, B.M. Economic Utility: Combinatorial Pharmacogenomics and Medication Cost Savings for Mental Health Care in a Primary Care Setting. *Clin. Ther.* **2017**, *39*, 592–602. [CrossRef]
52. Thorn, C.F.; Klein, T.E.; Altman, R.B. Codeine and morphine pathway. *Pharm. Genom.* **2009**, *19*, 556–558. [CrossRef]
53. Grond, S.; Sablotzki, A. Clinical Pharmacology of Tramadol. *Clin. Pharmacokinet.* **2004**, *43*, 879–923. [CrossRef]
54. Gong, L.; Stamer, U.M.; Tzvetkov, M.V.; Altman, R.B.; Klein, T.E. PharmGKB summary: Tramadol pathway. *Pharm. Genom.* **2014**, *24*, 374–380. [CrossRef]
55. Dayer, P.; Desmeules, J.; Leemann, T.; Striberni, R. Bioactivation of the narcotic drug codeine in human liver is mediated by the polymorphic monooxygenase catalyzing debrisoquine 4-hydroxylation (cytochrome P-450 dbl/bufI). *Biochem. Biophys. Res. Commun.* **1988**, *152*, 411–416. [CrossRef]
56. Kirchheiner, J.; Schmidt, H.; Tzvetkov, M.; A Keulen, J.-T.H.; Lötsch, J.; Roots, I.; Brockmöller, J. Pharmacokinetics of codeine and its metabolite morphine in ultra-rapid metabolizers due to CYP2D6 duplication. *Pharm. J.* **2006**, *7*, 257–265. [CrossRef]
57. Gasche, Y.; Daali, Y.; Fathi, M.; Chiappe, A.; Cottini, S.; Dayer, P.; Desmeules, J.A. Codeine Intoxication Associated with Ultrarapid CYP2D6 Metabolism. *N. Engl. J. Med.* **2004**, *351*, 2827–2831. [CrossRef] [PubMed]

58. Poulsen, L.; Brøsen, K.; Arendt-Nielsen, L.; Gram, L.F.; Elbaek, K.; Sindrup, S.H. Codeine and morphine in extensive and poor metabolizers of sparteine: Pharmacokinetics, analgesic effect and side effects. *Eur. J. Clin. Pharmacol.* **1996**, *51*, 289–295. [CrossRef] [PubMed]
59. Williams, D.G.; Hatch, D.J.; Howard, R.F. Codeine phosphate in paediatric medicine. *Br. J. Anaesth.* **2001**, *86*, 413–421. [CrossRef] [PubMed]
60. Medicines and Healthcare products Regulatory Agency. Codeine for analgesia: Restricted use in children because of reports of morphine toxicity. *Drug Saf. Update* **2013**, *6*, A1.
61. Safety Review Update of Codeine Use in Children; New Boxed Warning and Contraindication on Use after Tonsillectomy and/or Adenoidectomy. Available online: https://www.fda.gov/media/85072/download (accessed on 25 July 2020).
62. Kelly, L.E.; Rieder, M.; Anker, J.V.D.; Malkin, B.; Ross, C.; Neely, M.N.; Carleton, B.; Hayden, M.R.; Madadi, P.; Koren, G. More Codeine Fatalities After Tonsillectomy in North American Children. *Pediatrics* **2012**, *129*, e1343–e1347. [CrossRef] [PubMed]
63. MHRA. Codeine for Cough and Cold: Restricted Use in Children. Available online: https://www.gov.uk/drug-safety-update/codeine-for-cough-and-cold-restricted-use-in-children (accessed on 25 July 2020).
64. Baber, M.; Chaudhry, S.; Kelly, L.E.; Ross, C.J.; Carleton, B.C.; Berger, H.; Koren, G. The pharmacogenetics of codeine pain relief in the postpartum period. *Pharm. J.* **2015**, *15*, 430–435. [CrossRef] [PubMed]
65. Chen, T.-C.; Chen, L.-C.; Knaggs, R.D. A 15-year overview of increasing tramadol utilisation and associated mortality and the impact of tramadol classification in the United Kingdom. *Pharmacoepidemiol. Drug Saf.* **2018**, *27*, 487–494. [CrossRef] [PubMed]
66. Borlak, J.; Hermann, R.; Erb, K.; Thum, T. A rapid and simple CYP2D6 genotyping assay—Case study with the analgetic tramadol. *Metabolism* **2003**, *52*, 1439–1443. [CrossRef]
67. Kirchheiner, J.; Keulen, J.-T.H.; Bauer, S.; Roots, I.; Brockmöller, J. Effects of the CYP2D6 Gene Duplication on the Pharmacokinetics and Pharmacodynamics of Tramadol. *J. Clin. Psychopharmacol.* **2008**, *28*, 78–83. [CrossRef]
68. Stamer, U.M.; Stüber, F.; Muders, T.; Musshoff, F. Respiratory Depression with Tramadol in a Patient with Renal Impairment and CYP2D6 Gene Duplication. *Anesth. Analg.* **2008**, *107*, 926–929. [CrossRef]
69. Wen, Q.-H.; Zhang, Z.; Cai, W.-K.; Lin, X.-Q.; He, G.-H. The Associations between CYP2D6*10 C188T Polymorphism and Pharmacokinetics and Clinical Outcomes of Tramadol: A Systematic Review and Meta-analysis. *Pain Med.* **2020**. [CrossRef] [PubMed]
70. Parker, B.A.; Capizzi, J.A.; Grimaldi, A.S.; Clarkson, P.M.; Cole, S.M.; Keadle, J.; Chipkin, S.R.; Pescatello, L.S.; Simpson, K.; White, C.M.; et al. Effect of Statins on Skeletal Muscle Function. *Circulation* **2013**, *127*, 96–103. [CrossRef] [PubMed]
71. Alfirevic, A.; Neely, D.; Armitage, J.; Chinoy, H.; Cooper, R.G.; Laaksonen, R.; Carr, D.F.; Bloch, K.M.; Fahy, J.; Hanson, A.; et al. Phenotype Standardization for Statin-Induced Myotoxicity. *Clin. Pharmacol. Ther.* **2014**, *96*, 470–476. [CrossRef] [PubMed]
72. Hopewell, J.C.; Offer, A.; Haynes, R.; Bowman, L.; Li, J.; Chen, F.; Bulbulia, R.; Lathrop, M.; Baigent, C.; Landray, M.J.; et al. Independent risk factors for simvastatin-related myopathy and relevance to different types of muscle symptom. *Eur. Hear. J.* **2020**, *41*, 3336–3342. [CrossRef] [PubMed]
73. Kobie, J.; Guo, Z.; Cho, C.R.; Menzel, K.; McCrea, J.B.; Blanchard, R.; Shaw, P.M. Pharmacogenetic Analysis of OATP1B1, UGT1A1, and BCRP Variants in Relation to the Pharmacokinetics of Letermovir in Previously Conducted Clinical Studies. *J. Clin. Pharmacol.* **2019**, *59*, 1236–1243. [CrossRef]
74. Obaidat, A.; Roth, M.; Hagenbuch, B. The Expression and Function of Organic Anion Transporting Polypeptides in Normal Tissues and in Cancer. *Annu. Rev. Pharmacol. Toxicol.* **2012**, *52*, 135–151. [CrossRef]
75. Elsby, R.; Hilgendorf, C.; Fenner, K. Understanding the critical disposition pathways of statins to assess drug-drug interaction risk during drug development: It's not just about OATP1B1. *Clin. Pharmacol. Ther.* **2012**, *92*, 584–598. [CrossRef]
76. Wilhelmsen, L.; Link, E.M.; Parish, S.; Armitage, J.M.; Bowman, L.H.; Heath, S.; Matsuda, F.; Gut, I.; Lathrop, M.; A Collins, R. SLCO1B1Variants and Statin-Induced Myopathy—A Genomewide Study. *N. Engl. J. Med.* **2008**, *359*, 789–799. [CrossRef]
77. Donnelly, L.A.; Doney, A.S.F.; Tavendale, R.; Lang, C.C.; Pearson, E.R.; Colhoun, H.M.; McCarthy, M.I.; Hattersley, A.T.; Morris, A.D.; Palmer, C.N.A. Common Nonsynonymous Substitutions in SLCO1B1 Predispose to Statin Intolerance in Routinely Treated Individuals With Type 2 Diabetes: A Go-DARTS Study. *Clin. Pharmacol. Ther.* **2011**, *89*, 210–216. [CrossRef]

78. Turner, R.M.; Pirmohamed, M. Statin-Related Myotoxicity: A Comprehensive Review of Pharmacokinetic, Pharmacogenomic and Muscle Components. *J. Clin. Med.* **2019**, *9*, 22. [CrossRef]
79. Carr, D.F.; Francis, B.; Jorgensen, A.L.; Zhang, E.; Chinoy, H.; Heckbert, S.R.; Bis, J.C.; Brody, J.A.; Floyd, J.S.; Psaty, B.M.; et al. Genome-wide association study of statin-induced myopathy in patients recruited using the UK clinical practice research datalink. *Clin. Pharmacol. Ther.* **2019**. [CrossRef] [PubMed]
80. Skottheim, I.B.; Gedde-Dahl, A.; Hejazifar, S.; Hoel, K.; Åsberg, A. Statin induced myotoxicity: The lactone forms are more potent than the acid forms in human skeletal muscle cells in vitro. *Eur. J. Pharm. Sci.* **2008**, *33*, 317–325. [CrossRef] [PubMed]
81. Voora, D.; Shah, S.H.; Spasojevic, I.; Ali, S.; Reed, C.R.; Salisbury, B.A.; Ginsburg, G.S. The SLCO1B1*5Genetic Variant Is Associated With Statin-Induced Side Effects. *J. Am. Coll. Cardiol.* **2009**, *54*, 1609–1616. [CrossRef] [PubMed]
82. Puccetti, L.; Ciani, F.; Auteri, A. Genetic involvement in statins induced myopathy. Preliminary data from an observational case–control study. *Atherosclerosis* **2010**, *211*, 28–29. [CrossRef]
83. De Keyser, C.E.; Peters, B.J.; Becker, M.L.; Visser, L.E.; Uitterlinden, A.G.; Klungel, O.H.; Verstuyft, C.; Hofman, A.; Der Zee, A.-H.M.-V.; Stricker, B.H.C. The SLCO1B1 c.521T>C polymorphism is associated with dose decrease or switching during statin therapy in the Rotterdam Study. *Pharm. Genom.* **2014**, *24*, 43–51. [CrossRef]
84. Carr, D.F.; O'Meara, H.; Jorgensen, A.L.; Campbell, J.; Hobbs, M.; McCann, G.; Van Staa, T.; Pirmohamed, M. SLCO1B1 Genetic Variant Associated With Statin-Induced Myopathy: A Proof-of-Concept Study Using the Clinical Practice Research Datalink. *Clin. Pharmacol. Ther.* **2013**, *94*, 695–701. [CrossRef] [PubMed]
85. Xiang, Q.; Chen, S.-Q.; Ma, L.-Y.; Hu, K.; Zhang, Z.; Mu, G.-Y.; Xie, Q.-F.; Zhang, X.-D.; Cui, Y.-M. Association between SLCO1B1 T521C polymorphism and risk of statin-induced myopathy: A meta-analysis. *Pharm. J.* **2018**, *18*, 721–729. [CrossRef] [PubMed]
86. Santos, P.C.J.D.L.; Gagliardi, A.C.M.; Miname, M.H.; Chacra, A.P.; Santos, R.D.; Krieger, J.E.; Pereira, A.D.C. SLCO1B1 haplotypes are not associated with atorvastatin-induced myalgia in Brazilian patients with familial hypercholesterolemia. *Eur. J. Clin. Pharmacol.* **2011**, *68*, 273–279. [CrossRef] [PubMed]
87. Turner, R.M.; Fontana, V.; Zhang, J.E.; Carr, D.; Yin, P.; Fitzgerald, R.; Morris, A.P.; Pirmohamed, M. A Genome-wide Association Study of Circulating Levels of Atorvastatin and Its Major Metabolites. *Clin. Pharmacol. Ther.* **2020**, *108*, 287–297. [CrossRef]
88. Danik, J.S.; Chasman, D.I.; MacFadyen, J.G.; Nyberg, F.; Barratt, B.J.; Ridker, P.M. Lack of association between SLCO1B1 polymorphisms and clinical myalgia following rosuvastatin therapy. *Am. Hear. J.* **2013**, *165*, 1008–1014. [CrossRef]
89. Bai, X.; Zhang, B.; Wang, P.; Wang, G.-L.; Li, J.-L.; Wen, D.-S.; Long, X.-Z.; Sun, H.-S.; Liu, Y.-B.; Huang, M.; et al. Effects of SLCO1B1 and GATM gene variants on rosuvastatin-induced myopathy are unrelated to high plasma exposure of rosuvastatin and its metabolites. *Acta Pharmacol. Sin.* **2019**, *40*, 492–499. [CrossRef] [PubMed]
90. Floyd, J.S.; Bloch, K.M.; Brody, J.A.; Maroteau, C.; Siddiqui, M.K.; Gregory, R.; Carr, D.F.; Molokhia, M.; Liu, X.; Bis, J.C.; et al. Pharmacogenomics of statin-related myopathy: Meta-analysis of rare variants from whole-exome sequencing. *PLoS ONE* **2019**, *14*, e0218115. [CrossRef] [PubMed]
91. Siddiqui, M.K.; Maroteau, C.; Veluchamy, A.; Tornio, A.; Tavendale, R.; Carr, F.; Abelega, N.-U.; Carr, D.; Bloch, K.; Hallberg, P.; et al. A common missense variant of LILRB5 is associated with statin intolerance and myalgia. *Eur. Hear. J.* **2017**, *38*, 3569–3575. [CrossRef] [PubMed]
92. Statin Immune Study (ImmunoStat) NCT02984293. 2016. Available online: https://clinicaltrials.gov/ct2/show/NCT02984293 (accessed on 6 June 2020).
93. Kitzmiller, J.P.; Luzum, J.A.; Baldassarre, D.; Krauss, R.M.; Medina, M.W. CYP3A4*22 and CYP3A5*3 are associated with increased levels of plasma simvastatin concentrations in the cholesterol and pharmacogenetics study cohort. *Pharm. Genom.* **2014**, *24*, 486–491. [CrossRef] [PubMed]
94. Keskitalo, J.E.; Zolk, O.; Fromm, M.F.; Kurkinen, K.J.; Neuvonen, P.J.; Niemi, M. ABCG2 Polymorphism Markedly Affects the Pharmacokinetics of Atorvastatin and Rosuvastatin. *Clin. Pharmacol. Ther.* **2009**, *86*, 197–203. [CrossRef] [PubMed]
95. Becker, M.L.; Visser, L.E.; Van Schaik, R.H.; Hofman, A.; Uitterlinden, A.G.; Stricker, B.H. Influence of genetic variation in CYP3A4 and ABCB1 on dose decrease or switching during simvastatin and atorvastatin therapy. *Pharmacoepidemiol. Drug Saf.* **2009**, *19*, 75–81. [CrossRef]

96. Kivistö, K.T.; Niemi, M.; Schaeffeler, E.; Pitkälä, K.; Tilvis, R.; Fromm, M.F.; Schwab, M.; Eichelbaum, M.; Strandberg, T. Lipid-lowering response to statins is affected by CYP3A5 polymorphism. *Pharmacogenetics* **2004**, *14*, 523–525. [CrossRef]
97. Zuccaro, P.; Mombelli, G.; Calabresi, L.; Baldassarre, D.; Palmi, I.; Sirtori, C.R. Tolerability of statins is not linked to CYP450 polymorphisms, but reduced CYP2D6 metabolism improves cholesteraemic response to simvastatin and fluvastatin. *Pharmacol. Res.* **2007**, *55*, 310–317. [CrossRef]
98. Postmus, I.; Trompet, S.; Deshmukh, H.A.; Barnes, M.R.; Li, X.; Warren, H.R.; Chasman, D.; Zhou, K.; Arsenault, B.; Donnelly, L.A.; et al. Pharmacogenetic meta-analysis of genome-wide association studies of LDL cholesterol response to statins. *Nat. Commun.* **2014**, *5*, 5068. [CrossRef]
99. Miroševic Skvrce, N.M.; Božina, N.; Zibar, L.; Barisic, I.; Pejnović, L.; Macolic Šarinić, V.M. CYP2C9andABCG2polymorphisms as risk factors for developing adverse drug reactions in renal transplant patients taking fluvastatin: A case–control study. *Pharmacogenomics* **2013**, *14*, 1419–1431. [CrossRef]
100. Buzkova, H.; Pechandova, K.; Danzig, V.; Vareka, T.; Perlík, F.; Zák, A.; Slanar, O. Lipid-lowering effect of fluvastatin in relation to cytochrome P450 2C9 variant alleles frequently distributed in the Czech population. *Med. Sci. Monit.* **2012**, *18*, CR512–CR517. [CrossRef] [PubMed]
101. Pinal-Fernandez, I.; Casal-Dominguez, M.; Mammen, A.L. Immune-Mediated Necrotizing Myopathy. *Curr. Rheumatol. Rep.* **2018**, *20*, 1–10. [CrossRef] [PubMed]
102. Mohassel, P.; Mammen, A.L. Anti-HMGCR Myopathy. *J. Neuromuscul. Dis.* **2018**, *5*, 11–20. [CrossRef] [PubMed]
103. Limaye, V.; Bundell, C.; Hollingsworth, P.; Rojana-Udomsart, A.; Mastaglia, F.; Blumbergs, P.; Lester, S. Clinical and genetic associations of autoantibodies to 3-hydroxy-3-methyl-glutaryl-coenzyme a reductase in patients with immune-mediated myositis and necrotizing myopathy. *Muscle Nerve* **2015**, *52*, 196–203. [CrossRef]
104. Mammen, A.L.; Gaudet, D.; Brisson, D.; Christopher-Stine, L.; Lloyd, T.E.; Leffell, M.S.; Zachary, A.A. Increased frequency of DRB1*11:01 in anti-hydroxymethylglutaryl-coenzyme A reductase-associated autoimmune myopathy. *Arthritis Rheum.* **2012**, *64*, 1233–1237. [CrossRef]
105. Ramsey, L.B.; Johnson, S.G.; Caudle, K.E.; Haidar, C.E.; Voora, D.; Wilke, R.A.; Maxwell, W.D.; McLeod, H.L.; Krauss, R.M.; Roden, D.M.; et al. The Clinical Pharmacogenetics Implementation Consortium Guideline for SLCO1B1 and Simvastatin-Induced Myopathy: 2014 Update. *Clin. Pharmacol. Ther.* **2014**, *96*, 423–428. [CrossRef]
106. Dutch Pharmacogenetics Working Group (DPWG). Pharmacogenetic Recommendations. 2020. Available online: https://www.knmp.nl/downloads/pharmacogenetic-recommendations-may-2020.pdf (accessed on 5 June 2020).
107. Food & Drug Administration. FDA Drug Safety Communication: New Restrictions, Contraindications, and Dose Limitations for Zocor (Simvastatin) to Reduce the Risk of Muscle Injury. 2017. Available online: https://www.fda.gov/drugs/drug-safety-and-availability/fda-drug-safety-communication-new-restrictions-contraindications-and-dose-limitations-zocor (accessed on 5 June 2020).
108. Peyser, B.; Perry, E.P.; Singh, K.; Gill, R.D.; Mehan, M.R.; Haga, S.B.; Musty, M.D.; Milazzo, N.A.; Savard, D.; Li, Y.-J.; et al. Effects of Delivering SLCO1B1 Pharmacogenetic Information in Randomized Trial and Observational Settings. *Circ. Genom. Precis. Med.* **2018**, *11*. [CrossRef]
109. De Vera, M.A.; Bhole, V.; Burns, L.C.; Lacaille, D. Impact of statin adherence on cardiovascular disease and mortality outcomes: A systematic review. *Br. J. Clin. Pharmacol.* **2014**, *78*, 684–698. [CrossRef]
110. Turner, R.M.; Pirmohamed, M. Chapter 5—Pharmacogenetics and Pharmacogenomics in Cardiovascular Medicine and Surgery. In *Cardiovascular Genetics and Genomics*; Kumar, D., Elliott, P., Eds.; Springer: Cham, Switzerland, 2018; pp. 119–172.
111. Kazui, M.; Nishiya, Y.; Ishizuka, T.; Hagihara, K.; Farid, N.A.; Okazaki, O.; Ikeda, T.; Kurihara, A. Identification of the Human Cytochrome P450 Enzymes Involved in the Two Oxidative Steps in the Bioactivation of Clopidogrel to Its Pharmacologically Active Metabolite. *Drug Metab. Dispos.* **2010**, *38*, 92–99. [CrossRef]
112. Mega, J.L.; Close, S.L.; Wiviott, S.D.; Shen, L.; Hockett, R.D.; Brandt, J.T.; Walker, J.R.; Antman, E.M.; Macias, W.; Braunwald, E.; et al. Cytochrome P-450 Polymorphisms and Response to Clopidogrel. *N. Engl. J. Med.* **2009**, *360*, 354–362. [CrossRef]
113. Trenk, D.; Hochholzer, W. Genetics of platelet inhibitor treatment. *Br. J. Clin. Pharmacol.* **2014**, *77*, 642–653. [CrossRef] [PubMed]

114. Mega, J.L.; Simon, T.; Collet, J.P.; Anderson, J.L.; Antman, E.M.; Bliden, K.; Cannon, C.P.; Danchin, N.; Giusti, B.; Gurbel, P.; et al. Reduced-function CYP2C19 genotype and risk of adverse clinical outcomes among patients treated with clopidogrel predominantly for PCI: A meta-analysis. *JAMA* **2010**, *304*, 1821–1830. [CrossRef] [PubMed]
115. Holmes, M.V.; Perel, P.; Shah, T.; Hingorani, A.D.; Casas, J.P. CYP2C19 genotype, clopidogrel metabolism, platelet function, and cardiovascular events: A systematic review and meta-analysis. *JAMA* **2011**, *306*, 2704–2714. [CrossRef] [PubMed]
116. Johnson, J.A.; Roden, D.M.; Lesko, L.J.; Ashley, E.; Klein, T.E.; Shuldiner, A.R. Clopidogrel: A Case for Indication-Specific Pharmacogenetics. *Clin. Pharmacol. Ther.* **2012**, *91*, 774–776. [CrossRef] [PubMed]
117. Klein, M.D.; Williams, A.K.; Lee, C.R.; Stouffer, G.A. Clinical Utility of CYP2C19 Genotyping to Guide Antiplatelet Therapy in Patients With an Acute Coronary Syndrome or Undergoing Percutaneous Coronary Intervention. *Arter. Thromb. Vasc. Biol.* **2019**, *39*, 647–652. [CrossRef]
118. Pan, Y.; Chen, W.; Xu, Y.; Yi, X.; Han, Y.; Yang, Q.; Li, X.; Huang, L.; Johnston, S.C.; Zhao, X.; et al. Genetic Polymorphisms and Clopidogrel Efficacy for Acute Ischemic Stroke or Transient Ischemic Attack: A Systematic Review and Meta-Analysis. *Circulation* **2017**, *135*, 21–33. [CrossRef]
119. Guo, B.; Tan, Q.; Guo, D.; Shi, Z.; Zhang, C.; Guo, W. Patients carrying CYP2C19 loss of function alleles have a reduced response to clopidogrel therapy and a greater risk of in-stent restenosis after endovascular treatment of lower extremity peripheral arterial disease. *J. Vasc. Surg.* **2014**, *60*, 993–1001. [CrossRef]
120. Wang, C.C.L.; Blomster, J.I.; Heizer, G.; Berger, J.S.; Baumgartner, I.; Fowkes, F.G.R.; Held, H.; Katona, B.G.; Norgren, L.; Jones, W.S.; et al. Cardiovascular and Limb Outcomes in Patients With Diabetes and Peripheral Artery Disease: The EUCLID Trial. *J. Am. Coll. Cardiol.* **2018**, *72*, 3274–3284. [CrossRef]
121. Scott, S.A.; Sangkuhl, K.; Stein, C.M.; Hulot, J.-S.; Mega, J.L.; Roden, D.M.; Klein, T.E.; Sabatine, M.S.; Johnson, J.A.; Shuldiner, A.R. Clinical Pharmacogenetics Implementation Consortium Guidelines for CYP2C19 Genotype and Clopidogrel Therapy: 2013 Update. *Clin. Pharmacol. Ther.* **2013**, *94*, 317–323. [CrossRef]
122. Cavallari, L.H.; Lee, C.R.; Beitelshees, A.L.; Cooper-DeHoff, R.M.; Duarte, J.D.; Voora, D.; Kimmel, S.E.; McDonough, C.W.; Gong, Y.; Dave, C.V.; et al. Multisite Investigation of Outcomes With Implementation of CYP2C19 Genotype-Guided Antiplatelet Therapy After Percutaneous Coronary Intervention. *JACC Cardiovasc. Interv.* **2018**, *11*, 181–191. [CrossRef]
123. Turner, R.M.; Pirmohamed, M. Cardiovascular Pharmacogenomics: Expectations and Practical Benefits. *Clin. Pharmacol. Ther.* **2014**, *95*, 281–293. [CrossRef] [PubMed]
124. Owen, R.P.; Gong, L.; Sagreiya, H.; Klein, T.E.; Altman, R.B. VKORC1 Pharmacogenomics Summary. *Pharm. Genom.* **2010**, *20*, 642–644. [CrossRef] [PubMed]
125. Jones, M.; McEwan, P.; Morgan, C.L.; Peters, J.R.; Goodfellow, J.; Currie, C.J. Evaluation of the pattern of treatment, level of anticoagulation control, and outcome of treatment with warfarin in patients with non-valvar atrial fibrillation: A record linkage study in a large British population. *Heart* **2005**, *91*, 472–477. [CrossRef] [PubMed]
126. Hylek, E.M.; Evans-Molina, C.; Shea, C.; Henault, L.E.; Regan, S. Major Hemorrhage and Tolerability of Warfarin in the First Year of Therapy among Elderly Patients with Atrial Fibrillation. *Circulation* **2007**, *115*, 2689–2696. [CrossRef] [PubMed]
127. Bourgeois, S.; Jorgensen, A.L.; Zhang, E.J.; Hanson, A.; Gill, M.; Bumpstead, S.; Toh, C.-H.; Williamson, P.R.; Daly, A.K.; Kamali, F.; et al. A multi-factorial analysis of response to warfarin in a UK prospective cohort. *Genome Med.* **2016**, *8*, 1–12. [CrossRef] [PubMed]
128. Pirmohamed, M.; Kamali, F.; Daly, A.K.; Wadelius, M. Oral anticoagulation: A critique of recent advances and controversies. *Trends Pharmacol. Sci.* **2015**, *36*, 153–163. [CrossRef]
129. Borgiani, P.; Ciccacci, C.; Forte, V.; Sirianni, E.; Novelli, L.; Bramanti, P.; Novelli, G. CYP4F2genetic variant (rs2108622) significantly contributes to warfarin dosing variability in the Italian population. *Pharmacogenomics* **2009**, *10*, 261–266. [CrossRef]
130. Takeuchi, F.; McGinnis, R.; Bourgeois, S.; Barnes, C.; Eriksson, N.; Soranzo, N.; Whittaker, P.; Ranganath, V.; Kumanduri, V.; McLaren, W.; et al. A Genome-Wide Association Study Confirms VKORC1, CYP2C9, and CYP4F2 as Principal Genetic Determinants of Warfarin Dose. *PLoS Genet.* **2009**, *5*, e1000433. [CrossRef]
131. Yuan, H.-Y.; Chen, J.-J.; Lee, M.T.; Wung, J.-C.; Chen, Y.-F.; Charng, M.-J.; Lu, M.-J.; Hung, C.-R.; Wei, C.-Y.; Chen, C.-H.; et al. A novel functional VKORC1 promoter polymorphism is associated with inter-individual and inter-ethnic differences in warfarin sensitivity. *Hum. Mol. Genet.* **2005**, *14*, 1745–1751. [CrossRef]

132. Lee, M.T.M.; Klein, T.E. Pharmacogenetics of warfarin: Challenges and opportunities. *J. Hum. Genet.* **2013**, *58*, 334–338. [CrossRef]
133. Johnson, J.A.; Cavallari, L.H. Pharmacogenetics and Cardiovascular Disease—Implications for Personalized Medicine. *Pharmacol. Rev.* **2013**, *65*, 987–1009. [CrossRef] [PubMed]
134. Suarez-Kurtz, G.; Botton, M.R. Pharmacogenomics of warfarin in populations of African descent. *Br. J. Clin. Pharmacol.* **2013**, *75*, 334–346. [CrossRef] [PubMed]
135. Johnson, J.A.; Cavallari, L.H. Warfarin pharmacogenetics: An illustration of the importance of studies in minority populations. *Clin. Pharmacol. Ther.* **2014**, *95*, 242–244. [CrossRef]
136. Asiimwe, I.G.; Zhang, E.J.; Osanlou, R.; Krause, A.; Dillon, C.; Suarez-Kurtz, G.; Zhang, H.; Perini, J.A.; Renta, J.Y.; Duconge, J.; et al. Genetic Factors Influencing Warfarin Dose in Black-African Patients: A Systematic Review and Meta-Analysis. *Clin. Pharmacol. Ther.* **2020**, *107*, 1420–1433. [CrossRef] [PubMed]
137. Perera, M.A.; Cavallari, L.H.; Limdi, N.; Gamazon, E.R.; Konkashbaev, A.; Daneshjou, R.; Pluzhnikov, A.; Crawford, D.C.; Wang, J.; Liu, N.; et al. Genetic variants associated with warfarin dose in African-American individuals: A genome-wide association study. *Lancet* **2013**, *382*, 790–796. [CrossRef]
138. McDonald, M.G.; Rieder, M.J.; Nakano, M.; Hsia, C.K.; Rettie, A.E. CYP4F2 Is a Vitamin K1 Oxidase: An Explanation for Altered Warfarin Dose in Carriers of the V433M Variant. *Mol. Pharmacol.* **2009**, *75*, 1337–1346. [CrossRef]
139. Cha, P.-C.; Mushiroda, T.; Takahashi, A.; Kubo, M.; Minami, S.; Kamatani, N.; Nakamura, Y. Genome-wide association study identifies genetic determinants of warfarin responsiveness for Japanese. *Hum. Mol. Genet.* **2010**, *19*, 4735–4744. [CrossRef]
140. Shendre, A.; Brown, T.M.; Liu, N.; Hill, C.E.; Beasley, T.M.; Nickerson, D.A.; Limdi, N.A. Race-Specific Influence of CYP4F2 on Dose and Risk of Hemorrhage Among Warfarin Users. *Pharmacotherapy* **2016**, *36*, 263–272. [CrossRef]
141. Bress, A.; Patel, S.R.; Perera, M.A.; Campbell, R.T.; Kittles, R.A.; Cavallari, L.H. Effect of NQO1 and CYP4F2 genotypes on warfarin dose requirements in Hispanic–Americans and African–Americans. *Pharmacogenomics* **2012**, *13*, 1925–1935. [CrossRef]
142. Daneshjou, R.; Gamazon, E.R.; Burkley, B.; Cavallari, L.H.; Johnson, J.A.; Klein, T.E.; Limdi, N.; Hillenmeyer, S.; Percha, B.; Karczewski, K.J.; et al. Genetic variant in folate homeostasis is associated with lower warfarin dose in African Americans. *Blood* **2014**, *124*, 2298–2305. [CrossRef]
143. Johnson, J.A.; Caudle, K.E.; Gong, L.; Whirl-Carrillo, M.; Stein, C.M.; Scott, S.A.; Lee, M.T.M.; Gage, B.F.; Kimmel, S.E.; Perera, M.A.; et al. Clinical Pharmacogenetics Implementation Consortium (CPIC) Guideline for Pharmacogenetics-Guided Warfarin Dosing: 2017 Update. *Clin. Pharmacol. Ther.* **2017**, *102*, 397–404. [CrossRef] [PubMed]
144. Klein, T.E.; Altman, R.B.; Eriksson, N.; Gage, B.F.; Kimmel, S.E.; Lee, M.-T.M.; Limdi, N.A.; Page, D.; Roden, D.M.; Wagner, M.J.; et al. Estimation of the warfarin dose with clinical and pharmacogenetic data. *N. Engl. J. Med.* **2009**, *360*, 753–764. [PubMed]
145. Jorgensen, A.L.; Prince, C.; Fitzgerald, G.; Hanson, A.; Downing, J.; Reynolds, J.; Zhang, J.E.; Alfirevic, A.; Pirmohamed, M. Implementation of genotype-guided dosing of warfarin with point-of-care genetic testing in three UK clinics: A matched cohort study. *BMC Med.* **2019**, *17*, 76. [CrossRef] [PubMed]
146. Shendre, A.; Dillon, C.; Limdi, N.A. Pharmacogenetics of warfarin dosing in patients of African and European ancestry. *Pharmacogenomics* **2018**, *19*, 1357–1371. [CrossRef] [PubMed]
147. Hernandez, W.; Gaamzon, E.R.; Aquino-Michaels, K.; Patel, S.; O'Brien, T.J.; Harralson, A.F.; Kittles, R.A.; Barbour, A.; Tuck, M.; McIntosh, S.D.; et al. Ethnicity-specific pharmacogenetics: The case of warfarin in African Americans. *Pharm. J.* **2014**, *14*, 223–228. [CrossRef]
148. Tishkoff, S.A.; Reed, F.A.; Friedlaender, F.R.; Ehret, C.; Ranciaro, A.; Froment, A.; Hirbo, J.B.; Awomoyi, A.A.; Bodo, J.-M.; Doumbo, O.; et al. The Genetic Structure and History of Africans and African Americans. *Science* **2009**, *324*, 1035–1044. [CrossRef] [PubMed]
149. Hernandez, W.; Danahey, K.; Pei, X.; Yeo, K.-T.J.; Leung, E.; Volchenboum, S.L.; Ratain, M.J.; Meltzer, D.O.; Stranger, B.E.; Perera, M.A.; et al. Pharmacogenomic genotypes define genetic ancestry in patients and enable population-specific genomic implementation. *Pharm. J.* **2020**, *20*, 126–135. [CrossRef]
150. Ho, K.H.; Van Hove, M.; Leng, G. Trends in anticoagulant prescribing: A review of local policies in English primary care. *BMC Health Serv. Res.* **2020**, *20*, 1–8. [CrossRef]
151. Julia, S.; James, U. Direct Oral Anticoagulants: A Quick Guide. *Eur. Cardiol.* **2017**, *12*, 40–45.

152. Burn, J.; Pirmohamed, M. Direct oral anticoagulants versus warfarin: Is new always better than the old? *Open Heart* **2018**, *5*, e000712. [CrossRef]
153. Mega, J.L.; Walker, J.R.; Ruff, C.T.; Vandell, A.G.; Nordio, F.; Deenadayalu, N.; Murphy, S.A.; Lee, J.; Mercuri, M.F.; Giugliano, R.P.; et al. Genetics and the clinical response to warfarin and edoxaban: Findings from the randomised, double-blind ENGAGE AF-TIMI 48 trial. *Lancet* **2015**, *385*, 2280–2287. [CrossRef]
154. Ruff, C.T.; Giugliano, R.P.; Braunwald, E.; Hoffman, E.B.; Deenadayalu, N.; Ezekowitz, M.D.; Camm, A.J.; Weitz, J.I.; Lewis, B.S.; Parkhomenko, A.; et al. Comparison of the efficacy and safety of new oral anticoagulants with warfarin in patients with atrial fibrillation: A meta-analysis of randomised trials. *Lancet* **2014**, *383*, 955–962. [CrossRef]
155. Pirmohamed, M. Warfarin: The End or the End of One Size Fits All Therapy? *J. Pers. Med.* **2018**, *8*, 22. [CrossRef] [PubMed]
156. Johnson, J.A.; Burlew, B.S. Metoprolol metabolism via cytochrome P4502D6 in ethnic populations. *Drug Metab. Dispos.* **1996**, *24*, 350–355.
157. Rau, T.; Heide, R.; Bergmann, K.; Wuttke, H.; Werner, U.; Feifel, N.; Eschenhagen, T. Effect of the CYP2D6 genotype on metoprolol metabolism persists during long-term treatment. *Pharmacogenetics* **2002**, *12*, 465–472. [CrossRef]
158. Conrad, K.A. Comparison of the Inotropic and Chronotropic Effects of Metoprolol and Propranolol. *J. Clin. Pharmacol.* **1981**, *21*, 213–218. [CrossRef]
159. Rau, T.; Wuttke, H.; Michels, L.; Werner, U.; Bergmann, K.; Kreft, M.; Fromm, M.; Eschenhagen, T. Impact of the CYP2D6 Genotype on the Clinical Effects of Metoprolol: A Prospective Longitudinal Study. *Clin. Pharmacol. Ther.* **2009**, *85*, 269–272. [CrossRef]
160. Batty, J.A.; Hall, A.S.; White, H.L.; Wikstrand, J.; De Boer, R.A.; Van Veldhuisen, D.J.; Van Der Harst, P.; Waagstein, F.; Hjalmarson, Å.; Kjekshus, J.; et al. An Investigation of CYP2D6 Genotype and Response to Metoprolol CR/XL During Dose Titration in Patients With Heart Failure: A MERIT-HF Substudy. *Clin. Pharmacol. Ther.* **2014**, *95*, 321–330. [CrossRef]
161. Bijl, M.J.; Visser, L.E.; van Schaik, R.H.; Kors, J.A.; Witteman, J.C.M.; Hofman, A.; Vulto, A.G.; van Gelder, T.; Stricker, B.H.C. Genetic variation in the CYP2D6 gene is associated with a lower heart rate and blood pressure in beta-blocker users. *Clin. Pharmacol. Ther.* **2009**, *85*, 45–50. [CrossRef]
162. Meloche, M.; Khazaka, M.; Kassem, I.; Barhdadi, A.; Dubé, M.P.; De Denus, S. CYP2D6 polymorphism and its impact on the clinical response to metoprolol: A systematic review and meta-analysis. *Br. J. Clin. Pharmacol.* **2020**, *86*, 1015–1033. [CrossRef]
163. Shahabi, P.; Dubé, M.P. Cardiovascular pharmacogenomics; state of current knowledge and implementation in practice. *Int. J. Cardiol.* **2015**, *184*, 772–795. [CrossRef] [PubMed]
164. Zisaki, A.; Miskovic, L.; Hatzimanikatis, V. Antihypertensive Drugs Metabolism: An Update to Pharmacokinetic Profiles and Computational Approaches. *Curr. Pharm. Des.* **2014**, *21*, 806–822. [CrossRef] [PubMed]
165. Leopold, G. Balanced Pharmacokinetics and Metabolism of Bisoprolol. *J. Cardiovasc. Pharmacol.* **1986**, *8*, S16–S20. [CrossRef] [PubMed]
166. Scavone, C.; Di Mauro, C.; Ruggiero, R.; Bernardi, F.F.; Trama, U.; Aiezza, M.L.; Rafaniello, C.; Capuano, A. Severe Cutaneous Adverse Drug Reactions Associated with Allopurinol: An Analysis of Spontaneous Reporting System in Southern Italy. *Drugs Real World Outcomes* **2020**, *7*, 41–51. [CrossRef] [PubMed]
167. Bastuji-Garin, S.; Rzany, B.; Stern, R.S.; Shear, N.H.; Naldi, L.; Roujeau, J.C. Clinical classification of cases of toxic epidermal necrolysis, Stevens-Johnson syndrome, and erythema multiforme. *Arch. Dermatol.* **1993**, *129*, 92–96. [CrossRef] [PubMed]
168. Halevy, S.; Ghislain, P.-D.; Mockenhaupt, M.; Fagot, J.-P.; Bavinck, J.N.B.; Sidoroff, A.; Naldi, L.; Dunant, A.; Viboud, C.; Roujeau, J.-C. Allopurinol is the most common cause of Stevens-Johnson syndrome and toxic epidermal necrolysis in Europe and Israel. *J. Am. Acad. Dermatol.* **2008**, *58*, 25–32. [CrossRef] [PubMed]
169. Cho, Y.-T.; Chu, C.-Y. Treatments for Severe Cutaneous Adverse Reactions. *J. Immunol. Res.* **2017**, 1–9. [CrossRef]
170. Saito, Y.; Stamp, L.K.; Caudle, K.E.; Hershfield, M.; McDonagh, E.M.; Callaghan, J.T.; Tassaneeyakul, W.; Mushiroda, T.; Kamatani, N.; Goldspiel, B.R.; et al. Clinical Pharmacogenetics Implementation Consortium (CPIC) guidelines for human leukocyte antigen B (HLA-B) genotype and allopurinol dosing: 2015 update. *Clin. Pharmacol. Ther.* **2015**, *99*, 36–37. [CrossRef]
171. Lam, M.P.; Yeung, C.K.; Cheung, B.M.Y. Pharmacogenetics of Allopurinol-Making an Old Drug Safer. *J. Clin. Pharmacol.* **2013**, *53*, 675–679. [CrossRef]

172. Chiu, M.L.; Hu, M.; Ng, M.H.; Yeung, C.; Chan, J.-Y.; Chang, M.; Cheng, S.; Li, L.; Tomlinson, B. Association between HLA-B*58:01 allele and severe cutaneous adverse reactions with allopurinol in Han Chinese in Hong Kong. *Br. J. Dermatol.* **2012**, *167*, 44–49. [CrossRef]
173. Gomes, E.R.; Demoly, P. Epidemiology of hypersensitivity drug reactions. *Curr. Opin. Allergy Clin. Immunol.* **2005**, *5*, 309–316. [CrossRef] [PubMed]
174. Stamp, L.K.; Barclay, M.L. How to prevent allopurinol hypersensitivity reactions? *Rheumatology* **2017**, *57* (Suppl. 1), i35–i41. [CrossRef] [PubMed]
175. Ramasamy, S.; Korb-Wells, C.; Kannangara, D.R.W.; Smith, M.W.H.; Wang, N.; Roberts, D.M.; Graham, G.G.; Williams, K.M.; Day, R.O. Allopurinol Hypersensitivity: A Systematic Review of All Published Cases, 1950–2012. *Drug Saf.* **2013**, *36*, 953–980. [CrossRef]
176. Wang, C.-W.; Dao, R.-L.; Chung, W.-H. Immunopathogenesis and risk factors for allopurinol severe cutaneous adverse reactions. *Curr. Opin. Allergy Clin. Immunol.* **2016**, *16*, 339–345. [CrossRef] [PubMed]
177. Qurie, A.; Bansal, P.; Goyal, A.; Musa, A. Allopurinol. [Updated 2020 July 4]; In *StatPearls [Internet]*; StatPearls Publishing: Treasure Island, FL, USA, January 2020. Available online: https://www.ncbi.nlm.nih.gov/books/NBK499942/ (accessed on 12 August 2020).
178. Lin, C.-H.; Chen, J.-K.; Ko, T.-M.; Wei, C.-Y.; Wu, J.-Y.; Chung, W.-H.; Chen, S.-Y.; Liao, Y.-D.; Hung, S.-I.; Chen, Y.-T. Immunologic basis for allopurinol-induced severe cutaneous adverse reactions: HLA-B*58:01-restricted activation of drug-specific T cells and molecular interaction. *J. Allergy Clin. Immunol.* **2014**, *135*, 1063–1065.e5. [CrossRef]
179. Chung, W.-H.; Pan, R.-Y.; Chu, M.-T.; Chin, S.-W.; Huang, Y.-L.; Wang, W.-C.; Chang, J.-Y.; Hung, S.-I. Oxypurinol-Specific T Cells Possess Preferential TCR Clonotypes and Express Granulysin in Allopurinol-Induced Severe Cutaneous Adverse Reactions. *J. Investig. Dermatol.* **2015**, *135*, 2237–2248. [CrossRef]
180. Hershfield, M.S.; Callaghan, J.T.; Tassaneeyakul, W.; Mushiroda, T.; Thorn, C.F.; E Klein, T.; Lee, M.T.M. Clinical Pharmacogenetics Implementation Consortium Guidelines for Human Leukocyte Antigen-B Genotype and Allopurinol Dosing. *Clin. Pharmacol. Ther.* **2013**, *93*, 153–158. [CrossRef]
181. Accord-Uk Ltd via Electronic Medicines Compendium, Allopurinol 100mg Tablets BP. [Online]. Available online: https://www.medicines.org.uk/emc/product/5693/smpc (accessed on 24 July 2020).
182. Pirmohamed, M.; Ostrov, D.A.; Park, B.K. New genetic findings lead the way to a better understanding of fundamental mechanisms of drug hypersensitivity. *J. Allergy Clin. Immunol.* **2015**, *136*, 236–244. [CrossRef]
183. Gidal, B.E. Carbamazepine Hypersensitivity: Progress Toward Predicting the Unpredictable. *Epilepsy Curr.* **2011**, *11*, 189–191. [CrossRef]
184. McCormack, M.; Alfirevic, A.; Bourgeois, S.; Farrell, J.J.; Kasperavičiūtė, D.; Carrington, M.; Sills, G.J.; Marson, T.; Jia, X.; De Bakker, P.I.; et al. HLA-A*3101 and Carbamazepine-Induced Hypersensitivity Reactions in Europeans. *N. Engl. J. Med.* **2011**, *364*, 1134–1143. [CrossRef]
185. Daly, A.K.; Donaldson, P.T.; Bhatnagar, P.; Shen, Y.; Pe'Er, I.; Floratos, A.; Daly, M.J.; Goldstein, D.B.; John, S.L.; Graham, J.; et al. HLA-B*5701 genotype is a major determinant of drug-induced liver injury due to flucloxacillin. *Nat. Genet.* **2009**, *41*, 816–819. [CrossRef] [PubMed]
186. Mallal, S.; Phillips, E.; Carosi, G.; Molina, J.-M.; Workman, C.; Tomažič, J.; Jägel-Guedes, E.; Rugina, S.; Kozyrev, O.; Cid, J.F.; et al. HLA-B*5701 Screening for Hypersensitivity to Abacavir. *N. Engl. J. Med.* **2008**, *358*, 568–579. [CrossRef] [PubMed]
187. Mikat-Stevens, N.A.; Larson, I.A.; Tarini, B.A. Primary-care providers' perceived barriers to integration of genetics services: A systematic review of the literature. *Genet. Med.* **2015**, *17*, 169–176. [CrossRef] [PubMed]
188. De Denus, S.; Letarte, N.; Hurlimann, T.; Lambert, J.-P.; Lavoie, A.; Robb, L.; Sheehan, N.L.; Turgeon, J.; Vadnais, B. An evaluation of pharmacists' expectations towards pharmacogenomics. *Pharmacogenomics* **2013**, *14*, 165–175. [CrossRef] [PubMed]
189. Just, K.S.; Steffens, M.; Swen, J.J.; Patrinos, G.P.; Guchelaar, H.-J.; Stingl, J.C. Medical education in pharmacogenomics—Results from a survey on pharmacogenetic knowledge in healthcare professionals within the European pharmacogenomics clinical implementation project Ubiquitous Pharmacogenomics (U-PGx). *Eur. J. Clin. Pharmacol.* **2017**, *73*, 1247–1252. [CrossRef] [PubMed]
190. Rafi, I.; Crinson, I.; Dawes, M.; Rafi, D.; Pirmohamed, M.; Walter, F.M. The implementation of pharmacogenomics into UK general practice: A qualitative study exploring barriers, challenges and opportunities. *J. Community Genet.* **2020**, *11*, 269–277. [CrossRef]

191. Rigter, T.; Jansen, M.E.; De Groot, J.M.; Janssen, S.W.; Rodenburg, W.; Cornel, M.C. Implementation of Pharmacogenetics in Primary Care: A Multi-Stakeholder Perspective. *Front. Genet.* **2020**, *11*, 10. [CrossRef]
192. Van Der Wouden, C.H.; Cambon-Thomsen, A.; Cecchin, E.; Cheung, K.C.; Dávila-Fajardo, C.L.; Deneer, V.H.; Dolžan, V.; Ingelman-Sundberg, M.; Jönsson, S.; O Karlsson, M.; et al. Implementing Pharmacogenomics in Europe: Design and Implementation Strategy of the Ubiquitous Pharmacogenomics Consortium. *Clin. Pharmacol. Ther.* **2017**, *101*, 341–358. [CrossRef]
193. Robinson, J. Everything you need to know about the NHS genomic medicine service. *Pharm. J.* **2020**. Available online: https://www.pharmaceutical-journal.com/news-and-analysis/features/everything-you-need-to-know-about-the-nhs-genomic-medicineservice/20207495.article?firstPass=false (accessed on 5 July 2020). [CrossRef]
194. Plumpton, C.; Roberts, D.; Pirmohamed, M.; Hughes, D.A. A Systematic Review of Economic Evaluations of Pharmacogenetic Testing for Prevention of Adverse Drug Reactions. *Pharmacoeconomics* **2016**, *34*, 771–793. [CrossRef]
195. Dong, O.M.; Wheeler, S.B.; Cruden, G.; Lee, C.R.; Voora, D.; Dusetzina, S.B.; Wiltshire, T. Cost-Effectiveness of Multigene Pharmacogenetic Testing in Patients With Acute Coronary Syndrome After Percutaneous Coronary Intervention. *Value Health* **2019**, *23*, 61–73. [CrossRef] [PubMed]
196. Fargher, E.A.; Eddy, C.; Newman, W.G.; Qasim, F.; Tricker, K.; Elliott, R.; Payne, K. Patients' and healthcare professionals' views on pharmacogenetic testing and its future delivery in the NHS. *Pharmacogenomics* **2007**, *8*, 1511–1519. [CrossRef] [PubMed]
197. Powell, K.P.; Christianson, C.A.; Cogswell, W.A.; Dave, G.; Verma, A.; Eubanks, S.; Henrich, V.C. Educational Needs of Primary Care Physicians Regarding Direct-to-Consumer Genetic Testing. *J. Genet. Couns.* **2011**, *21*, 469–478. [CrossRef] [PubMed]
198. McInnes, G.M.; Altman, R.B. Drug Response Pharmacogenetics for 200,000 UK Biobank Participants. *bioRxiv* **2020**. [CrossRef]
199. Manolio, T.A.; Collins, F.S.; Cox, N.J.; Goldstein, D.B.; Hindorff, L.A.; Hunter, D.J.; McCarthy, M.I.; Ramos, E.M.; Cardon, L.R.; Chakravarti, A.; et al. Finding the missing heritability of complex diseases. *Nat. Cell Biol.* **2009**, *461*, 747–753. [CrossRef] [PubMed]
200. Baudou, E.; Lespine, A.; Durrieu, G.; André, F.; Gandia, P.; Durand, C.; Cunat, S. Correspondence: Serious Ivermectin Toxicity and Human ABCB1 Nonsense Mutations. *N. Engl. J. Med.* **2020**, *383*, 787–789. [CrossRef]
201. Lauschke, V.M.; Zhou, Y.; Ingelman-Sundberg, M. Novel genetic and epigenetic factors of importance for inter-individual differences in drug disposition, response and toxicity. *Pharmacol. Ther.* **2019**, *197*, 122–152. [CrossRef]
202. Kalinin, A.A.; Higgins, G.A.; Reamaroon, N.; Soroushmehr, S.; Allyn-Feuer, A.; Dinov, I.D.; Najarian, K.; Athey, B.D. Deep learning in pharmacogenomics: From gene regulation to patient stratification. *Pharmacogenomics* **2018**, *19*, 629–650. [CrossRef]
203. Van Der Lee, M.; Allard, W.G.; Vossen, R.H.A.M.; Baak-Pablo, R.F.; Menafra, R.; Deiman, B.A.; Deenen, M.J.; Neven, P.; Johansson, I.; Gastaldello, S.; et al. A unifying model to predict variable drug response for personalised medicine. *bioRxiv* **2020**, *2020*. [CrossRef]

3

Pharmacogenomic Biomarkers and their Applications in Psychiatry

Heejin Kam and Hotcherl Jeong *

College of Pharmacy, Ewha Womans University, Seoul 03760, Korea; ladykam@ewhain.net
* Correspondence: hotcherl@ewha.ac.kr

Abstract: Realizing the promise of precision medicine in psychiatry is a laudable and beneficial endeavor, since it should markedly reduce morbidity and mortality and, in effect, alleviate the economic and social burden of psychiatric disorders. This review aims to summarize important issues on pharmacogenomics in psychiatry that have laid the foundation towards personalized pharmacotherapy and, in a broader sense, precision medicine. We present major pharmacogenomic biomarkers and their applications in a variety of psychiatric disorders, such as depression, attention-deficit/hyperactivity disorder (ADHD), narcolepsy, schizophrenia, and bipolar disorder. In addition, we extend the scope into epilepsy, since antiepileptic drugs are widely used to treat psychiatric disorders, although epilepsy is conventionally considered to be a neurological disorder.

Keywords: precision medicine; personalized medicine; pharmacogenomics; pharmacogenomic biomarkers; psychiatry; psychiatric disorders; epilepsy

1. Introduction

The World Health Organization (WHO) estimates that about 25% of the population around the world will suffer from at least one mental disorder at some time in their lives [1,2]. Depression and anxiety are among the most common disorders, and these can affect people regardless of age, gender, ethnicity, or background. We do not fully understand what causes most cases of mental health impairment, but it is known that both genetic and environmental factors can often contribute to an individual's predisposition to a particular disorder. In other cases, serious injuries or traumatic events cause psychological symptoms that persist for a long period of time [3].

Medications can be used in order to reduce the intensity of symptoms or treat several psychiatric disorders. A patient's response to the many medications used to treat various psychiatric disorders can be highly variable [4]. Drug response is dependent on personal health risk factors (e.g., gender, age, liver and renal function, blood pressure, body fat, alcohol and drugs, and drug–drug interactions). In addition, genetic factors, i.e., individual's unique genetic makeup, can affect drug response influencing both pharmacokinetic parameters by causing variable activity of the systems that are responsible for the absorption, distribution, metabolism, and excretion of the drug and pharmacodynamic parameters, like the mechanisms of action of the drug [5,6]. Pharmacogenomics (PGx) refers to the study of drug response as it relates to potential individual genetic variations.

For an increasing number of drugs, pharmacogenomic testing is available and used to pre-screen patients and help them in selecting drug choice and drug dose accordingly [4,7]. Now, more than 10% of medications that are approved by the U.S. Food and Drug Administration (FDA) provide pharmacogenomic information (PGx information) in their drug labeling. This proportion is gradually increasing as more pharmacogenomic biomarkers (PGx biomarkers) are discovered and validated.

There are solid reasons for pharmacogenomic testing (PGx testing). Some drugs are only effective for specific genotypes and the testing can avoid unpredictable, severe, and potentially fatal drug reactions. Furthermore, for some drugs, a patient's ancestry is the essential consideration. For example, for carbamazepine, a commonly used antiepileptic drug, the FDA recommends that, if patients are descendants of genetically high-risk populations, they should take PGx testing for the presence of *HLA-B*15:02* before treatment [8–10]. Carriers of this variant, which is frequently found in Han Chinese descendants, are highly susceptible to the development of Stevens–Johnson syndrome and toxic epidermal necrolysis, which often lead to serious conditions, during the course of carbamazepine therapy. The *HLA-B* variant alleles are just one example of such adverse drug reactions (ADRs). In fact, there is a plethora of genetic variants that are associated with ADRs. As an evident example, carriers of a variant of MT-RNR1 (mitochondrially encoded 12S rRNA), an RNA-coding gene, are at high risk of irreversible hearing loss by a single dose of gentamicin [11,12].

For a growing number of drugs, PGx testing provide a means of optimizing the drug choice and drug dose. Drug labels include not only standard dosing information, but also guidelines for adjusting the drug dose or selecting an alternative drug, when necessary, based on a patient's genetic makeup if gene-drug interrelationships are well understood. Dosing adjustment requirements or recommendations are mostly in variants of genes that encode drug-metabolizing enzymes or drug transporters [13]. Thus, PGx biomarkers in genetic variants that are important for interindividual variations in PK and PD have been very useful in the optimization of pharmacotherapy. Several independent institutions, including the FDA [14], the European Medicines Agency (EMA), the Clinical Pharmacogenetics Implementation Consortium (CPIC) [15], the Canadian Pharmacogenomics Network for Drug Safety (CPNDS) [16,17], and the Dutch Pharmacogenetics Working Group (DPWG), have provided instructions on how PGx testing results can be interpreted in terms of the drug choice and the drug dose [18–20].

Accumulated data are then noted to FDA and its Table of Pharmacogenomic Biomarkers in Drug Labeling is widely used as a standard guideline [14]. PGx information is only included on labels when it is useful to inform clinicians of the impact of genotype on phenotype—gene–drug interrelationships—or to indicate whether a PGx test is available for a particular medication. As of now, the Table of PGx Biomarkers includes 431 drug-biomarker pairs for 298 drugs across therapeutic areas. In addition, PharmGKB provides a comprehensive resource, in which evidence-based PGx knowledges are curated and disseminated by scientific team about how our body responds to medications [21]. Pharmacogenomic information is important: it can maximize drug efficacy and reduce/avoid drug toxicity. Currently, FDA's Table of PGx Biomarkers describes PGx information for 35 psychiatric medications, as in Table 1. In addition, the Table of PGx Biomarkers includes PGx information for eight antiepileptic drugs (AEDs), as in Table 2.

Table 1. Food and Drug Administration (FDA) pharmacogenomic biomarkers in drug labeling in psychiatry.

Drug	Type	Indication	Biomarker	FDA	FDA Labeling Sections	EMA
			Antidepressants			
Amitriptyline	TCA	Depression	CYP2D6	Actionable	Precautions	
Amoxapine	TCA	Depression	CYP2D6	Actionable	Precautions	
Bupropion	NDRI	Depression	CYP2D6	Informative	Clinical Pharmacology	
Citalopram	SSRI	Depression	CYP2C19	Actionable	Dosage and Administration Warnings Clinical Pharmacology	
			CYP2D6	Informative	Clinical Pharmacology	

Table 1. *Cont.*

Drug	Type	Indication	Biomarker	FDA	FDA Labeling Sections	EMA
Clomipramine	TCA	Depression	CYP2D6	Actionable	Precautions	
Desipramine	TCA	Depression	CYP2D6	Actionable	Precautions	
Desvenlafaxine	SNRI	Depression	CYP2D6	Informative	Clinical Pharmacology	
Doxepin	TCA	Depression	CYP2C19	Actionable	Clinical Pharmacology	
			CYP2D6		Clinical Pharmacology	
Duloxetine	SNRI	Depression	CYP2D6	Actionable	Drug Interactions	Actionable
Escitalopram	SSRI	Depression	CYP2C19	Actionable	Adverse Reactions	
			CYP2D6	Informative	Drug Interactions	
Fluoxetine	SSRI	Depression	CYP2D6	Informative	Precautions Clinical Pharmacology	
Fluvoxamine	SSRI	Depression	CYP2D6	Actionable	Drug Interactions	
Imipramine	TCA	Depression	CYP2D6	Actionable	Precautions	
Nefazodone	SARI	Depression	CYP2D6	Informative	Precautions	
Nortriptyline	TCA	Depression	CYP2D6	Actionable	Precautions	
Paroxetine	SSRI	Depression	CYP2D6	Informative	Drug Interactions Clinical Pharmacology	
Protriptyline	TCA	Depression	CYP2D6	Actionable	Precautions	
Trimipramine	TCA	Depression	CYP2D6	Actionable	Precautions	
Venlafaxine	SNRI	Depression	CYP2D6	Actionable	Drug Interactions Use in Specific Populations Clinical Pharmacology	
Vortioxetine	SSRI	Depression	CYP2D6	Actionable	Dosage and Administration Clinical Pharmacology	Actionable
Stimulants and non-stimulants						
Amphetamine	Stimulant	ADHD	CYP2D6	Informative	Clinical Pharmacology	
Atomoxetine	Non-stimulant	ADHD	CYP2D6	Actionable	Dosage and Administration Warnings and Precautions Adverse Reactions Drug Interactions Use in Specific Populations Clinical Pharmacology	
Modafinil	WPA	Narcolepsy	CYP2D6	Actionable	Clinical Pharmacology	
Pitolisant	H_3R antagonist	Narcolepsy	CYP2D6	Actionable	Dosage and Administration Use in Specific Populations Clinical Pharmacology	

Table 1. *Cont.*

Drug	Type	Indication	Biomarker	FDA	FDA Labeling Sections	EMA
			Antipsychotics			
Aripiprazole	Atypical	Schizophrenia Bipolar disorder	CYP2D6	Actionable	Dosage and Administration Use in Specific Populations Clinical Pharmacology	Actionable
Aripiprazole lauroxil	Atypical	Schizophrenia	CYP2D6	Actionable	Dosage and Administration Use in Specific Populations Clinical Pharmacology	
Brexpiprazole	Atypical	Schizophrenia Very severe depression	CYP2D6	Actionable	Dosage and Administration Use in Specific Populations Clinical Pharmacology	Actionable
Cariprazine	Atypical	Schizophrenia Bipolar disorder	CYP2D6	Informative	Clinical Pharmacology	
Clozapine	Atypical	Schizophrenia	CYP2D6	Actionable	Dosage and Administration Use in Specific Populations Clinical Pharmacology	
Iloperidone	Atypical	Schizophrenia	CYP2D6	Actionable	Dosage and Administration Warnings and Precautions Drug Interactions Clinical Pharmacology	
Paliperidone	Atypical	Schizophrenia	CYP2D6	Informative	Clinical Pharmacology	
Perphenazine	Typical	Schizophrenia	CYP2D6	Actionable	Precautions Clinical Pharmacology	
Pimozide	Typical	Tourette syndrome	CYP2D6	Testing Required	Dosage and Administration Precautions	
Risperidone	Atypical	Schizophrenia Bipolar disorder	CYP2D6	Informative	Clinical Pharmacology	
Thioridazine	Typical	Schizophrenia Other psychotic disorders	CYP2D6	Actionable	Contraindications Warnings Precautions	

H_3R antagonist = histamine H_3 receptor antagonist; NDRI = norepinephrine-dopamine reuptake inhibitor; SARI = serotonin antagonist and reuptake inhibitor; SNRI = serotonin and norepinephrine reuptake inhibitor; SSRI = selective serotonin reuptake inhibitor; TCA = tricyclic and tetracyclic antidepressant; WPA = wakefulness promoting agent.

Table 2. FDA pharmacogenomic biomarkers in drug labeling in epilepsy.

Drug	Type	Indication	Biomarker	FDA	FDA Labeling Sections	EMA
Brivaracetam	Inhibits synaptic vesicle SV2A protein	Epilepsy	CYP2C19	Actionable	Clinical Pharmacology	Actionable
Carbamazepine	Enhances sodium channel (rapid inactivation) Inhibits L-type calcium channel	Epilepsy Bipolar disorder	HLA-B	Testing Required	Boxed Warning Warnings Precautions	
			HLA-A	Actionable	Warnings	
Clobazam	$GABA_A$ receptor agonist	Epilepsy	CYP2C19	Actionable	Dosage and Administration Use in Specific Populations Clinical Pharmacology	
Diazepam	$GABA_A$ receptor agonist	Epilepsy	CYP2C19	Actionable	Clinical Pharmacology	
Lacosamide	Enhances sodium channel (slow inactivation)	Epilepsy	CYP2C19	Informative	Clinical Pharmacology	Informative
Oxcarbazepine	Enhances sodium channel (rapid inactivation) Inhibits N/P- and R-type calcium channel	Epilepsy Bipolar disorder	HLA-B	Testing recommended	Warnings and Precautions	
Phenytoin	Enhances sodium channel (rapid inactivation)	Epilepsy	CYP2C9	Actionable	Clinical Pharmacology	
			CYP2C19		Clinical Pharmacology	
			HLA-B		Warnings	
Valproic Acid	Inhibits voltage-dependent sodium and T-type calcium channels Enhances GABA transmission	Epilepsy	POLG	Testing Required	Boxed Warning Contraindications Warnings and Precautions	
			Nonspecific (Urea cycle disorders)	Actionable	Contraindications Warnings and Precautions	

2. CYP2D6 and CYP2C9 Genes

The cytochrome P450s (CYPs) comprise a large superfamily of a variety of enzymes that serve as major workhorses for metabolizing steroid hormones, lipids, toxins, and xenobiotics. The CYP superfamily genes encode enzymes that function as monooxygenases and catalyze the modification of about 25–30% commonly used drugs [22,23]. The *CYP* genes are quite polymorphic and they can lead to increased, decreased, or completely absent drug metabolism activity. Among these genes, *CYP2D6* is particularly important and heavily studied. More than 100 *CYP2D6* variants have been reported and catalogued at the Pharmacogene Variation Consortium database [24]. In addition to large numbers of single nucleotide polymorphisms (SNPs), other types of variations—gene deletions, duplications, copy-number variants, and pseudogenes that are close to the gene—make genotyping very challenging.

Many of these variants cause the enzyme to change activity at different levels. The level of CYP2D6 activity decides how an individual responds to the substrate drugs. A standard dosage of the drug may show inadequate efficacy in some individuals and serious toxicity in others. To name a few, the drug substrates of CYP2D6 include atomoxetine (a non-stimulant for ADHD), clozapine (an antipsychotic for schizophrenia), and venlafaxine (an antidepressant), among psychiatric medications, as in Table 1 [4,25]. For these drugs, standard doses will result in higher-than-optimal active levels when individuals have absent or deficient CYP2D6 activity. Thus, the risk of ADRs increases and it may result in treatment failure.

There are substantial variations in *CYP2D6* allele frequencies among different populations [26,27]. The wild-type CYP2D6*1 allele shows normal enzyme activity and the extensive or normal metabolizer phenotype. The CYP2D6*2, -*33, and -*35 alleles also belong to this group. Other alleles contain non-functional variant(s), which produce a non-functioning enzyme (*3, *4, *5, *6, *7, and *8) or a decreased-activity enzyme (*10, *17, *29, and *41) [28]. Intermediate and poor metabolizers are individuals who carry decreased and null CYP2D6 alleles, respectively. Notably, approximately 30% of Asians and Asian descendants are intermediate metabolizers. In these populations, the *10 allele with decreased activity is very common: about 40%, when compared with about 2% in Caucasians [29]. Thus, a large proportion of Asians belong to intermediate metabolizers than Caucasians [30]. The African and African American populations also show a large proportion of CYPD6 alleles having sub-optimal activity. The frequencies of the remaining alleles vary depending on the population [30–32]. In Caucasians, only small proportions (less than 10%) are poor metabolizers [30]. In contrast, approximately 40% are extensive/normal metabolizers who carry two copies of *1 allele [33–35]. CYP2D6 poor metabolizers show higher levels of amitriptyline (as an example of drug substrates) in the plasma, when compared with extensive metabolizers, after standard doses of amitriptyline are taken [36]. When individuals carry a CYP2D6 null variant, their risk of developing ADRs becomes, at least, moderately increased [37]. Because standard dosages may cause to ADRs in poor metabolizers, it is recommended to avoid many tricyclic antidepressants (TCAs) and, instead, take an alternative option, a drug that is not a substrate of CYP2D6 [38].

Interestingly, copy-number variants were also found in *CYP2D6* genes [24]. In other words, individuals who carry more than two copies of functional CYP2D6 alleles—three to 13 copies of *CYP2D6* active allele—have been reported. These carriers are CYP2D6 ultrarapid metabolizers. In the case of 13 functional copies, the rate was up to 17 times higher than for individuals with no active CYP2D6 enzyme [39]. If the drug substrate has increased rate of metabolism, then its active form will not be available and, thus, the therapeutic response will become poor.

3. Antidepressants—Depression

Depression (also known as major depressive disorder) is a common and serious psychiatric disorder that affects more than 350 million people each year across the world [1]. People with disabilities face high risk for depression and, inversely, this disorder is a major cause of disability. Antidepressants are medications for treating depression [40]. They regulate neurotransmitters, such as serotonin, norepinephrine, and dopamine, which are linked to mood and emotion. Antidepressants can also be used for other indications, such as pain, anxiety, and insomnia. Even if their FDA approval is not designated to treat attention-deficit/hyperactivity disorder (ADHD), antidepressants are often used in order to treat the ADHD of adults.

Depending on the drug target, the neurotransmitter and/or its metabolizing enzyme, antidepressants can be categorized into four major classes—two older ones, tricyclic antidepressants (TCAs) and monoamine oxidase inhibitors (MAOIs), and two newer ones, selective serotonin reuptake inhibitors (SSRIs) and serotonin norepinephrine reuptake inhibitors (SNRIs) Table 1 [41,42]. SSRIs include citalopram, escitalopram, fluoxetine, paroxetine, and sertraline. SNRIs include duloxetine and venlafaxine. Bupropion is another newer antidepressant that is widely used, which, as a norepinephrine-dopamine reuptake inhibitor, works in a different mechanism of action than either SSRIs or SNRIs. These newer antidepressants, SSRIs, SNRIs, and bupropion, make fewer ADRs than older antidepressants and they can be used to treat a broader class of depressive or anxiety disorders.

Individual response to some antidepressants varies for reasons not yet well understood. Once a patient starts to take antidepressants, it is advisable not to stop taking them without the recommendation of a doctor. Therefore, it is necessary to know which medicine works for them beforehand. Some antidepressants may result in more adverse effects than others. Common ADRs include diarrhea, nausea and vomiting, weight gain, sleepiness, and sexual problems.

SLC6A4, the serotonin transporter gene, is a well-characterized gene that is associated with the treatment outcome of depression [43–46]. The serotonin transporter has twelve transmembrane helices and one extracellular loop located between helices 3 and 4. This transporter functions to reuptake serotonin (5HT) into the presynaptic neurons. The 5′ promoter region, called 5HT-transporter-linked polymorphic region (5-HTTLPR), of the *SLC6A4* gene is polymorphic in its length [47]. 5-HTTLPR locates approximately 1,000 bp upstream from the start site of transcription and comprises of repetitions of 16 imperfect 22-bp repeat units. 5-HTTLPR produces either a short (*s*) allele or the long (*l*) allele, respectively, depending on the occurrence of a deletion or an insertion of 6–8 units. The *l* allele is 44 bp shorter than the *s* allele and it is associated with higher levels of transcription of the *SLC6A4* gene in human cell lines. Some studies suggest that the *l*-allele patients respond better to antidepressants, even if this needs to be further investigated [48,49].

3.1. *Amitriptyline*

Amitriptyline (brand name Elavil) is a TCA that is used to treat many psychiatric disorders, including obsessive-compulsive disorder [50]. TCAs mostly mediate their therapeutic effects through inhibiting reuptake of serotonin and norepinephrine and, thus, hold more neurotransmitters around the synaptic cleft. The main drawback of TCAs is that their side effects are common, since they can also inhibit other receptors, such as α1-adrenergic, histamine H1, and muscarinic acetylcholine receptors. Additionally, this is the reason why TCAs have been replaced by SSRIs, which are more specific. Nonetheless, TCAs remain very useful in treating specific classes of depression and other psychiatric disorders. Amitriptyline is mostly metabolized by the CYP2C19 and CYP2D6 pathways [37]. Whereas CYP2C19 converts amitriptyline to active metabolites, such as nortriptyline, which is also a TCA, CYP2D6-mediated metabolism results in the less active 10-hydroxy metabolite.

The FDA's guideline on amitriptyline states that CYP2D6 poor metabolizers will have higher plasma levels of the medication than expected when normal doses are given. The FDA also recommends that monitoring TCA plasma levels is necessary whenever a TCA is co-administered with another medication, which is known to be a CYP2D6 inhibitor. The CPIC has also made recommendations that the dosages of TCAs need to be adjusted, depending on CYP2C19 and CYP2D6 genotypes [38]. CYP2D6 poor metabolizers need to avoid any TCA due to the potential risk of ADRs. For CYP2D6 intermediate metabolizers, it is recommended to reduce the dosage up to about 75% of the usual dose. CYP2D6 ultrarapid metabolizers are recommended for avoiding TCAs, because of the potential lack of therapeutic effect and to take an alternative medication that is not a CYP2D6 substrate. CYP2C19 poor metabolizers need to avoid tertiary amine drugs due to the potential risk of ADRs and to consider a drug substitute that is not metabolized via the CYP2C19 pathway [51]. For CYP2C19 ultrarapid metabolizers, it is recommended to avoid amitriptyline, as this tertiary amine drug is expected to make an insufficient therapeutic effect, and to take an alternative medication that is not a CYP2C19 substrate, such as nortriptyline or desipramine.

One important precaution in increasing amitriptyline dose for CYP2D6 metabolizers is the fact that, when the level of hydroxyl-metabolites increases, it can lead to cardiotoxicity [52,53]. Presently, the optimal range of hydroxy-metabolite levels in the plasma and how the overall effects of CYP2D6 and CYP2C19 genotypes can be expressed as an individual's treatment outcome of amitriptyline are poorly understood [38].

3.2. *Venlafaxine*

Venlafaxine (brand name Effexor) is an antidepressant that is used to treat the depression, anxiety, and panic disorder [54,55]. Both venlafaxine and its major metabolite, desvenlafaxine, belong to the drug class of SNRIs. As the CYP2D6 enzyme catalyzes the transformation of venlafaxine into its active metabolite, O-desmethylvenlafaxine (ODV), individuals with reduced or absent CYP2D6 activity will have high levels of venlafaxine, but low levels of ODV in the plasma. This situation can occur if a concomitant drug is a CYP2D6 inhibitor or the *CYP2D6* gene contains decreased-function allele(s).

The FDA's guideline on venlafaxine indicates that neither specific dose recommendations for CYP2D6 poor metabolizers nor dose adjustment in the case of coadministration of venlafaxine and any CYP2D6 inhibitor. Instead, the drug label includes the statement that imipramine partially inhibits the metabolism of venlafaxine, but the total concentration of active compounds (both venlafaxine and

ODV) remains unchanged. On the other hand, the DPWG provides recommendations on venlafaxine dosing based on the CYP2D6 genotype. According to the guideline, CYP2D6 poor and intermediate metabolizers needs to use an alternative drug. When ADRs occur and an alternative medication is not available, then venlafaxine can be used after a dose reduction based on clinical progress. The DPWG recommends that CYP2D6 ultrarapid metabolizers need to take an increased dose of venlafaxine up to 50% from the standard dose or use an alternative drug when treatment effects of dose adjustment cannot be monitored, as they will have lower plasma levels in the sum of venlafaxine and ODV [56].

CYP2D6 genotype can affect individual's risk of ADRs from taking venlafaxine. CYP2D6 poor metabolizers have higher levels of venlafaxine and lower levels of ODV, and this can be interpreted as a higher risk of side effects and a reduced efficacy of the medication, respectively [57]. Old people tend to be at high risk [58–60]. For poor metabolizers receiving venlafaxine, ADRs are reported to occur more frequently in the gastrointestinal system (e.g., diarrhea and vomiting) or in cardiovascular system (e.g., hypertension, tachycardia, and prolonged QTc interval) [61,62]. Preemptive CYP2D6 genotyping before venlafaxine administration can make a decision on personalized dosing, which, in combination with therapeutic drug monitoring, could shorten the time taken to find an optimal maintenance dose and prevent potential ADRs [60,61,63–65]. However, there are discrepancies in the benefits of routine CYP2D6 genotyping. Some studies suggest that changes of drug metabolism that are rooted from CYP2D6 genetic variants make insufficient effects on the therapeutic levels of venlafaxine and that CYP2D6 genotyping would not forecast the treatment efficacy of venlafaxine in patients with depression [66–69].

4. Anti-Anxiety Medications—Anxiety Disorder

Anti-anxiety medications help to alleviate the symptoms of anxiety, such as intense and persistent fear and worry and panic attacks [70]. Benzodiazepines are the most commonly used anti-anxiety medications for treating anxiety disorders [71]. In the case of social anxiety disorder (also known as social phobia), benzodiazepines are a common second-line treatment option (its first-line treatment option is SSRIs or other antidepressants). Short half-life benzodiazepines include β-blockers and lorazepam, and they are used for the short-term anxiety. β-Blockers make the effects on physical symptoms of anxiety. For the long-term treatment of chronic anxiety, buspirone is an option, rather than benzodiazepines. Like other medications, some anti-anxiety medications also result in serious ADRs. However, we do not understand what causes these side effects and, thus, none of these anti-anxiety medications are currently included in either FDA's Table of PGx Biomarkers or PharmGKB drug label annotations.

5. Stimulants and Non-Stimulants—ADHD and Narcolepsy

Attention-deficit/hyperactivity disorder (ADHD) is a common psychiatric and neurodevelopmental disorder in children, which is estimated to affect 5% of children and 2.5% of adults around the world [72–75]. According to the Diagnostics and Statistical Manual of Mental Disorders, Fifth Edition (DSM-5) [76], which is widely used in the United States, ADHD is marked as age-inappropriate pattern of inattention and/or hyperactive-impulsive symptoms [77]. On the other hand, the International Classification of Diseases, Eleventh Edition (ICD-11), which is widely accepted outside the United States, refers to ADHD as a hyperkinetic disorder and defines it as impairment in all three domains of inattention, hyperactivity, and impulsivity. This definition is a more narrow scope than the DSM-5 definition [72,78]. Currently, there are five ADHD medications that are approved by FDA, which can be dichotomized into stimulants (methylphenidate and amphetamine) and non-stimulants (atomoxetine, clonidine, and guanfacine) [79,80]. In this section, amphetamine and atomoxetine are examined due to their significance in PGx, as in Table 1.

Narcolepsy is a psychiatric disorder of hypersomnolence, which is characterized by disturbed sleep, sleep paralysis, hallucinations, and direct onset of REM sleep from wakefulness [63–65]. Narcolepsy is categorized into type 1 and type 2. Type 1 narcolepsy is characterized by the presence of cataplexy and loss of orexin (hypocretin) neurons that activate histaminergic neuron, which control wakefulness [66], whereas type 2 narcolepsy is characterized by the absence of cataplexy and normal cerebrospinal fluid hypocretin levels. For narcolepsy treatment, modafinil, antidepressants, and psychostimulants, such as pitolisant and methylphenidate, are applied, depending on patient's symptoms [66]. In this section, modafinil and pitolisant, which are relevant with PGx, are examined.

5.1. *Amphetamine*

Amphetamine is a central nervous system stimulant that is approved for the treatment of ADHD and it is also used to treat narcolepsy as a third-line therapy [81–83]. Amphetamine has two enantiomers (*d*-amphetamine and *l*-amphetamine) and it can be composed of various types of salts, including *d*-methamphetamine salts, dexamfetamine, and a *d*-amphetamine prodrug, lisdexamfetamine dimesylate. In the 1930s, it was first noted that amphetamine relaxes hyperactivity, despite its stimulant nature [84]. Later, Cochrane Database of Systematic Reviews investigated 19 studies and concluded that patients rated that all amphetamines alleviated the severity of ADHD symptoms, while physicians evaluated lisdexamfetamine and mixed amphetamine salts alleviated the severity [85]. Amphetamine increases synaptic levels of monoamines, such as dopamines and noradrenalines in the brain, by inhibiting reuptake and releasing them into the synaptic cleft [86]. Although metabolism of amphetamine has not been thoroughly studied, it is known that CYP2D6 catalyzes the ring hydroxylation in order to produce 4-hydroxy-amphetamine [82,87]. Therefore, it is possible that amphetamine metabolism may vary in populations [82].

5.2. *Atomoxetine*

Atomoxetine is a non-stimulant, which is approved to treat ADHD [88]. Although its mechanism is not clear, as atomoxetine is a SNRI, it is thought that atomoxetine increases the synaptic levels of monoamines, including norepinephrine and dopamine in the brain by inhibiting reuptake [86]. Atomoxetine is mainly metabolized by CYP2D6 and, thus, CYP2D6 poor metabolizers have higher exposure to atomoxetine than the extensive metabolizers due to higher plasma concentrations and slower elimination [89]. Although atomoxetine has a wide therapeutic window, CYP2D6 poor metabolizers or patients who are taking a CYP2D6 inhibitor, such as paroxetine, fluoxetine, and quinidine, may benefit from improved therapeutic outcomes or suffer from an increased risk of adverse effects [88,90]. Therefore, atomoxetine dosing should be adjusted and carefully monitored for CYP2D6 poor metabolizers or patients concomitantly administering a CYP2D6 inhibitor.

5.3. *Modafinil*

Modafinil is approved for improving wakefulness in adult patients with excessive sleepiness that is related to narcolepsy, obstructive sleep apnea (OSA), or shift work sleep disorder (SWSD) [91]. It is commonly used in narcolepsy to treat daytime sleepiness [66]. Modafinil inhibits dopamine transporters and norepinephrine transporters, and these catecholamine effects are thought to give the cognitive and behavioral effects, including arousal and activity-promoting effects [92]. According to in vitro studies, modafinil and its metabolite, modafinil sulfone, are CYP2C19 reversible inhibitors. Therefore, modafinil may increase CYP2C19 substrate drugs, such as phenytoin, diazepam, propranolol, omeprazole, and clomiphene [91]. CYP2C19 also provides an ancillary route for certain CYP2D6 substrates, such as TCAs (clomipramine and desipramine) and SSRIs. CYP2D6 poor metabolizers on medications, which are metabolized by CYP2C19 ancillary pathway, may increase the plasma level of CYP2D6 substrates [91].

5.4. *Pitolisant*

Pitolisant (brand name WAKIX®) is approved for the treatment of excessive daytime sleepiness (EDS) in adult patients with narcolepsy. As a psychostimulant, pitolisant is a histamine-3 (H3) receptor antagonist and inverse agonist, which activates histamine release [93,94]. Pitolisant is majorly metabolized by CYP2D6 and minorly by CYP3A4 to inactive 5-amino-valeric acid and then further metabolized by glucuronidation or conjugation with glycine [94,95]. The main metabolic enzyme CYP2D6 affects plasma concentration. CYP2D6 poor metabolizers are less able to metabolize pitolisant into an inactive metabolite, so they have higher plasma concentrations of active pitolisant. Therefore, dose reduction is recommended for CYP2D6 poor metabolizers [94]. According to the pitolisant FDA-approved drug label, for CYP2D6 poor metabolizers, pitolisant should be titrated to a maximum dose of 17.8 mg once daily after seven days of treatment, while the recommended dosage range for normal metabolizers is 17.8 to 35.6 mg daily [94].

6. Antipsychotics—Psychosis with Schizophrenia or Bipolar Disorder

Antipsychotic medications are used to treat psychosis with schizophrenia and bipolar disorder [96,97]. The word "psychosis" means a condition that affects how the brain processes. Patients might see and hear things that do not exist (hallucinations) and/or believe unrealistic things (delusions). Psychosis can be a physical symptom, such as substance abuse, or a mental disorder with extreme stress or trauma, such as schizophrenia, bipolar disorder, or very severe depression (also known as psychotic depression). Antipsychotic medications do not cure these conditions, but, instead, can alleviate these symptoms and improve quality of life.

Typical antipsychotic medications are also called neuroleptics or first-generation antipsychotics [98]. They were first developed in the 1950s and still remain useful in the treatment of many psychosis symptoms, especially when other medications do not function. However, typical antipsychotics have a high risk of ADRs. Atypical antipsychotic medications are also called as second-generation antipsychotics. Both typical and atypical antipsychotics function as dopamine antagonists, but atypical antipsychotics show weaker affinity for dopamine receptors and, instead, strong affinity for serotonin receptors, particularly 5-HT2A [98]. The first atypical antipsychotic drug, clozapine, was first identified in 1958, but its development and approval in the US took a long time and, in the 1990s, clozapine finally emerged as a successful medication of schizophrenia, regardless of its high cost. Common atypical antipsychotics show a broad range of action and include aripiprazole, olanzapine, paliperidone, risperidone, and ziprasidone, as in Table 1.

Dopaminergic receptors are predominant G protein-coupled receptors in the vertebrate central nervous systems and they are involved in a variety of neurological processes [99]. These processes affect motivation, cognitive behavior, memory and learning, pleasure, and coordination of voluntary movements. Thus, dopaminergic receptors are common neuropsychiatric drug targets and, in fact, many antipsychotics are dopaminergic receptor antagonists. Many atypical antipsychotics inhibit serotonin (5-HT) receptors in the brain, the 5-HT2A receptor in particular, which play a critical role in schizophrenia.

Inter-individual differences in response to antipsychotic medications vary in a wide range and it often takes several trials to find the best medication that fits. In addition, antipsychotics can cause many ADRs, including weight gain, low blood pressure, and uncontrollable movements. Typical antipsychotics can cause a condition, called tardive dyskinesia (TD), when taken in the long term [100]. TD causes stiff, jerky muscle movements of the face, mainly at the mouth, which a person cannot control. TD rarely occurs while taking atypical antipsychotics.

According to the WHO, schizophrenia is a chronic and severe neurodevelopmental disorder, and it affects 20 million people worldwide. Etiology of schizophrenia remains unclear, but genetic and environmental factors seem to work together [101]. The pathogenesis involves a variety of neurotransmitter systems, which include dopamine, noradrenaline, glutamate, GABA, and acetylcholine. Schizophrenia can lead to substantial morbidity and mortality. Although antipsychotics are a mainstay of schizophrenia treatment, its treatment outcomes are inadequate for many patients. Antipsychotics exert their therapeutic actions by blocking D2 dopamine receptors on the post-synaptic membrane in the brain. The heritability of schizophrenia is very high, as demonstrated by family, twin, and adoption studies. For example, twin studies show that, if one identical twin develops schizophrenia, then there is a 40–50% chance that the other twin also has it. However, the search for "schizophrenia genes" has been elusive [102,103].

One genome-wide association study in 2014 identified 108 SNPs that were associated with schizophrenia, 83 of which were new. Not surprisingly, most of these SNPs occurred in genes that are highly expressed in the brain. However, surprisingly, some associated SNPs were found in genes that are expressed in tissues that are involved in the immune system [104].

Dysbindin-1 regulates the transport and release of synaptic vesicles and is encoded by the *DTNBP1* gene. Its genetic variants can affect the availability of dopamine D2 receptors. Recently, one study revealed that some genetic variants in the *DTNBP1* gene are associated with individual cognitive response to antipsychotics [105,106]. PGx association studies focused on pharmacodynamic genes in psychiatry are in progress and these should allow for better prediction of drug efficacy and potential ADRs.

6.1. Aripiprazole

Aripiprazole is an atypical antipsychotic that is used for managing schizophrenia, bipolar disorder, major depressive disorder, and Tourette's disorder. Two enzymes, CYP2D6 and CYP3A4, are the mainstay of its metabolism and elimination. The FDA's Table of PGx Biomarkers for aripiprazole states that CYP2D6 poor metabolizers need to take half of the usual dose [26]. When CYP2D6 poor metabolizers are taking concomitant strong CYP3A4 inhibitors (e.g., clarithromycin and itraconazole), the dosage should be adjusted as only one-quarter of the usual dose.

6.2. Clozapine

Clozapine is among the most effective antipsychotics available in treating schizophrenia and, in treatment-resistant schizophrenia, this is the only option to be effective. Schizophrenia patients show high risk of recurrent suicidal behavior and clozapine can function to reduce this condition [107]. When compared with typical antipsychotics, clozapine is much less likely to cause extrapyramidal side effects, which are severe movement disorders, but clozapine is administered to only the most severely ill, since there are substantial risks that are associated with clozapine therapy. Clozapine-induced agranulocytosis is one example and treatment with clozapine requires monitoring white blood and absolute neutrophil counts through enrollment requirements in a computer-based registry [108] Clozapine is mainly metabolized in the liver by CYP1A2 [109]. CYP2D6 and CYP3A4 enzymes are also involved in clozapine metabolism. CYP2D6 poor metabolizers may cause higher plasma levels of clozapine from usual doses than others. The FDA's Table of PGx Biomarkers for clozapine states that a dose needs to be reduced for patients who are CYP2D6 poor metabolizers.

6.3. Risperidone

Risperidone, which is an atypical antipsychotic, is the most commonly prescribed among antipsychotics in the US [110,111]. It is used in treating schizophrenia, bipolar disorder, and severe dementia. CYP2D6 enzyme metabolizes risperidone to an active metabolite 9-hydroxyrisperidone. This reaction is also catalyzed by CYP3A4 to a lesser extent. Thus, CYP2D6 poor metabolizers would show a decreased ability to metabolize risperidone and be at a higher risk of ADRs due to an increased plasma level of risperidone than normal metabolizers who carry two active *CYP2D6* alleles. In contrast, CYP2D6 ultrarapid metabolizers may show a decreased response to therapy. The FDA's Table of PGx Biomarkers for risperidone states that poor and extensive/normal metabolizers show no significant differences in the rates of adverse effects. Additionally, the DPWG recently revised its dosing guidelines as "no action is needed" for CYP2D6 poor metabolizers taking risperidone.

A recent association study of *KCNH7* variants reveals that two SNPs in the *KCNH7/Kv11.3* gene were significantly associated with risperidone responses [112,113]. The *KCNH7/Kv11.3* gene encodes one subunit of the potassium voltage-gated channel Kv11 family.

6.4. Thioridazine

Thioridazine is particularly used for patients who have failed to respond to, or cannot tolerate, other antipsychotics [114]. Thioridazine tends to lengthen the QT interval in a dose-dependent manner. Drugs showing this potential are associated with life-threatening ventricular tachycardia, called "torsades de pointes". The CYP2D6 enzyme mainly metabolizes thioridazine [115]. Given standard doses of thioridazine, individuals with reduced levels of CYP2D6 activity may cause higher drug levels in the plasma and increase the potential of cardiac arrhythmias. The FDA's Table of PGx Biomarkers for thioridazine states that thioridazine is contraindicated in patients who have low levels of CYP2D6 activity and in co-administration with other drugs that inhibit CYP2D6, such as fluoxetine and paroxetine, or inhibit the metabolism of thioridazine.

7. Mood Stabilizers—Bipolar Disorder

Mood stabilizers are used mainly in treating bipolar disorder and mood swings and in augmenting the treatment effect of antidepressants, through decreasing abnormal activity in the brain [116,117]. Lithium is approved for treating mania and bipolar disorder and it provides anti-suicide benefits to individuals on long-term maintenance. Anticonvulsant medications were originally developed to treat seizures, but were found to also help control unstable moods. These can be used as mood stabilizers and valproic acid is an example of anticonvulsants commonly used as a mood stabilizer. Mood stabilizers can lead to several ADRs, including excessively high blood levels.

Epileptic seizures are a malfunction of the brain, like major depression, anxiety disorders, and other psychoses. Thus, epilepsy has psychiatric aspects, and some psychiatric disorders are highly associated with epilepsy. Patients with mood disorders tend to experience seizures of both kinds—epileptic seizures and non-epileptic seizures. This relationship seems to flow in both directions: mood disorders increase the risk of seizures and seizures increase the risk of mood disorders. This is why some mood stabilizers are also used as antiepileptic drugs, and these will be described in the next section.

8. Antiepileptic Drugs—Epilepsy

According to the International League Against Epilepsy (ILAE) and the International Bureau for Epilepsy [118], epilepsy is defined as "a disorder of the brain characterized by an enduring predisposition to generate epileptic seizures and by the neurobiological, cognitive, psychological, and social consequences of this condition. The definition of epilepsy requires the occurrence of at least one epileptic seizure". Being characterized by recurrent seizures, epilepsy affected 65 million people worldwide [119]. Although epilepsy can be controlled by epileptic drugs, the response to antiepileptic treatment varies highly, depending on a patient due to genetic variation in genes causing or related with the epilepsy in pharmacokinetics and pharmacodynamics, as in Table 2 [120].

8.1. Brivaracetam

Brivaracetam is approved for partial-onset seizures in patients four years of age and older [121]. It binds to the synaptic vesicle glycoprotein 2A (SV2A) with high affinity. It regulates the release of neurotransmitters at the presynaptic terminal and reduces neuronal excitability [122]. The amide moiety is hydrolyzed in primary metabolism and then CYP2C19 further metabolizes in order to form the hydroxy metabolite [121]. CYP2C19 intermediate or poor metabolizers are less able to metabolize the drug, resulting in a high plasma concentration of Brivaracetam, which may increase the risk of adverse effects, including sedation, fatigue, dizziness, and nausea. Therefore, patients who are CYP2C19 poor metabolizers or patients using CYP2C19 inhibitors may require a dose reduction [121].

8.2. Carbamazepine

Carbamazepine is approved for partial seizures, tonic-clonic seizures, mixed seizures patterns, and pain control for trigeminal neuralgia [123]. It is a tricyclic compound, and it binds to voltage-dependent sodium channels, which blocks the repetitive firing of an action potential by reducing polysynaptic responses [88]. Blocking the sodium channels and L-type calcium channel inhibits the action potential generated in the epileptic seizures [88]. Although carbamazepine is widely used as the first-line treatment, adverse reactions, such as hypersensitivity, occur to 10% of patients [88]. Hypersensitivity reactions are largely cutaneous, ranging from mild reactions, such as maculopapular exanthema (MPE) to life-threatening reactions, such as Stevens–Johnson syndrome (SJS), toxic epidermal necrolysis (TEN), and drug reaction with eosinophilia and systemic symptoms (DRESS) [88]. The risk of hypersensitivity is known to be correlated by specific human leukocyte antigen (HLA) alleles, such as HLA-B and HLA-A [124]. Particularly, the HLA-B*15:02 allele, which is known to mediate the activation of cytotoxic T-lymphocytes, mainly contributes to causing carbamazepine-induced SJS/TEN [120]. When compared with the HLA-B*15:02 allele, the HLA-A*31:01 allele shows a weaker association with causing SJS/TEN, yet it is identified to induce all carbamazepine hypersensitivity phenotypes, including MPE, DRESS, and SJS/TEN [88]. While HLA-B*15:02 is mainly found in Southeast Asia, HLA-A*31:01 is widely distributed across the world [88]. Because of these side effects, the FDA requires HLA-B*15:02 for patients in which HLA-B* may be present like Asian-descent patients. As of HLA-A*31:01, patients that are known to carry HLA-A*31:01 should weigh the risks and benefits before starting the medication [123].

8.3. Clobazam

Clobazam is approved for adjunctive treatment of seizures associated with Lennox–Gastaut syndrome (LGS) in patients two years of age or older [125]. LGS is a complex, rare, and severe childhood-onset epilepsy with multiple and concurrent seizures, cognitive retardation, and slow spike-wave activity in electroencephalogram (EEG) [88]. Clobazam is a 1,5-benzodiazepine and $GABA_A$ receptor agonist, which binds to postsynaptic $GABA_A$ receptors in the brain, causes hyperpolarization, and creates an inhibitory signal [126]. It is primarily metabolized by CYP3A4 and, minorly, by CYP2C19 and CYP2B6 to an active metabolite, N-desmethyl clobazam (norclobazam). Norclobazam is further metabolized to 4′-hydroxy-N-desmethylclobazam mainly by CYP2C19 [125,127]. Thus, poor CYP2C19 metabolizers have a long-term effect as the effects of norclobazam continue. Moreover, it is known that clobazam clearance is decreased in poor metabolizers, which increases the level of norclobazam [127,128]. Thirty-eight different CYP2C19 alleles have been identified so far that can affect the enzyme's activity [129,130]. Clobazam poor metabolizers are required in order to adjust dosage [125].

8.4. Diazepam

Diazepam is approved for various clinical uses, including anxiety disorders, symptomatic relief of acute agitation, tremor, hallucinosis, and skeletal muscle spasm. It is also indicated for use as an adjunctive therapy for convulsive disorder [131]. It is a benzodiazepine and $GABA_A$ receptor agonist, which creates an inhibitory signal in the vertebrate central nervous system [131,132]. CYP3A4 and CYP2C19 primarily metabolizes diazepam to an active metabolite, N-desmethyldiazepam [131]. It is further hydroxylated by CYP3A4 to another active metabolite oxazepam [131]. Both active metabolites are mainly eliminated by glucuronidation [131]. Genetic polymorphisms on CYP2C19 and CYP3A4 can affect the clearance of the drug, creating inter-individual variation, according to the FDA-approved drug label for diazepam gel (Diastat) [131]. On the other hand, the label for diazepam oral formulations (Valium) does not indicate pharmacogenomic relationship and only states that there is a potentially relevant interaction between diazepam and compounds that inhibit certain hepatic enzymes (particularly, CYP3A and CYP2C19) [131].

8.5. Lacosamide

Lacosamide is a third-generation anticonvulsant, which is approved for partial-onset seizures in patients four years of age and older [133]. As a functionalized amino acid, lacosamide is believed to amplify the slow inactivation of voltage-gated sodium channels in order to stabilize hyperexcited neuronal membranes and suppress the repetitive neuronal firing [134]. CYP3A4, CYP2C9, and CYP2C19 are involved in metabolism to form a major inactive O-desmethyl metabolite [88]. Amongst them, the role of CYP2C19 is extensively studied that CYP2C19 poor metabolizers have lower plasma concentration of the inactive O-desmethyl metabolite and similar concentration of active lacosamide. Consequently, CYP2C19 poor and normal metabolizers showed similar clinical effects in lacosamide pharmacokinetics [133].

8.6. Oxcarbazepine

As a structural analogue of carbamazepine, oxcarbazepine shows a similar mechanism of action with carbamazepine by blocking voltage-gated sodium channels [135,136]. Oxcarbazepine is metabolized to its monohydroxy derivative (MHD), which is an active metabolite, while carbamazepine is rapidly reduced to an epoxide metabolite [137]. In addition, oxcarbazepine inhibits N/P- and R-type calcium channels, whereas carbamazepine inhibits L-type calcium channels [135]. In terms of PGx testing, similar to carbamazepine, potential patients of oxcarbazepine should get tested for HLA-B*15:02 due to the risk of SJS/TEN [99]. However, HLA-A testing is not required, as oxcarbazepine is known to have fewer adverse reactions than carbamazepine due to their distinct pharmacokinetic characteristics [138].

8.7. Phenytoin

Phenytoin is approved for the control of generalized-onset tonic-clonic (grand mal) and complex partial (psychomotor and temporal lobe) seizures and the prevention and treatment of seizures occurring during or following neurosurgery [139]. It reduces brain stem centers' maximal activity, which are responsible for tonic phase by stabilizing excessive stimulation induced hyperexcitability and reducing post-tetanic potentiation at synapses [139]. Phenytoin has a narrow therapeutic range of serum concentration between 10–20 μg/mL [88]. If the serum concentration exceeds the therapeutic range, then the risks of side effects increase and so therapeutic drug monitoring (TDM) of phenytoin is necessary [88,140]. It is known that CYP2C9 and CYP2C19 affect the serum concentration of phenytoin, as both of the enzymes are involved in the metabolism of phenytoin [88]. CYP2C9 poor metabolizers have reduced clearance rates, which may increase the serum level of phenytoin, increasing the risk of side effects. Similar to carbamazepine and oxcarbazepine, HLA-B*15:02 allele carriers have high risk of phenytoin-induced SJS/TEN, and so they should avoid phenytoin as an alternative for carbamazepine [139].

8.8. Valproic Acid

Valproic acid is approved for monotherapy and adjunctive therapy of complex partial seizures, simple and complex absence seizures, and adjunctive therapy of multiple seizure types that include absence seizures [141]. It is a fatty acid and enhances GABA transmission by inhibiting reabsorption of GABA and inhibits voltage dependent sodium and T-type calcium channels [132,142]. Valproic acid is contraindicated for patients with *polymerase-*γ-producing mitochondrial disease, as the genetic mutations in mitochondrial DNA polymerase γ (*POLG*) gene is strongly associated with acute liver failure and consequent death [141,142]. Valproic acid overexpresses *POLG1* gene and it changes several mitochondria genes, which affect mitochondria genesis [142]. Therefore, POLG mutation screening should be performed prior to valproic acid treatment [141]. Additionally, valproic acid is contraindicated for patients with urea cycle disorders (UCD) due to an increased risk of hyperammonemic encephalopathy, which can be fatal. Therefore, patients should be evaluated for UCD if they have a history of unexplained encephalopathy or coma, or cyclic vomiting and lethargy, or a family history of UCD, or show symptoms of UCD [141].

9. Beyond Pharmacogenomic Testing

Precision medicine targets providing the optimal diagnoses and treatments for each patient based on the categorization of biomarkers [143–146]. PGx is one of the main research areas of precision medicine. Nowadays, advances in artificial intelligence (AI), machine learning, multi-omics, and neuroimaging allow for analyzing and integrating complex genomic and clinical data in psychiatry and neurology. Artificial intelligence is the field of computing science that produces an algorithm based on available data to create predictive outcomes, even for unknown data in the future [147–150]. Particularly, state-of-the-art technology of deep learning revolutionized bioinformatics and medical imaging by yielding helpful software tools [151,152]. Whereas cancer therapy has routine clinical settings with well-established genomic data, in neuropsychiatry, the relationship between PGx data and their clinical significances has not been fully studied. Thus, the usage of artificial intelligence remains limited in the field.

AI has been used in predicting diagnosis, treatment outcome, and prognosis. As of psychiatry and neurology, multiple studies have used models, including deep learning architecture, random forest, tree-based ensemble, elastic net, and linear regression in order to evaluate and predict lithium treatment response on major depressive disorder [153]. To predict prognosis of major depressive disorder, there are algorithms, such as Gaussian process algorithm, Deep Patient, DeepCare, and Doctor AI, which utilize electronic health records. For example, Deep Patient has forecasted psychiatric disorders, including ADHD or schizophrenia with high accuracy (AUC = 0.863 and AUC = 0.853, respectively) [154]. However, the technology is still at an infancy phase and there are many obstacles and limitations to overcome in order to apply it clinically. For example, each algorithm is developed and assigned for each disease and so it is difficult to apply it to other diseases. Moreover, the sample size of each algorithm is too small to apply to public [153].

Various research efforts are ongoing in order to improve diagnosis, prognosis, and treatment in neuropsychiatry: PGx data and their treatment outcomes have been collected to support data-driven clinical decision-making for the patient. To this end, relations between genetic variation and variable drug responses to psychiatric medications should be well established [153]. The use of AI and machine learning analyses to predict individual-specific responses to psychiatric medications is challenging, but well worth pursuing [153].

Author Contributions: H.J. designed and supervised the study. H.K. and H.J. analyzed the reference articles and wrote the manuscript. All authors have read and agreed to the published version of the manuscript.

References

1. World Health Organization. Mental Health. Available online: https://www.who.int/health-topics/mental-health (accessed on 25 November 2020).
2. Wainberg, M.L.; Scorza, P.; Shultz, J.M.; Helpman, L.; Mootz, J.J.; Johnson, K.A.; Neria, Y.; Bradford, J.-M.E.; Oquendo, M.A.; Arbuckle, M.R.; et al. Challenges and opportunities in global mental health: A research-to-practice perspective. *Curr. Psychiatry Rep.* **2017**, *19*, 28. [CrossRef]
3. Clous, E.; Beerthuizen, K.; Ponsen, K.J.; Luitse, J.; Olff, M.; Goslings, C. Trauma and psychiatric disorders: A systematic review. *J. Trauma Acute Care Surg.* **2017**, *82*, 794–801. [CrossRef]
4. Lozupone, M.; Seripa, D.; Stella, E.; La Montagna, M.; Solfrizzi, V.; Quaranta, N.; Veneziani, F.; Cester, A.; Sardone, R.; Bonfiglio, C. Innovative biomarkers in psychiatric disorders: A major clinical challenge in psychiatry. *Expert Rev. Proteom.* **2017**, *14*, 809–824. [CrossRef]
5. Eichelbaum, M.; Ingelman-Sundberg, M.; Evans, W.E. Pharmacogenomics and individualized drug therapy. *Annu. Rev. Med.* **2006**, *57*, 119–137. [CrossRef] [PubMed]

6. Lauschke, V.M.; Zhou, Y.; Ingelman-Sundberg, M. Novel genetic and epigenetic factors of importance for inter-individual differences in drug disposition, response and toxicity. *Pharmacol. Ther.* **2019**, *197*, 122–152. [CrossRef] [PubMed]
7. Sullivan, P.F.; Agrawal, A.; Bulik, C.M.; Andreassen, O.A.; Børglum, A.D.; Breen, G.; Cichon, S.; Edenberg, H.J.; Faraone, S.V.; Gelernter, J.; et al. Psychiatric genomics: An update and an agenda. *Am. J. Psychiatry* **2018**, *175*, 15–27. [CrossRef] [PubMed]
8. Hung, S.-I.; Chung, W.-H.; Jee, S.-H.; Chen, W.-C.; Chang, Y.-T.; Lee, W.-R.; Hu, S.-L.; Wu, M.-T.; Chen, G.-S.; Wong, T.-W.; et al. Genetic susceptibility to carbamazepine-induced cutaneous adverse drug reactions. *Pharm. Genom.* **2006**, *16*, 297–306. [CrossRef] [PubMed]
9. Dean, L. Carbamazepine Therapy and HLA Genotype. In *Medical Genetics Summaries*; National Center for Biotechnology Information: Bethesda, MD, USA, 2012.
10. Fricke-Galindo, I.; LLerena, A.; Jung-Cook, H.; López-López, M. Carbamazepine adverse drug reactions. *Expert Rev. Clin. Pharmacol.* **2018**, *11*, 705–718. [CrossRef]
11. Barbarino, J.M.; McGregor, T.L.; Altman, R.B.; Klein, T.E. PharmGKB summary: Very important pharmacogene information for MT-RNR1. *Pharm. Genom.* **2016**, *26*, 558. [CrossRef]
12. Rahman, S.; Ecob, R.; Costello, H.; Sweeney, M.G.; Duncan, A.J.; Pearce, K.; Strachan, D.; Forge, A.; Davis, A.; Bitner-Glindzicz, M.; et al. Hearing in 44–45 year olds with m.1555A > G, a genetic mutation predisposing to aminoglycoside-induced deafness: A population based cohort study. *BMJ Open* **2012**, *2*. [CrossRef]
13. Van der Wouden, C.H.; van Rhenen, M.H.; Jama, W.O.; Ingelman-Sundberg, M.; Lauschke, V.M.; Konta, L.; Schwab, M.; Swen, J.J.; Guchelaar, H.J. Development of the PGx-passport: A panel of actionable germline genetic variants for pre-emptive pharmacogenetic testing. *Clin. Pharmacol. Ther.* **2019**, *106*, 866–873. [CrossRef] [PubMed]
14. U.S. Food & Drug Administration. Table of Pharmacogenomic Biomarkers in Drug Labeling. Available online: https://www.fda.gov/drugs/science-and-research-drugs/table-pharmacogenomic-biomarkers-drug-labeling (accessed on 1 November 2020).
15. The Clinical Pharmacogenetics Implementation Consortium. Guidelines. Available online: https://web.archive.org/web/20201101003826/ (accessed on 1 November 2020).
16. The Canadian Pharmacogenomics Network for Drug Safety (CPNDS). Available online: https://web.archive.org/web/20201125025807/ (accessed on 25 November 2020).
17. Ross, C.J.; Visscher, H.; Sistonen, J.; Brunham, L.R.; Pussegoda, K.; Loo, T.T.; Rieder, M.J.; Koren, G.; Carleton, B.C.; Hayden, M.R.; et al. The canadian pharmacogenomics network for drug safety: A model for safety pharmacology. *Thyroid* **2010**, *20*, 681–687. [CrossRef] [PubMed]
18. Swen, J.J.; Huizinga, T.W.; Gelderblom, H.; De Vries, E.G.; Assendelft, W.J.; Kirchheiner, J.; Guchelaar, H.-J. Translating pharmacogenomics: Challenges on the road to the clinic. *PLoS Med.* **2007**, *4*, e209. [CrossRef] [PubMed]
19. Ehmann, F.; Caneva, L.; Prasad, K.; Paulmichl, M.; Maliepaard, M.; Llerena, A.; Ingelman-Sundberg, M.; Papaluca-Amati, M. Pharmacogenomic information in drug labels: European medicines agency perspective. *Pharm. J.* **2015**, *15*, 201–210. [CrossRef] [PubMed]
20. Drozda, K.; Pacanowski, M.A.; Grimstein, C.; Zineh, I. Pharmacogenetic labeling of FDA-approved drugs: A regulatory retrospective. *JACC Basic Transl. Sci.* **2018**, *3*, 545–549. [CrossRef]
21. The Pharmacogenomics Knowledgebase. Clinical Guideline Annotations. Available online: https://www.pharmgkb.org/guidelineAnnotations (accessed on 1 November 2020).
22. Guengerich, F.P. Cytochrome P450 research and the journal of biological chemistry. *J. Biol. Chem.* **2019**, *294*, 1671–1680. [CrossRef]
23. Manikandan, P.; Nagini, S. Cytochrome P450 structure, function and clinical significance: A review. *Curr. Drug Targets* **2018**, *19*, 38–54. [CrossRef]
24. Pharmacogene Variation Consortium. CYP2D6 Allele Nomenclature. Available online: https://web.archive.org/web/20201031133042/ (accessed on 31 October 2020).
25. El-Mallakh, R.S.; Roberts, R.J.; El-Mallakh, P.L.; Findlay, L.J.; Reynolds, K.K. Pharmacogenomics in psychiatric practice. *Clin. Lab. Med.* **2016**, *36*, 507–523. [CrossRef]
26. Gaedigk, A.; Sangkuhl, K.; Whirl-Carrillo, M.; Klein, T.; Leeder, J.S. Prediction of CYP2D6 phenotype from genotype across world populations. *Genet. Med.* **2017**, *19*, 69–76. [CrossRef]

27. LLerena, A.; Naranjo, M.E.G.; Rodrigues-Soares, F.; Penas-LLedo, E.M.; Farinas, H.; Tarazona-Santos, E. Interethnic variability of CYP2D6 alleles and of predicted and measured metabolic phenotypes across world populations. *Expert Opin. Drug Metab. Toxicol.* **2014**, *10*, 1569–1583. [CrossRef]
28. Oshiro, C.; Thorn, C.F.; Roden, D.M.; Klein, T.E.; Altman, R.B. KCNH2 pharmacogenomics summary. *Pharm. Genom.* **2010**, *20*, 775. [CrossRef] [PubMed]
29. Gaedigk, A.; Gotschall, R.R.; Forbes, N.S.; Simon, S.D.; Kearns, G.L.; Leeder, J.S. Optimization of cytochrome P4502D6 (CYP2D6) phenotype assignment using a genotyping algorithm based on allele frequency data. *Pharm. Genom.* **1999**, *9*, 669–682. [CrossRef] [PubMed]
30. Bradford, L.D. CYP2D6 allele frequency in european caucasians, Asians, Africans and their descendants. *Pharmacogenomics* **2002**, *3*, 229–243. [CrossRef] [PubMed]
31. Yokota, H.; Tamura, S.; Furuya, H.; Kimura, S.; Watanabe, M.; Kanazawa, I.; Kondo, I.; Gonzalez, F.J. Evidence for a new variant CYP2D6 allele CYP2D6J in a japanese population associated with lower In Vivo rates of sparteine metabolism. *Pharmacogenetics* **1993**, *3*, 256–263. [CrossRef]
32. Sistonen, J.; Sajantila, A.; Lao, O.; Corander, J.; Barbujani, G.; Fuselli, S. CYP2D6 worldwide genetic variation shows high frequency of altered activity variants and no continental structure. *Pharm. Genom.* **2007**, *17*, 93–101.
33. Ingelman-Sundberg, M. Genetic polymorphisms of cytochrome P 450 2D6 (CYP2D6): Clinical consequences, evolutionary aspects and functional diversity. *Pharm. J.* **2005**, *5*, 6–13.
34. Ingelman-Sundberg, M.; Sim, S.C.; Gomez, A.; Rodriguez-Antona, C. Influence of cytochrome P450 polymorphisms on drug therapies: Pharmacogenetic, pharmacoepigenetic and clinical aspects. *Pharmacol. Ther.* **2007**, *116*, 496–526. [CrossRef]
35. Schroth, W.; Hamann, U.; Fasching, P.A.; Dauser, S.; Winter, S.; Eichelbaum, M.; Schwab, M.; Brauch, H. CYP2D6 polymorphisms as predictors of outcome in breast cancer patients treated with tamoxifen: Expanded polymorphism coverage improves risk stratification. *Clin. Cancer Res.* **2010**, *16*, 4468–4477. [CrossRef]
36. De Vos, A.; Van Der Weide, J.; Loovers, H. Association between CYP2C19* 17 and metabolism of amitriptyline, citalopram and clomipramine in Dutch hospitalized patients. *Pharm. J.* **2011**, *11*, 359–367. [CrossRef]
37. Steimer, W.; Zopf, K.; von Amelunxen, S.; Pfeiffer, H.; Bachofer, J.; Popp, J.; Messner, B.; Kissling, W.; Leucht, S. Amitriptyline or not, that is the question: Pharmacogenetic testing of CYP2D6 and CYP2C19 identifies patients with low or high risk for side effects in amitriptyline therapy. *Clin. Chem.* **2005**, *51*, 376–385. [CrossRef]
38. Hicks, J.; Swen, J.; Thorn, C.; Sangkuhl, K.; Kharasch, E.; Ellingrod, V.; Skaar, T.; Müller, D.; Gaedigk, A.; Stingl, J.; et al. Clinical pharmacogenetics implementation consortium guideline for CYP2D6 and CYP2C19 genotypes and dosing of tricyclic antidepressants. *Clin. Pharmacol. Ther.* **2013**, *93*, 402–408. [CrossRef] [PubMed]
39. Ma, M.K.; Woo, M.H.; Mcleod, H.L. Genetic basis of drug metabolism. *Am. J. Health-Syst. Pharm.* **2002**, *59*, 2061–2069. [CrossRef] [PubMed]
40. Błaszczyk, B.; Czuczwar, S.J. Epilepsy coexisting with depression. *Pharmacol. Rep.* **2016**, *68*, 1084–1092. [CrossRef] [PubMed]
41. Feighner, J.P. Mechanism of action of antidepressant medications. In *Proceedings of the Assessing Antidepressant Efficacy: A Reexamination*; American Psychological Association: Phoenix, AZ, USA, 1998.
42. Sheffler, Z.M.; Abdijadid, S. *Antidepressants*; StatPearls: Treasure Island, FL, USA, 2020.
43. Ramamoorthy, S.; Leibach, F.; Mahesh, V.; Ganapathy, V. Partial purification and characterization of the human placental serotonin transporter. *Placenta* **1993**, *14*, 449–461. [CrossRef]
44. Lesch, K.-P.; Wolozin, B.; Estler, H.; Murphy, D.; Riederer, P. Isolation of a cDNA encoding the human brain serotonin transporter. *J. Neural Transm. Gen. Sect. JNT* **1993**, *91*, 67–72. [CrossRef] [PubMed]
45. Lesch, K.-P.; Bengel, D.; Heils, A.; Sabol, S.Z.; Greenberg, B.D.; Petri, S.; Benjamin, J.; Müller, C.R.; Hamer, D.H.; Murphy, D.L. Association of anxiety-related traits with a polymorphism in the serotonin transporter gene regulatory region. *Science* **1996**, *274*, 1527–1531. [CrossRef] [PubMed]
46. Clarke, H.; Flint, J.; Attwood, A.; Munafo, M. Association of the 5-HTTLPR genotype and unipolar depression: A meta-analysis. *Psychol. Med.* **2010**, *40*, 1767–1778. [CrossRef]
47. Heils, A.; Teufel, A.; Petri, S.; Stöber, G.; Riederer, P.; Bengel, D.; Lesch, K.P. Allelic variation of human serotonin transporter gene expression. *J. Neurochem.* **1996**, *66*, 2621–2624. [CrossRef]
48. Taylor, M.J.; Sen, S.; Bhagwagar, Z. Antidepressant response and the serotonin transporter gene-linked polymorphic region. *Biol. Psychiatry* **2010**, *68*, 536–543. [CrossRef] [PubMed]

49. Kato, M.; Serretti, A. Review and meta-analysis of antidepressant pharmacogenetic findings in major depressive disorder. *Mol. Psychiatry* **2010**, *15*, 473–500. [CrossRef] [PubMed]
50. Mellström, B.; Säwe, J.; Bertilsson, L.; Sjöqvist, F. Amitriptyline metabolism: Association with debrisoquin hydroxylation in nonsmokers. *Clin. Pharmacol. Ther.* **1986**, *39*, 369–371. [CrossRef]
51. Hicks, J.K.; Sangkuhl, K.; Swen, J.J.; Ellingrod, V.L.; Müller, D.J.; Kazu, S.; Bishop, J.R.; Kharasch, E.D.; Skaar, T.C.; Gaedigk, A. Clinical Pharmacogenetics Implementation Consortium Guideline (CPIC®) for CYP2D6 and CYP2C19 Genotypes and Tricyclic Antidepressants: 2016 Update. *Clin. Pharmacol. Ther.* **2017**, *102*, 37–44. [CrossRef] [PubMed]
52. Stern, S.L.; Ribner, H.S.; Cooper, T.B.; Nelson, L.D.; Johnson, M.H.; Suckow, R.F. 2-Hydroxydesipramine and desipramine plasma levels and electrocardiographic effects in depressed younger adults. *J. Clin. Psychopharmacol.* **1991**, *11*, 93–98. [CrossRef] [PubMed]
53. Schneider, L.S.; Cooper, T.B.; Severson, J.A.; Zemplenyi, T.; Sloane, R.B. Electrocardiographic changes with nortriptyline and 10-hydroxynortriptyline in elderly depressed outpatients. *J. Clin. Psychopharmacol.* **1988**, *8*, 402–408. [CrossRef] [PubMed]
54. Suwała, J.; Machowska, M.; Wiela-Hojeńska, A. Venlafaxine pharmacogenetics: V comprehensive review. *Pharmacogenomics* **2019**, *20*, 829–845. [CrossRef]
55. Venlafaxine, Desvenlafaxine. In *LiverTox: Clinical and Research Information on Drug-Induced Liver Injury*; National Institute of Diabetes and Digestive and Kidney Diseases: Bethesda, MD, USA, 2012.
56. Royal Dutch Pharmacists Association (KNMP). Venlafaxine-CYP2D. Available online: https://kennisbank.knmp.nl/login?destination= (accessed on 25 November 2020).
57. Sangkuhl, K.; Stingl, J.C.; Turpeinen, M.; Altman, R.B.; Klein, T.E. PharmGKB summary: Venlafaxine pathway. *Pharm. Genom.* **2014**, *24*, 62. [CrossRef]
58. Berm, E.; Kok, R.; Hak, E.; Wilffert, B. Relation between CYP2D6 genotype, phenotype and therapeutic drug concentrations among nortriptyline and venlafaxine users in old age psychiatry. *Pharmacopsychiatry* **2016**, *49*, 186–190. [CrossRef]
59. Berm, E.J.; Hak, E.; Postma, M.; Boshuisen, M.; Breuning, L.; Brouwers, J.R.; Dhondt, T.; Jansen, P.A.; Kok, R.M.; Maring, J.G.; et al. Effects and cost-effectiveness of pharmacogenetic screening for CYP2D6 among older adults starting therapy with nortriptyline or venlafaxine: Study protocol for a pragmatic randomized controlled trial (CYSCEtrial). *Trials* **2015**, *16*, 37. [CrossRef]
60. Waade, R.B.; Hermann, M.; Moe, H.L.; Molden, E. Impact of age on serum concentrations of venlafaxine and escitalopram in different CYP2D6 and CYP2C19 genotype subgroups. *Eur. J. Clin. Pharmacol.* **2014**, *70*, 933–940. [CrossRef]
61. Shams, M.; Arneth, B.; Hiemke, C.; Dragicevic, A.; Müller, M.; Kaiser, R.; Lackner, K.; Härtter, S. CYP2D6 polymorphism and clinical effect of the antidepressant venlafaxine. *J. Clin. Pharm. Ther.* **2006**, *31*, 493–502. [CrossRef]
62. Johnson, E.M.; Whyte, E.; Mulsant, B.H.; Pollock, B.G.; Weber, E.; Begley, A.E.; Reynolds, C.F. Cardiovascular changes associated with venlafaxine in the treatment of late-life depression. *Am. J. Geriatr. Psychiatry* **2006**, *14*, 796–802. [CrossRef]
63. Montané Jaime, L.K.; Paul, J.; Lalla, A.; Legall, G.; Gaedigk, A. Impact of CYP2D6 on venlafaxine metabolism in trinidadian patients with major depressive disorder. *Pharmacogenomics* **2018**, *19*, 197–212. [CrossRef]
64. Olson, M.C.; Maciel, A.; Gariepy, J.F.; Cullors, A.; Saldivar, J.-S.; Taylor, D.; Centeno, J.; Garces, J.A.; Vaishnavi, S. Clinical impact of pharmacogenetic-guided treatment for patients exhibiting neuropsychiatric disorders: A randomized controlled trial. *Prim. Care Companion CNS Disord.* **2017**, *19*. [CrossRef] [PubMed]
65. Lloret-Linares, C.; Daali, Y.; Chevret, S.; Nieto, I.; Molière, F.; Courtet, P.; Galtier, F.; Richieri, R.-M.; Morange, S.; Llorca, P.-M.; et al. Exploring venlafaxine pharmacokinetic variability with a phenotyping approach, a multicentric french-swiss study (MARVEL study). *BMC Pharmacol. Toxicol.* **2017**, *18*, 1–12. [CrossRef]
66. Burke, W.; Thummel, K. Telling it like it is: A call for accurate pharmacogenetic labeling. *JAMA Intern. Med.* **2014**, *174*, 1945. [CrossRef]
67. Watanabe, Y.; Asami, Y.; Hirano, Y.; Kuribayashi, K.; Itamura, R.; Imaeda, T. Factors impacting the efficacy of venlafaxine extended release 75–225 mg/day in patients with major depressive disorder: Exploratory post hoc subgroup analyses of a randomized, double-blind, placebo-controlled study in Japan. *Neuropsychiatr. Dis. Treat.* **2018**, *14*, 1261. [CrossRef] [PubMed]

68. Taranu, A.; Colle, R.; Gressier, F.; El Asmar, K.; Becquemont, L.; Corruble, E.; Verstuyft, C. Should a routine genotyping of CYP2D6 and CYP2C19 genetic polymorphisms be recommended to predict venlafaxine efficacy in depressed patients treated in psychiatric settings? *Pharmacogenomics* **2017**, *18*, 639–650. [CrossRef]
69. Van der Schans, J.; Hak, E.; Postma, M.; Breuning, L.; Brouwers, J.R.; Ditters, K.; Jansen, P.A.; Kok, R.M.; Maring, J.G.; van Marum, R.; et al. Effects of pharmacogenetic screening for CYP2D6 among elderly starting therapy with nortriptyline or venlafaxine: A pragmatic randomized controlled trial (CYSCE Trial). *J. Clin. Psychopharmacol.* **2019**, *39*, 583–590. [CrossRef] [PubMed]
70. Maron, E.; Nutt, D. Biological markers of generalized anxiety disorder. *Dialogues Clin. Neurosci.* **2017**, *19*, 147. [CrossRef]
71. Riss, J.; Cloyd, J.; Gates, J.; Collins, S. Benzodiazepines in epilepsy: Pharmacology and pharmacokinetics. *Acta Neurol. Scand.* **2008**, *118*, 69–86. [CrossRef]
72. Agrawal, N.; Faruqui, R.; Bodani, M. *Oxford Textbook of Neuropsychiatry*; Oxford University Press: Oxford, UK, 2020.
73. Polanczyk, G.; De Lima, M.S.; Horta, B.L.; Biederman, J.; Rohde, L.A. The worldwide prevalence of ADHD: A systematic review and metaregression analysis. *Am. J. Psychiatry* **2007**, *164*, 942–948. [CrossRef] [PubMed]
74. Polanczyk, G.V.; Willcutt, E.G.; Salum, G.A.; Kieling, C.; Rohde, L.A. ADHD prevalence estimates across three decades: An updated systematic review and meta-regression analysis. *Int. J. Epidemiol.* **2014**, *43*, 434–442. [CrossRef]
75. Simon, V.; Czobor, P.; Bálint, S.; Mészáros, A.; Bitter, I. Prevalence and correlates of adult attention-deficit hyperactivity disorder: Meta-analysis. *Br. J. Psychiatry* **2009**, *194*, 204–211. [CrossRef] [PubMed]
76. *Diagnostic and Statistical Manual of Mental Disorders: DSM-5*; American Psychiatric: Washington, DC, USA; London, UK, 2013.
77. Moreira-Maia, C.R.; Massuti, R.; Tessari, L.; Campani, F.; Akutagava-Martins, G.C.; Cortese, S.; Rohde, L.A. Are ADHD medications under or over prescribed worldwide?: Protocol for a systematic review and meta-analysis. *Medicine* **2018**, *97*. [CrossRef] [PubMed]
78. World Health Organization. International Classification of Diseases (ICD-11) for Mortality and Morbidity Statistics, Eleventh Revision. Available online: https://icd.who.int/browse11/l-m/en (accessed on 31 October 2020).
79. Subcommittee on Attention-Deficit/Hyperactivity Disorder; Steering Committee on Quality Improvement and Management. ADHD: Clinical practice guideline for the diagnosis, evaluation, and treatment of attention-deficit/hyperactivity disorder in children and adolescents. *Am. Acad. Pediatrics* **2011**, *128*, 1007–1022.
80. Hutchison, S.L.; Ghuman, J.K.; Ghuman, H.S.; Karpov, I.; Schuster, J.M. Efficacy of atomoxetine in the treatment of attention-deficit hyperactivity disorder in patients with common comorbidities in children, adolescents and adults: A review. *Ther. Adv. Psychopharmacol.* **2016**, *6*, 317–334. [CrossRef]
81. Arbor Pharmaceuticals. EVEKEO ODT (Amphetamine Sulfate). Available online: https://www.accessdata.fda.gov/drugsatfda_docs/label/2019/209905s000lbl.pdf (accessed on 31 October 2020).
82. Neos Therapeutics. ADZENYS ER (Amphetamine). Available online: https://www.accessdata.fda.gov/drugsatfda_docs/label/2017/204325s000lbl.pdf (accessed on 31 October 2020).
83. Barateau, L.; Lopez, R.; Dauvilliers, Y. Treatment options for narcolepsy. *CNS Drugs* **2016**, *30*, 369–379. [CrossRef]
84. Bradley, C. The Behavior of Children Receiving Benzedrine. *Am. J. Psychiatry* **1937**, *94*, 577–585. [CrossRef]
85. Castells, X.; Blanco-Silvente, L.; Cunill, R. Amphetamines for attention deficit hyperactivity disorder (ADHD) in adults. *Cochrane Database Syst. Rev.* **2018**, *8*. [CrossRef]
86. Hodgkins, P.; Shaw, M.; McCarthy, S.; Sallee, F.R. The pharmacology and clinical outcomes of amphetamines to treat ADHD. *CNS Drugs* **2012**, *26*, 245–268. [CrossRef]
87. Bach, M.V.; Coutts, R.T.; Baker, G.B. Involvement of CYP2D6 in the in vitro metabolism of amphetamine, two N-alkylamphetamines and their 4-methoxylated derivatives. *Xenobiotica* **1999**, *29*, 719–732. [CrossRef] [PubMed]
88. Pratt, V.M.; McLeod, H.L.; Rubinstein, W.S.; Scott, S.A.; Dean, L.C.; Kattman, B.L.; Malheiro, A.J. *Medical Genetics Summaries [Internet]*; National Center for Biotechnology Information: Bethesda, MD, USA, 2012.
89. Garnock-Jones, K.P.; Keating, G.M. Spotlight on atomoxetine in attention-deficit hyperactivity disorder in children and adolescentsy. *CNS Drugs* **2010**, *24*, 85–88. [CrossRef] [PubMed]

90. Brown, J.T.; Bishop, J.R. Atomoxetine pharmacogenetics: Associations with pharmacokinetics, treatment response and tolerability. *Pharmacogenomics* **2015**, *16*, 1513–1520. [CrossRef] [PubMed]
91. Teva Pharmaceuticals. PROVIGIL® (Modafinil). Available online: https://www.accessdata.fda.gov/drugsatfda_docs/label/2015/020717s037s038lbl.pdf (accessed on 1 November 2020).
92. Minzenberg, M.J.; Carter, C.S. Modafinil: A review of neurochemical actions and effects on cognition. *Neuropsychopharmacology* **2008**, *33*, 1477–1502. [CrossRef] [PubMed]
93. Schwartz, J.C. The histamine H3 receptor: From discovery to clinical trials with pitolisant. *Br. J. Pharmacol.* **2011**, *163*, 713–721. [CrossRef] [PubMed]
94. Harmony Biosciences. WAKIX® (Pitolisant). Available online: https://www.accessdata.fda.gov/drugsatfda_docs/label/2019/211150s000lbl.pdf (accessed on 1 November 2020).
95. Syed, Y.Y. Pitolisant: First global approval. *Drugs* **2016**, *76*, 1313–1318. [CrossRef] [PubMed]
96. Hudepohl, N.S.; Nasrallah, H.A. Antipsychotic drugs. In *Handbook of Clinical Neurology*; Elsevier: Amsterdam, The Netherlands, 2012; Volume 106, pp. 657–667.
97. Lally, J.; MacCabe, J.H. Antipsychotic medication in schizophrenia: A review. *Br. Med. Bull.* **2015**, *114*, 169–179. [CrossRef] [PubMed]
98. Nandra, K.S.; Agius, M. The differences between typical and atypical antipsychotics: The effects on neurogenesis. *Psychiatr. Danub.* **2012**, *24*, S95–S99.
99. Beaulieu, J.-M.; Gainetdinov, R.R. The physiology, signaling, and pharmacology of dopamine receptors. *Pharmacol. Rev.* **2011**, *63*, 182–217. [CrossRef]
100. Salem, H.; Pigott, T.; Zhang, X.Y.; Zeni, C.P.; Teixeira, A.L. Antipsychotic-induced Tardive dyskinesia: From biological basis to clinical management. *Expert Rev. Neurother.* **2017**, *17*, 883–894. [CrossRef]
101. Dean, K.; Murray, R.M. Environmental risk factors for psychosis. *Dialogues Clin. Neurosci.* **2005**, *7*, 69.
102. Allen, N.C.; Bagade, S.; McQueen, M.B.; Ioannidis, J.P.; Kavvoura, F.K.; Khoury, M.J.; Tanzi, R.E.; Bertram, L. Systematic meta-analyses and field synopsis of genetic association studies in schizophrenia: The SzGene database. *Nat. Genet.* **2008**, *40*, 827. [CrossRef] [PubMed]
103. Farrell, M.; Werge, T.; Sklar, P.; Owen, M.J.; Ophoff, R.; O'Donovan, M.C.; Corvin, A.; Cichon, S.; Sullivan, P.F. Evaluating historical candidate genes for schizophrenia. *Mol. Psychiatry* **2015**, *20*, 555–562. [CrossRef] [PubMed]
104. Ripke, S.; Neale, B. Schizophrenia working group of the psychiatric genomics consortium. Biological insights from 108 schizophrenia-associated genetic loci. *Nature* **2014**, *511*, 421–427.
105. Scheggia, D.; Mastrogiacomo, R.; Mereu, M.; Sannino, S.; Straub, R.E.; Armando, M.; Managò, F.; Guadagna, S.; Piras, F.; Zhang, F. Variations in Dysbindin-1 are associated with cognitive response to antipsychotic drug treatment. *Nat. Commun.* **2018**, *9*, 1–11. [CrossRef] [PubMed]
106. Leggio, G.; Torrisi, S.; Mastrogiacomo, R.; Mauro, D.; Chisari, M.; Devroye, C.; Scheggia, D.; Nigro, M.; Geraci, F.; Pintori, N.; et al. The epistatic interaction between the dopamine D3 receptor and dysbindin-1 modulates higher-order cognitive functions in mice and humans. *Mol. Psychiatry* **2019**, *24*, 1–4. [CrossRef]
107. Sriretnakumar, V.; Huang, E.; Müller, D.J. Pharmacogenetics of clozapine treatment response and side-effects in schizophrenia: An update. *Expert Opin. Drug Metab. Toxicol.* **2015**, *11*, 1709–1731. [CrossRef]
108. Oliver Freudenreich, J.M. Guidelines for Prescribing Clozapine in Schizophrenia. Available online: https://www.uptodate.com/contents/guidelines-for-prescribing-clozapine-in-schizophrenia?search=guidelines-for-prescribing-clozapinein-schizophrenia&source=search_result&selectedTitle=2~{}150&usage_type=default&display_rank=2 (accessed on 31 October 2020).
109. Van Troostwijk, L.J.D.; Koopmans, R.P.; Vermeulen, H.D.; Guchelaar, H.-J. CYP1A2 activity is an important determinant of clozapine dosage in schizophrenic patients. *Eur. J. Pharm. Sci.* **2003**, *20*, 451–457. [CrossRef]
110. Sampson, S.; Hosalli, P.; Furtado, V.A.; Davis, J.M. Risperidone (depot) for schizophrenia. *Cochrane Database Syst. Rev.* **2016**. [CrossRef]
111. Puangpetch, A.; Vanwong, N.; Nuntamool, N.; Hongkaew, Y.; Chamnanphon, M.; Sukasem, C. CYP2D6 polymorphisms and their influence on risperidone treatment. *Pharm. Pers. Med.* **2016**, *9*, 131. [CrossRef]
112. Heide, J.; Zhang, F.; Bigos, K.L.; Mann, S.A.; Carr, V.J.; Shannon Weickert, C.; Green, M.J.; Weinberger, D.R.; Vandenberg, J.I. Differential response to risperidone in schizophrenia patients by KCNH2 genotype and drug metabolizer status. *Am. J. Psychiatry* **2016**, *173*, 53–59. [CrossRef] [PubMed]

113. Wang, X.; Su, Y.; Yan, H.; Huang, Z.; Huang, Y.; Yue, W. Association study of KCNH7 polymorphisms and individual responses to risperidone treatment in schizophrenia. *Front. Psychiatry* **2019**, *10*, 633. [CrossRef] [PubMed]
114. Thanacoody, R.H. Thioridazine: The good and the bad. *Recent Pat. Anti-Infect. Drug Discov.* **2011**, *6*, 92–98. [CrossRef] [PubMed]
115. Dean, L. Thioridazine Therapy and CYP2D6 Genotypes. In *Medical Genetics Summaries [Internet]*; National Center for Biotechnology Information: Bethesda, MD, USA, 2017.
116. Grande, I.; Berk, M.; Birmaher, B.; Vieta, E. Bipolar disorder. *Lancet* **2016**, *387*, 1561–1572. [CrossRef]
117. Miller, T.H. Bipolar Disorder. *Prim. Care* **2016**, *43*, 269–284. [CrossRef] [PubMed]
118. Fisher, R.S.; Boas, W.V.E.; Blume, W.; Elger, C.; Genton, P.; Lee, P.; Engel, J., Jr. Epileptic seizures and epilepsy: Definitions proposed by the international league against epilepsy (ILAE) and the International bureau for epilepsy (IBE). *Epilepsia* **2005**, *46*, 470–472. [CrossRef] [PubMed]
119. Thurman, D.J.; Beghi, E.; Begley, C.E.; Berg, A.T.; Buchhalter, J.R.; Ding, D.; Hesdorffer, D.C.; Hauser, W.A.; Kazis, L.; Kobau, R.; et al. Standards for epidemiologic studies and surveillance of epilepsy. *Epilepsia* **2011**, *52* (Suppl. 7), 2–26. [CrossRef] [PubMed]
120. Balestrini, S.; Sisodiya, S.M. Pharmacogenomics in epilepsy. *Neurosci. Lett.* **2018**, *667*, 27–39. [CrossRef]
121. UCB. BRIVIACT® (Brivaracetam). Available online: https://www.accessdata.fda.gov/drugsatfda_docs/label/2018/205836s005,205837s004,205838s003lbl.pdf (accessed on 1 November 2020).
122. Niespodziany, I.; Rigo, J.M.; Moonen, G.; Matagne, A.; Klitgaard, H.; Wolff, C. Brivaracetam does not modulate ionotropic channels activated by glutamate, γ-aminobutyric acid, and glycine in hippocampal neurons. *Epilepsia* **2017**, *58*, e157–e161. [CrossRef]
123. Novartis Pharmaceuticals Corporation. Tegretol® (Carbamazepine). Available online: https://www.accessdata.fda.gov/drugsatfda_docs/label/2009/016608s101,018281s048lbl.pdf (accessed on 1 November 2020).
124. Chung, W.-H.; Hung, S.-I.; Hong, H.-S.; Hsih, M.-S.; Yang, L.-C.; Ho, H.-C.; Wu, J.-Y.; Chen, Y.-T. A marker for Stevens-Johnson syndrome. *Nature* **2004**, *428*, 486. [CrossRef]
125. Lundbeck. ONFI® (Clobazam). Available online: https://www.accessdata.fda.gov/drugsatfda_docs/label/2016/203993s005lbl.pdf (accessed on 1 November 2020).
126. Nakamura, F.; Suzuki, S.; Nishimura, S.; Yagi, K.; Seino, M. Effects of clobazam and its active metabolite on GABA-activated currents in rat cerebral neurons in culture. *Epilepsia* **1996**, *37*, 728–735. [CrossRef] [PubMed]
127. Kosaki, K.; Tamura, K.; Sato, R.; Samejima, H.; Tanigawara, Y.; Takahashi, T. A major influence of CYP2C19 genotype on the steady-state concentration of N-desmethylclobazam. *Brain Dev.* **2004**, *26*, 530–534. [CrossRef] [PubMed]
128. Seo, T.; Nagata, R.; Ishitsu, T.; Murata, T.; Takaishi, C.; Hori, M.; Nakagawa, K. Impact of CYP2C19 polymorphisms on the efficacy of clobazam therapy. *Pharmacogenomics* **2008**, *9*. [CrossRef]
129. Pharmacogene Variation Consortium. CYP2C19 Allele Nomenclature. Available online: https://www.pharmvar.org/gene/CYP2C19 (accessed on 1 November 2020).
130. Huddart, R.; Leeder, J.S.; Altman, R.B.; Klein, T.E. PharmGKB summary: Clobazam pathway, pharmacokinetics. *Pharm. Genom.* **2018**, *28*, 110. [CrossRef]
131. Roche. VALIUM (Diazepam). Available online: https://www.accessdata.fda.gov/drugsatfda_docs/label/2016/013263s094lbl.pdf (accessed on 1 November 2020).
132. Vossler, D.G.; Weingarten, M.; Gidal, B.E.; Committee, A.E.S.T. Summary of antiepileptic drugs available in the United States of America. *Epilepsy Curr.* **2018**, *18*, 1–26. [CrossRef]
133. VIMPAT® (Lacosamide). Available online: https://www.accessdata.fda.gov/drugsatfda_docs/label/2018/022253s042lbl.pdf (accessed on 1 November 2020).
134. Errington, A.C.; Stöhr, T.; Heers, C.; Lees, G. The investigational anticonvulsant lacosamide selectively enhances slow inactivation of voltage-gated sodium channels. *Mol. Pharmacol.* **2008**, *73*, 157–169. [CrossRef]
135. Abou-Khalil, B.W. Oxcarbazepine and carbamazepine: Expected and unexpected differences and similarities. *Epilepsy Curr.* **2007**, *7*, 74–76. [CrossRef]
136. Susan, M.; Faulds, D. Oxcarbazepine, a revidw of its pharmacology and the rapeutic potential in epilepsy, trigeminal neuralgia and affectire disorders. *Drugs* **1992**, *43*, 873–888.
137. Grant, S.M.; Faulds, D. Oxcarbazepine. *Drugs* **1992**, *43*, 873–888. [CrossRef] [PubMed]

138. Novartis Pharmaceuticals Corporation. TRILEPTAL® (Oxcarbazepine). Available online: https://www.accessdata.fda.gov/drugsatfda_docs/label/2017/021014s036lbl.pdf (accessed on 1 November 2020).
139. Pfizer Inc. DILANTIN® (Phenytoin Sodium). Available online: https://www.accessdata.fda.gov/drugsatfda_docs/label/2017/084349s080lbl.pdf (accessed on 1 November 2020).
140. Sutrisna, E. Personalized medicine phenytoin therapy. *J. Pharm. Biomed. Sci.* **2017**, *7*, 3–5. [CrossRef]
141. AbbVie Inc. DEPAKENE (Valproic Acid). Available online: https://www.accessdata.fda.gov/drugsatfda_docs/label/2016/018081s065_018082s048lbl.pdf (accessed on 1 November 2020).
142. Zhu, M.-M.; Li, H.-L.; Shi, L.-H.; Chen, X.-P.; Luo, J.; Zhang, Z.-L. The pharmacogenomics of valproic acid. *J. Hum. Genet.* **2017**, *62*, 1009–1014. [CrossRef] [PubMed]
143. Weinshilboum, R.; Wang, L. Pharmacogenomics: Bench to bedside. *Nat. Rev. Drug Discov.* **2004**, *3*, 739–748. [CrossRef] [PubMed]
144. Lazaridis, K.N.; Mcallister, T.M.; Babovic-Vuksanovic, D.; Beck, S.A.; Borad, M.J.; Bryce, A.H.; Chanan-Khan, A.A.; Ferber, M.J.; Fonseca, R.; Johnson, K.J.; et al. Implementing individualized medicine into the medical practice. *Am. J. Med. Genet. Part C Semin. Med. Genet.* **2014**, *166C*, 15–23. [CrossRef] [PubMed]
145. Evans, W.E.; Relling, M.V. Moving towards individualized medicine with pharmacogenomics. *Nature* **2004**, *429*, 464–468. [CrossRef]
146. Collins, F.S.; Varmus, H. A new initiative on precision medicine. *N. Engl. J. Med.* **2015**, *372*, 793–795. [CrossRef]
147. Iniesta, R.; Stahl, D.; McGuffin, P. Machine learning, statistical learning and the future of biological research in psychiatry. *Psychol. Med.* **2016**, *46*, 2455–2465. [CrossRef]
148. Lane, H.-Y.; Tsai, G.E.; Lin, E. Assessing gene-gene interactions in pharmacogenomics. *Mol. Diagn. Ther.* **2012**, *16*, 15–27. [CrossRef]
149. Lin, E.; Hwang, Y.; Liang, K.-H.; Chen, E.Y. Pattern-recognition techniques with haplotype analysis in pharmacogenomics. *Pharmacogenomics* **2007**, *8*. [CrossRef]
150. Russell, S.J.; Norvig, P. *Artificial Intelligence: A Modern Approach. Malaysia*; Pearson Education Limited: London, UK, 2016.
151. Bzdok, D.; Meyer-Lindenberg, A. Machine learning for precision psychiatry: Opportunities and challenges. *Biol. Psychiatry Cogn. Neurosci. Neuroimaging* **2018**, *3*, 223–230. [CrossRef]
152. Fernandes, B.S.; Williams, L.M.; Steiner, J.; Leboyer, M.; Carvalho, A.F.; Berk, M. The new field of "precision psychiatry". *BMC Med.* **2017**, *15*, 1–7. [CrossRef]
153. Lin, E.; Lin, C.-H.; Lane, H.-Y. Precision psychiatry applications with pharmacogenomics: Artificial intelligence and machine learning approaches. *Int. J. Mol. Sci.* **2020**, *21*, 969. [CrossRef] [PubMed]
154. Miotto, R.; Li, L.; Kidd, B.A.; Dudley, J.T. Deep patient: An unsupervised representation to predict the future of patients from the electronic health records. *Sci. Rep.* **2016**, *6*, 1–10. [CrossRef] [PubMed]

4

MicroRNAs Mediated Regulation of Expression of Nucleoside Analog Pathway Genes in Acute Myeloid Leukemia

Neha S. Bhise [1,2], Abdelrahman H. Elsayed [1], Xueyuan Cao [3], Stanley Pounds [4] and Jatinder K. Lamba [1,*]

1 Department of Pharmacotherapy and Translational Research, Center for Pharmacogenomics, University of Florida, Gainesville, FL 32610, USA; Neha.bhise@gmail.com (N.S.B.); aelsayed@ufl.edu (A.H.E.)

2 Department of Experimental and Clinical Pharmacology, University of Minnesota, Minneapolis, MN 55455, USA

3 Department of Acute and Tertiary Care, University of Tennessee Health Science Center, Memphis, TN 38163, USA; xcao12@uthsc.edu

4 Department of Biostatistics, St. Jude Children's Research Hospital, Memphis, TN 38105, USA; stanley.pounds@stjude.org

* Correspondence: jlamba@cop.ufl.edu

Abstract: Nucleoside analog, cytarabine (ara-C) is the mainstay of acute myeloid leukemia (AML) chemotherapy. Cytarabine and other nucleoside analogs require activation to the triphosphate form (ara-CTP). Intracellular ara-CTP levels demonstrate significant inter-patient variation and have been related to therapeutic response in AML patients. Inter-patient variation in expression levels of drug transporters or enzymes involved in the activation or inactivation of cytarabine and other analogs is a prime mechanism contributing to development of drug resistance. Since microRNAs (miRNAs) are known to regulate gene-expression, the aim of this study was to identify miRNAs involved in regulation of messenger RNA expression levels of cytarabine pathway genes. We evaluated miRNA and gene-expression levels of cytarabine metabolic pathway genes in 8 AML cell lines and The Cancer Genome Atlas (TCGA) data base. Using correlation analysis and functional validation experiments, our data demonstrates that miR-34a-5p and miR-24-3p regulate DCK, an enzyme involved in activation of cytarabine and DCTD, an enzyme involved in metabolic inactivation of cytarabine expression, respectively. Further our results from gel shift assays confirmed binding of these mRNA-miRNA pairs. Our results show miRNA mediated regulation of gene expression levels of nucleoside metabolic pathway genes can impact interindividual variation in expression levels which in turn may influence treatment outcomes.

Keywords: nucleoside analogs; microRNAs; gene expression; drug resistance; AML

1. Introduction

Nucleoside analogs (NA) are a class of chemotherapeutic agents that structurally resemble the endogenous purine or pyrimidine nucleosides. These therapeutic agents mimic the endogenous nucleosides with respect to their uptake and metabolism and are incorporated into the newly synthesized DNA leading to inhibition of DNA synthesis and chain termination. Some of the nucleoside analogs also inhibit or block the enzymes that are required for the synthesis of purine or pyrimidine nucleotides and RNA synthesis, leading to the activation of the caspase cascade and cell death. The nucleoside analogs are extensively used for the treatment of both hematological malignancies and solid tumors.

The pyrimidine nucleoside analog, cytarabine, is one of the most widely used chemotherapeutic drugs for the treatment of acute myeloid leukemia (AML).

One of the major obstacles in the treatment of AML is development of resistance to nucleoside analogs. There is a growing need to understand the mechanisms that lead to development of resistance to these nucleoside analogs in order to help identify strategies that would effectively treat patients with relapsing or refractory diseases. One of the primary mechanisms of resistance to nucleoside analogs is insufficient intracellular concentration of the active triphosphate metabolite. This insufficient triphosphate levels could be due to inefficient cellular uptake of the drug, reduced levels of the activating enzyme, increased levels of inactivating enzymes and/or due to increased levels of endogenous deoxynucleotide (dNTP) pools [1–4]. Resistance could also develop due to inability to achieve sufficient alterations in the DNA strands or the dNTP pools, either due to altered interaction with DNA polymerases or by a lack of inhibition of ribonucleotide reductases, or due to inadequate p53 exonuclease activity. Since the expression and activity of drug transporters and metabolizing enzymes in the activation pathway of nucleoside analogs plays an important role in development of resistance to the NAs, it is essential to understand the factors influencing the expression and activity of these proteins.

MicroRNAs (miRNAs) are a group of novel gene regulators, which have been recently recognized to play an important role in cancers due to their tumor suppressive and oncogenic functions [5]. MiRNAs are known to regulate the expression of the target genes by binding to the specific sequence mainly on the 3′ untranslated region on the genes. Role of miRNAs in regulating the expression of various drug-metabolizing enzymes like cytochrome P450 3A4 (CYP3A4) etc., drug transporters like BCRP and various drug targets [6–8] have been established. However, there have not been any studies that have comprehensively evaluated the effect of miRNAs on the important genes involved in the transport, activation and inactivation of nucleoside analogs. Hence, the aim of this study was to assess the effect of miRNAs on the expression of nucleoside analog pharmacokinetic (PK) and pharmacodynamic (PD) pathway genes and in turn assessing their potential impact on resistance to nucleoside analogs.

2. Materials and Methods

2.1. Cell culture and Reagents

The AML cell lines HL-60, MV-4-11, Kasumi-1, THP-1, AML-193 and KG-1 cell lines were obtained from American Type Culture Collection (ATCC) (Manassas, VA, USA), while MOLM-16 and ME-1 cell lines were obtained from DSMZ (Braunschweig, Germany). Kasumi-1, ME-1 and MOLM-16 cell lines were cultured in Roswell Park Memorial Institute (RMPI)-1640 medium supplemented with 20% fetal bovine serum (FBS), THP-1 cell line was cultured in RPMI-1640 medium supplemented with 10% FBS, HL-60 and KG-1 cell lines were cultured in IMDM medium supplemented with 20% FBS, while AML-193 cell lines was cultured in IMDM medium supplemented with 5% FBS, 0.005 mg/mL insulin, 0.005 mg/mL transferrin and 5 ng/mL granulocyte/macrophage colony stimulating factor (GM-CSF). All the cell lines were maintained in a 37 °C humidified incubator with 5% CO_2. The cells were passaged every two to three days in order to maintain them in logarithmic growth phase.

2.2. RNA Isolation

Total RNA was isolated from the AML cell pellets using RNeasy Plus Mini Kit (Qiagen, Valencia, CA, USA) according to the manufacturer's protocol and stored in −80 °C until further analysis. The RNA quality and concentration were measured using NanoDrop 2000 UV-Vis spectrophotometer (Thermo Scientific, Wilmington, DE, USA). The ratio of absorbance at 260 nm and 280 nm was used to assess RNA sample purity and A260/A280 ratio of 1.8–2.1 was considered to be indicative of highly purified RNA. RNA was normalized to 0.2 µg/µL with nuclease-free water before being used for performing reverse transcription reactions, as recommended by the manufacturer. The total RNA was reverse transcribed to complementary DNA (cDNA) using High Capacity cDNA Reverse Transcription Kit (Applied Biosystems, Foster City, CA, USA) according to manufacturer's protocol.

2.3. Gene Expression Analysis

The expression of nucleoside analog genes was determined using the TaqMan® Low Density Array (TLDA) cards (Applied Biosystems). Each TLDA card was custom designed with pre-loaded gene expression assays for measuring the messenger RNA (mRNA) expression of selected nucleoside analog metabolic pathway genes- ($n = 14$) deoxycytidine kinase (*DCK*), cytidine deaminase (*CDA*), solute carrier family 29, member 1 (*SLC29A1*), solute carrier family 28, member 1 (SLC28A1), solute carrier family 28, member 3 (SLC28A3), deoxycytidylate deaminase (*DCTD*), 5′-nucleotidase, cytosolic II (*NT5C2*), 5′-nucleotidase cytosolic III (*NT5C3*), cytidine 5′-triphosphate synthase (CTPS), cytidine monophosphate kinase (*CMPK*), nucleoside diphosphate kinase 1 (*NME1*), ribonucleotide reductase M1 (*RRM1*), ribonucleotide reductase M2 (*RRM2*), ribonucleotide reductase M2B (*RRM2B*). Each TLDA card consists of eight separate loading ports that fill into 48 separate wells, for a total of 384 wells per card. Thus, each card could analyze the expression of 24 different genes for eight different samples in duplicates. Each cDNA sample was added to equal volume of 2X TaqMan Universal PCR Master Mix (Thermo Scientific) and 100 µL of the sample-specific PCR mix was added to the fill reservoir on the TLDA card. The card was centrifuged twice for one minute at 1200 rpm to distribute the sample-specific PCR reaction mix to the reaction wells. The card was sealed using the TaqMan Array Micro Fluidic Card Sealer (Thermo Scientific) and placed on microfluidic card thermal cycling block of Applied Biosystems 7900HT Fast Real-time PCR System (Applied Biosystems). Thermal cycling conditions were as follows: 2 min at 50 °C, 10 min at 94.5 °C, 30 s at 97 °C, 1 min at 59.7 °C for 40 cycles. The target mRNA expression levels were normalized to GAPDH and the expression values of nucleoside analogs pathway genes were calculated using $\Delta\Delta C_T$ method [9].

2.4. MicroRNA Expression Analysis

For determination of miRNA expression, total RNA was isolated using mirVana™ miRNA Isolation kit (Life Technologies, Carlsbad, CA, USA) as per the manufacturer's protocol. The RNA quality and concentration were measured using NanoDrop 2000 UV-Vis spectrophotometer (Thermo Scientific). A total of 100 ng of purified total RNA was used for nCounter miRNA sample preparation reactions according to manufacturer's instructions and was assayed for determination of 800 human miRNA expression using the nCounter Human v2 miRNA Expression Assay kit (Nanostring Technologies, Seattle, WA, USA). Preparation of small RNA samples involved multiplexed ligation of specific tags (miRtags) to the target miRNAs that provide unique identification for each miRNA species. After ligation, the detection was done by hybridization to microRNA: tag specific nCounter capture and barcoded reporter probes. Data collection was carried out using the nCounter Digital Analyzer (Nanostring Technologies) at The University of Minnesota Genomics Center, following manufacturer's instructions to count individual fluorescent barcodes and quantify the target miRNA molecules present in each sample. MiRNA expression data normalization was performed using the nSolver™ Analysis Software (Nanostring Technologies) according to the manufacturer's instructions. In particular, initially the data was normalized using the expression of the top 100 code sets. Further, to account for the background correction, mean of negative controls plus two-standard deviation (SD) method was used. In order to avoid using the miRNAs with a very low expression, we further filtered out the miRNAs with expression counts < 30 (2 times the mean $\pm$ 2 SD of negative control value), in order to account for the background noise. Total 412 miRNAs with expression counts > 30 were included for further analysis.

2.5. Acute Myeloid Leukemia Patient Sample Data from The Cancer Genome Atlas

The miRNA expression and mRNA expression of the nucleoside analog pathway genes in AML patients was extracted from The Cancer Genome Atlas (TCGA) Data Portal (cancergenome.nih.gov) [10].

Out of the 200 AML patients in TCGA database, 197 patients had gene expression profiling data available and 187 patients had miRNA expression data available. 186 patients had both gene expression and miRNA expression data available.

2.6. Electrophoretic Mobility Shift Assays

The functional validation for binding efficiencies between miRNAs and mRNAs was performed using the electrophoretic mobility shift assays (EMSAs). The binding free energy between the respective mRNA and miRNA pair was predicted using the RNAhybrid software. The miRNA oligonucleotides were labeled with cy5™ dye on their 5′ ends. The 2′ O-methyl-modified mRNA oligonucleotides were labeled with IRDye®800 (LI-COR Biosciences, Lincoln, NE, USA) dye on their 5′ ends. The labeled oligonucleotides were synthesized by Integrated DNA Technologies (Coralville, IA, USA). RNA EMSA experiment was performed using the LightShift Chemiluminescent RNA EMSA Kit (Thermo Scientific) according to the manufacturer's protocol. The mRNA oligonucleotide was heated for 10 min at 80 °C and then placed on ice in order to relax the secondary structures. In each 20 μL binding reaction, 200 nM miRNA oligonucleotide and/or mRNA oligonucleotide were mixed with RNA EMSA binding buffer and incubated at 25 °C for 25 min. The reaction mixtures were separated on a 12% polyacrylamide gel by electrophoresis at 4 °C. The binding reactions were transferred onto nylon membrane and the resulting mobility shifts were imaged using and Odyssey CLx Infrared System (LI-COR Biosciences).

2.7. Bioinformatic Analysis

Prediction of miRNA binding sites was performed using multiple prediction programs, which use different criteria for prediction of binding sites: TargetScan (www.targetscan.org), miRanda (www.microRNA.org), PICTAR (pictar.mdc-berlin.de), miRWalk (www.umm.uni-heidelberg.de/apps/zmf/mirwalk). Binding free energy calculations were performed using RNAhybrid software [11]. The 3′UTR (3′ untranslated region) sequence of mRNA was obtained from the UCSC Genome browser (https://genome.ucsc.edu/) and miRNA sequence was obtained from miRBase software (http://www.mirbase.org/).

2.8. Statistical Analysis

The nonparametric Spearman correlation was used to measure the correlation of mRNA expression with miRNA expression. Statistical significance was determined when p-value was < 0.01.

3. Results

3.1. Effect of Micro RNA on the Expression of Nucleoside Analog Pathway Genes in Acute Myeloid Leukemia Cell Lines

We determined expression of 800 miRNAs and 13 genes involved in PK/PD pathway of nucleoside analogs (Figure 1) in cytogenetically different AML cell lines ($n = 8$). In order to identify the miRNAs associated with the expression of nucleoside analog pathway genes, we correlated the miRNA expression and mRNA expression using the spearman correlation analysis. Table 1 lists the negative correlations of nucleoside analog pathway genes and respective miRNAs at p <0.01. We further used CyTargetLinker software [12] to establish the network of miRNAs correlated with the respective PK/PD pathway genes of the nucleoside analogs. Figure 2 shows the miRNA-mRNA pairs identified by CyTargetLinker.

The expression of *DCK* (the rate-limiting enzyme in the nucleoside analog pathway) correlated with the expression of miR-34a-5p expression (spearman $r = -0.88$; p-value < 0.01) and miR-96-5p expression (spearman $r = -0.91$; p-value < 0.01). The expression of deactivating enzyme *DCTD* was found to be correlated with miR-24-3p expression (spearman $r = -0.93$; p-value < 0.01). Interestingly, in our previous study, we identified that expression of miRNA miR-24-3p was correlated with cytarabine-induced cell cytotoxicity (spearman $r = -0.81$, p-value < 0.05) [13] which is in agreement with the current observation. The expression of *CMPK*, a kinase responsible for phosphorylation of the monophosphate form of nucleoside analog was negatively correlated with the expression of miR-1301, miR-1323, miR-320e, miR-381, miR-507, miR-584-5p, miR-605, miR-762, miR-769-3p, miR-891a (all p-values < 0.01). RRM2 expression was found to be negatively associated with the expression of miR-151a-3p (p-value < 0.01). Figure 3 shows correlation plots between *DCTD*-miR-24, *DCK*-miR34 and *NT5C3*-miR149 pairs.

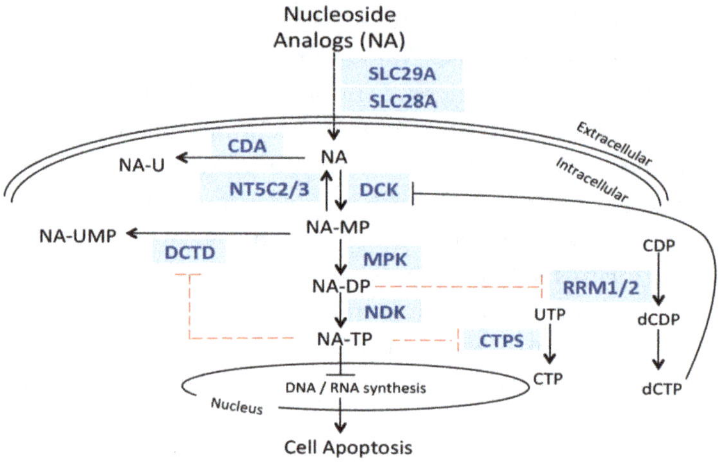

Figure 1. Disposition pathway of nucleoside analogs, cytarabine and clofarabine. DCTD: Deoxycytidylate deaminase, DCK: Deoxycytidine kinase, CDA: Cytidine deaminase, NT5C2/3: 5′-Nucleotidase, cytoplasmic, CTPS: CTP synthase, RRM1/2: Ribonucleotide reductase, SLC29A: Solute carrier family 29, SLC28A: Solute carrier family 28, MPK: Monophosphate kinase, NDK: Nucleoside diphosphate kinase

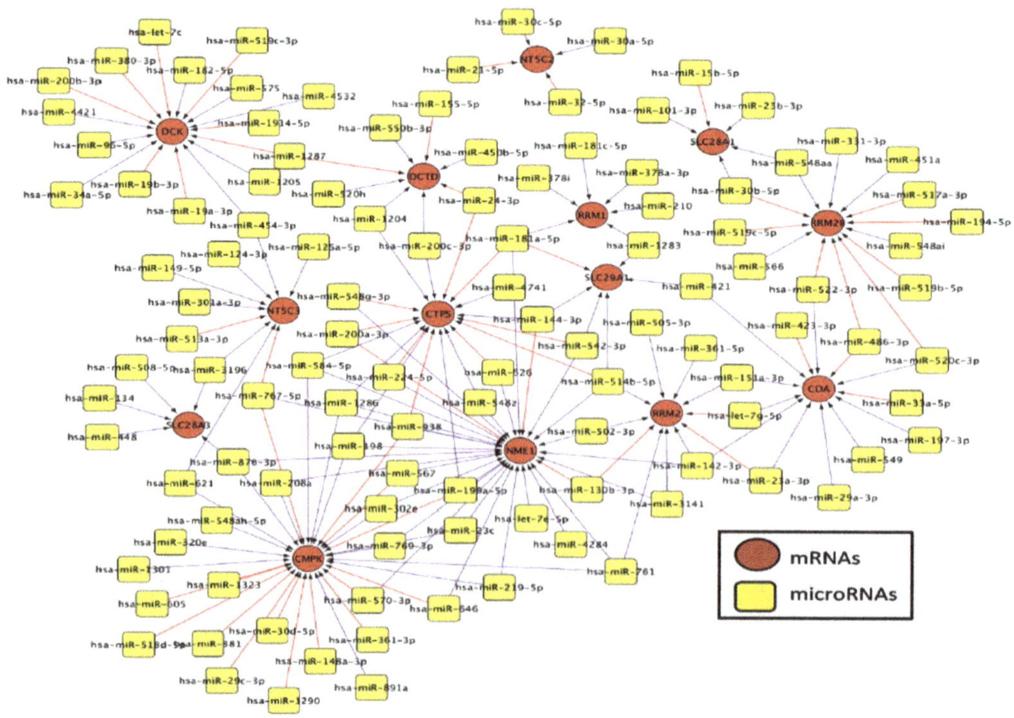

Figure 2. MicroRNA-mRNA network constructed using CyTargetLinker [12]. MiRNAs associated with the nucleoside analog metabolic pathway genes are shown in yellow and the mRNAs are depicted in red. Blue lines indicated positive and red indicated negative associations.

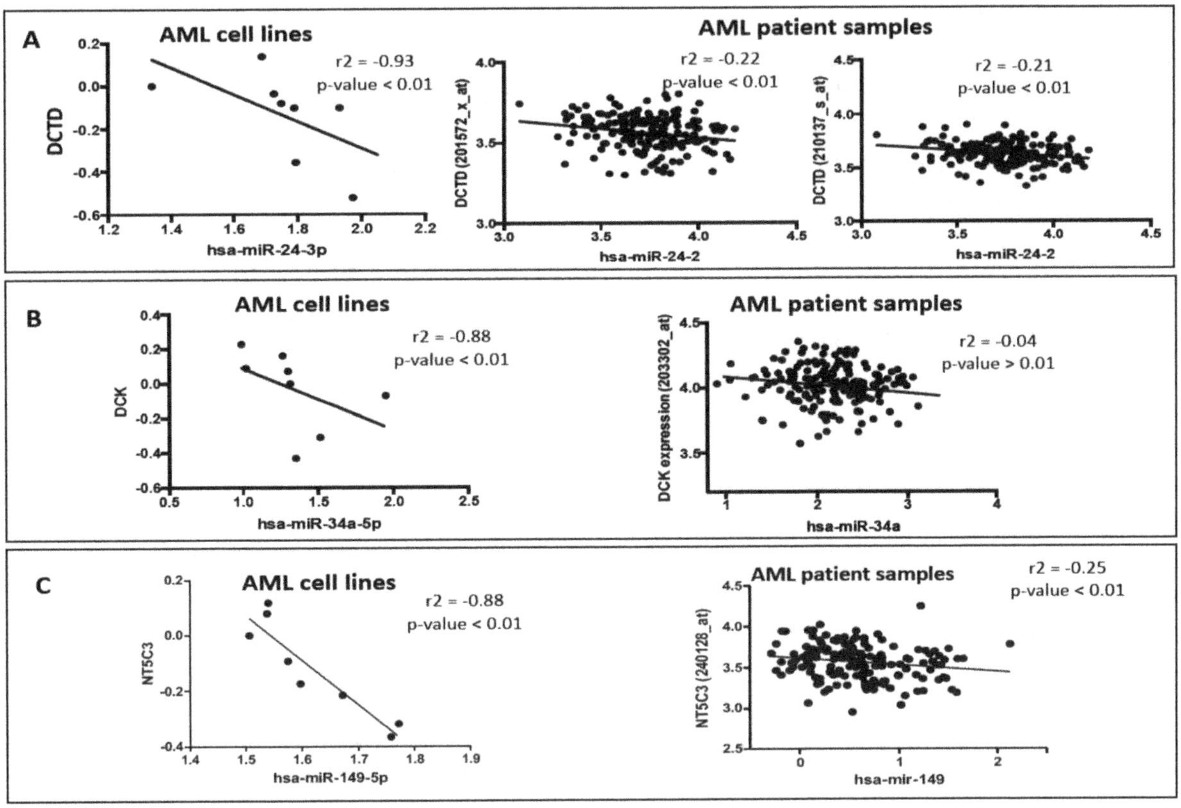

Figure 3. Correlation of miRNAs with nucleoside analog pathway gene expression in acute myeloid leukemia (AML) cell lines and patient samples from The Cancer Genome Atlas (TCGA) database. (**A**) Correlation between DCTD and hsa-miR-24a-3p. (**B**) Correlation between DCK and hsa-miR-34a-5p. (**C**) Correlation between NT5C3 and hsa-miR-149.

3.2. Bioinformatic Prediction of Binding of Micro RNAs and Messenger RNAs

MiRNAs are known to guide the RNA-induced silencing complex (RISC) to the specific sequence (usually in located in the 3′UTR) on the target mRNA. Using various bioinformatic prediction programs (TargetScan, miRanda, PICTAR, miRWalk) we determined if the miRNAs that were correlated with gene expression had binding sites on 3′-UTR of target genes. MiRNAs miR-1323, miR-30d-5p, miR-381, and miR-605 were predicted to have binding sites on *CMPK* gene, while miRNA miR-24-3p was found to have binding site on *DCTD* by multiple prediction programs. Supplementary Figure S1 shows comparisons of different miRNA prediction programs for genes involved in nucleoside analog pathways.

3.3. Effect of Micro RNAs on the Expression of Nucleoside Analog Pathway Genes in Acute Myeloid Leukemia Patients

In order to validate the significant correlations between miRNAs and mRNAs identified in AML cell lines, we evaluated the correlation between miRNA expression and nucleoside analog pathway gene expression in AML patient samples from TCGA database (n = 186). We extracted the miRNA expression data and nucleoside analog pathway gene expression data for AML patients from TCGA database and performed spearman correlation to identify the significant mRNA-miRNA pairs. Consistent with results from AML cell lines miR-24-3p was inversely correlated with the expression of both the probes for *DCTD* in AML patient samples ($r = -0.22$; p-value < 0.01 and $r = -0.21$; p-value < 0.01, Figure 3A). *DCK*-mir-34a pair unfortunately did not show significant association within the TCGA data-set. miR-149 was significantly correlated with expression of *NT5C3* in AML patients ($r = -0.25$; p-value < 0.01, Figure 3C).

Validation of Binding Efficiencies between Messenger RNAs and Micro RNAs

MiRNAs are known to bind to the specific seed sequence on the 3'UTR of the mRNAs, thereby regulating the expression of their target genes. In order to validate the binding between the mRNA-miRNAs identified from the in vitro studies and in AML patient samples, we performed RNA EMSA assays. We validated the interaction between *DCTD* and miR-24, since we identified this mRNA-miRNA pair to be significantly inversely correlated in both AML cell line and AML patient samples. In addition, various prediction databases predicted miRNA miR-24 to have binding site on the 3'UTR of *DCTD* mRNA. In silico analysis predicted miR-24-3p and miR-34a-5p might form complexes with target sequences in the 3'UTR of *DCTD* and *DCK* respectively with minimum free energies of binding of −27.2 kcal/mol for *DCTD* and miR-24-3p (Figure 4A and Table 1) and -25.6 kcal/mol for *DCK* and miR-34a-5p (Figure 5A and Table 1). The RNA EMSA results for IRD-800®-labeled *DCTD* and Cy-5-labeled miR-24-3p show miR-24a-3p was able to bind to its target sequence on *DCTD* 3'UTR (Figure 4B, lane 3) as seen by the band shift. The thermodynamic stability of this complex correlated with binding observed in the RNA EMSA assays. In addition, we found that mRNA-miRNA complex formed by *DCTD* and miR-24a-3p could be eliminated by adding excess unlabeled hsa-miR-24a-3p probe (Figure 4B, lane 4), but not by adding excess unlabeled non-specific probe (Figure 4B, lane 6). Adding excess unlabeled mRNA probe resulted in binding of all the labeled miRNA giving a greater intensity signal (Figure 4B, lane 5).

Similar to the interaction observed between *DCTD* and miR-24a-3p, we observed that miR-34a-5p binds to *DCK* 3'UTR as seen by shift in the band (Figure 5B, lane 3) and this interaction was eliminated by addition of unlabeled probe (Figure 5B, lane 4). Since the minimum free energy of binding for *NT5C3*- miR-149 pair was not strong (Table 1), we did not pursue EMSA assays for this pair.

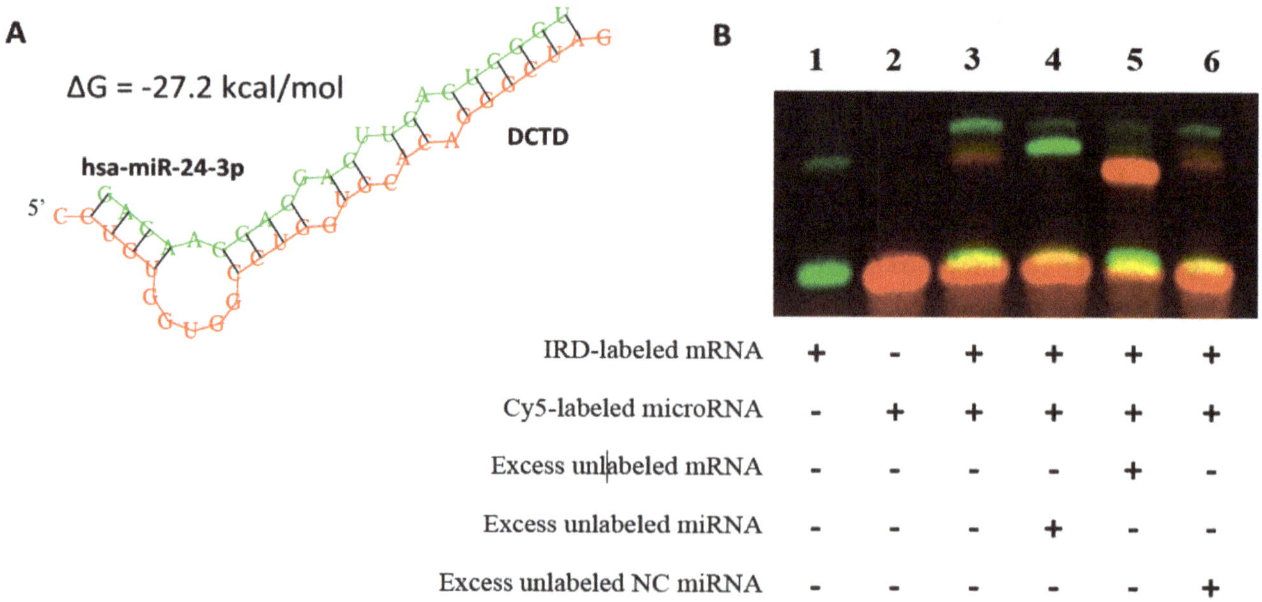

Figure 4. Validation of binding interaction between DCTD mRNA and has-miR-24-3p by RNA electrophoretic mobility shift assays (EMSAs). RNA EMSA with cy5-labeled has-miR-24-3p oligonucleotide and 2'-O-methyl modified and IRD-800 labeled DCTC mRNA oligonucleotide. Lanes 1 and 2 show the mobility of the labeled mRNA or miRNA oligonucleotide. Lane 3 shows the mobility of the labeled has-miR-24-3p oligonucleotide with *DCTD* mRNA oligonucleotide. Lanes 4 and 6 show the mobility of labeled *DCTD* mRNA oligonucleotide in presence of unlabeled excess specific competitor (has-miR-24-3p) ad excess unlabeled non-specific competitor (NC).

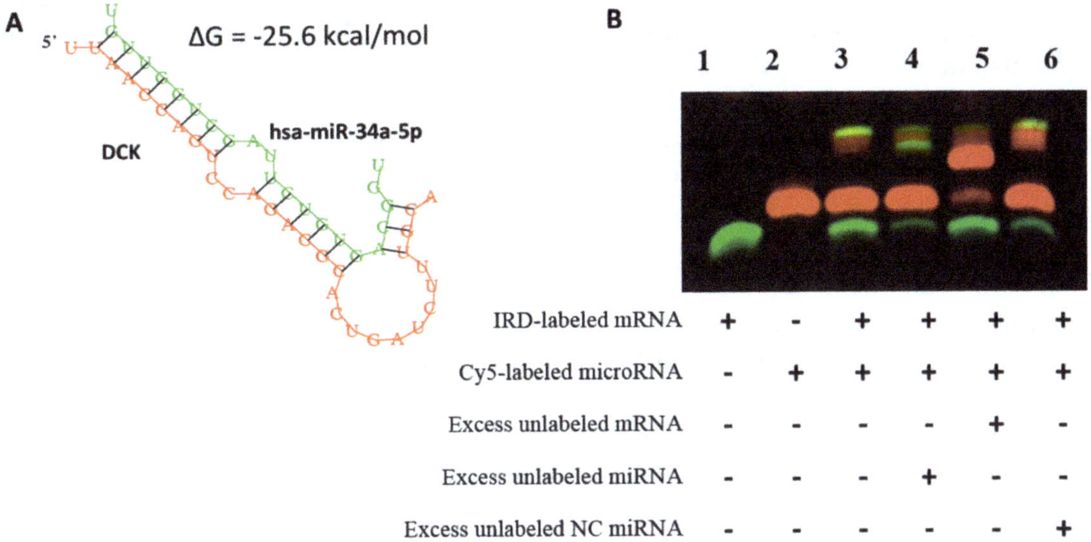

Figure 5. Validation of binding interactions between *DCK* and mRNA and has-miR-34a-5p by RNA EMSAs. RNA EMSA with cys5-labeled has-miR-34a-5p oligonucleotide and 2′-O-methyl modified and IRD-800 labeled DCK mRNA oligonucleotide. Lanes 1 and 2 show the mobility of the labeled mRNA or miRNA oligonucleotide. Lane 3 shows the mobility of the labeled has-miR-34a-5p oligonucleotide with DCK mRNA oligonucleotide. Lanes 4 and 6 show the mobility of labeled DCK mRNA oligonucleotide in presence of unlabeled excess specific competitor (has-miR-34a-5p) and excess unlabeled non-specific competitor (NC).

Table 1. MiRNAs with significant negative association (as reflected by *r* value) with nucleoside analog pathway genes in AML Cell lines.

Pathway Genes	MiRNAs	Spearman *r*	*p* Value	Minimum Free Energy (mfe) mRNA-miRNA Pair (kcal/mol)
DCTD	hsa-miR-24-3p	−0.9341	0.0011	−27.2
DCK	hsa-miR-96-5p	−0.9048	0.0046	−25.6
DCK	hsa-miR-34a-5p	−0.881	0.0072	−24.3
NT5C3	hsa-miR-149-5p	−0.881	0.0072	−21.4
RRM2	hsa-miR-151a-3p	−0.9524	0.0011	−26.4
RRM2B	hsa-miR-194-5p	−0.881	0.0072	−21.6
CMPK	hsa-miR-1301	−0.9762	0.0004	−23.6
CMPK	hsa-miR-320e	−0.9524	0.0011	−20.1
CMPK	hsa-miR-1323	−0.9286	0.0022	−22.3
CMPK	hsa-miR-584-5p	−0.9286	0.0022	−23.7
CMPK	hsa-miR-381	−0.881	0.0072	−25.8
CMPK	hsa-miR-507	−0.881	0.0072	−19.1
CMPK	hsa-miR-605	−0.881	0.0072	−23.1
CMPK	hsa-miR-762	−0.881	0.0072	−29.2
CMPK	hsa-miR-769-3p	−0.881	0.0072	−27.6
CMPK	hsa-miR-891a	−0.881	0.0072	−22.9
NME1	hsa-miR-514b-5p	−0.9286	0.0022	−22
NME1	hsa-miR-542-3p	−0.9286	0.0022	−19.3
NME1	hsa-miR-570-3p	−0.9048	0.0046	−22.2
NME1	hsa-miR-646	−0.9048	0.0046	−25.9
NME1	hsa-miR-224-5p	−0.881	0.0072	−17.9
NME1	hsa-miR-761	−0.881	0.0072	−24.3
NME1	hsa-miR-767-5p	−0.881	0.0072	−28.8
SLC28A1	hsa-miR-548aa	−0.9643	0.0028	−16.3
SLC28A3	hsa-miR-448	−0.9643	0.0028	−23.8

We further evaluated the association of the in vitro chemosensitivity of ara-C (defined previously Bhise et al, 2015 [13] with the three top miRNAs in the AML cell lines. As shown in Supplementary Figure S2. consistent with our results of miR-24-*DCTD* pair, we observed cell lines that were sensitive to ara-C has significantly higher levels of miR-24 as compared to cell lines that are resistant to ara-C ($p = 0.03$). These results suggest that high miR-24 in ara-C sensitive cell lines might be resulting in lowering *DCTD* levels and given that *DCTD* is involved in inactivation of ara-C, its low levels will result in better response.

4. Discussion

Nucleoside analogs are synthetic analogs of endogenous nucleosides that largely used for the treatment of hematological malignancies and solid tumors. Cytarabine, a pyrimidine nucleoside analog is the backbone of AML chemotherapy, while clofarabine is a second-generation purine nucleoside analog that is currently being investigated for treatment of AML in various clinical trials. Both cytarabine and clofarabine require active transport into the cell by nucleoside transporters, followed by activation by various kinases to form active di- and tri-phosphate metabolites that are incorporated in growing DNA strand and/or inhibit various enzymes involved in synthesis of endogenous nucleotides (Figure 1). However, despite being the backbone of treatment regimen used in AML patients, there is variability in response to cytarabine and other nucleoside analogs. In our previous study, we have demonstrated that miRNA expression is predictive of response to cytarabine therapy in AML patients and is also significantly associated with in vitro chemosensitivity of cytarabine in AML cell lines [13]. Recent studies are expanding on therapeutic relevance of miRNAs in AML. Recent review article by Wallace et al, 2017, have summarized the miRNAs that are deregulated in AML and thus hold potential as AML biomarkers. Further, mimics for miR-22, miR29b and miR-181 and antagomiRs for miR-21/miR-196b and miR-126 are currently under investigation for their therapeutic potential in AML [14]. However, given that cytarabine a nucleoside analog is the mainstay of AML chemotherapy for decades, in the current study, we wanted to determine if miRNA mediated regulation of expression of the transporters, activating and inactivating genes involved in the metabolic pathway of nucleoside analogs, could contribute to development of resistance to nucleoside analogs in AML patients. We hypothesized that miRNAs could bind to the 3′UTR of the mRNAs of nucleoside analog metabolic pathway genes, thereby altering their expression, which in turn would result in lower intracellular levels of active nucleoside analog triphosphate, resulting in chemo-resistance.

In our current study, DCK expression was negatively correlated with the expression of hsa-miR-34a-5p and hsa-miR-96-5p in AML cell lines (p-value < 0.01). DCK is a rate-limiting enzyme that is involved in activation of cytarabine and clofarabine. Studies have reported that decreased or complete loss of DCK activity results in cellular resistance to cytarabine [15–17]. Also, *DCK* mRNA expression has been shown to be positively associated with AML patient outcome, AML patients with higher *DCK* mRNA expression demonstrated longer event-free survival than those with lower *DCK* mRNA expression [18]. Using EMSA, we were able to show that hsa-miR-34a-5p by binding to the 3′-UTR regulates expression of *DCK*. MiRNA hsa-miR-34a has been extensively studied in various cancers [19–23] and it has been shown to play an important role as a tumor suppressor by targeting various genes. However, the effect of miR-34a on *DCK* expression has not yet been studied. Identification of this additional regulatory mechanism for an important enzyme in the activation of nucleoside analogs could help in better prediction of chemosensitivity of these drugs. Unfortunately, we did not observe any significant correlation between *DCK* mRNA and miR-34a levels in TCGA dataset.

We also identified hsa-miR-24-3p to be negatively correlated with the expression of *DCTD* in both AML cell lines and in AML patient samples (p-value < 0.01). In addition, multiple bioinformatic prediction programs identified a binding site for hsa-miR-24-3p on the 3′UTR of DCTD. Our

RNA EMSA results confirmed the binding interaction between DCTD and miR-24-3p. DCTD is an enzyme involved in deamination of the monophosphate form of the nucleoside analog, thus inactivating the drug. The levels of DCTD could thus affect the levels of the intracellular active triphosphate metabolites of nucleoside analogs. However, the role of *DCTD* in chemosensitivity of nucleoside analogs is poorly defined. Various studies have demonstrated a significant role of *DCTD* in metabolism of the monophosphate metabolite of the nucleoside analogs in human leukemia cells [24–26]. Sequencing of this gene identified a nonsynonymous SNP affecting the activity of *DCTD* in vitro [27]. Hence, the limited data on the regulation of *DCTD* gene warrants the need to evaluate additional mechanism regulating gene-expression. MiRNA miR-24 is has also been extensively studied in various cancers [28–34] and has been shown to enhance metastasis and invasion. Increased expression of miR-24 has been associated with increased risk of relapse and poor survival in acute lymphoblastic leukemia (ALL) [32]. In addition to miR-24 and hsa-miR-34a-5p, we also identified multiple other miRNAs that correlated with multiple genes in the PK/PD pathway (Table 1). We acknowledge the limitation of use of different platforms of miRNA and mRNA quantification between cell lines and the TCGA data-set which warrant the need for future prospective study to validate our results. Additionally, given that gel-shift assays do not consider interactions with argonaute which can impact thermodynamics of target recognition future in-depth mechanistic validation considering these factors are needed to establish miRNA-mRNA regulatory pairs of significant therapeutic implications in AML.

In summary, we identified several miRNAs, which were significantly associated with the expression of nucleoside analog pathway genes. Identification of these additional mechanisms of regulation would help provide a better understanding of the variability in the expression of these enzymes and transporters and in turn, help in better prediction of therapeutic response in AML patients. While additional functional studies are required to gain mechanistic understanding of these miRNA-mRNA interactions and its effect on the protein levels and activity, this study helps identify candidate miRNAs for further studies.

Supplementary Materials:
Figure S1: Comparison of microRNA prediction programs for predicting binding sites on nucleoside analog pathway genes. Figure S2: A) Eight AML cell lines were treated with varying concentration of ara-C for 48 hrs followed by measuring cell viability using MTT assays using as described previously (Bhise et al, 2015). Area under the survival was calculated using Graphpad Prism and cell lines were classified as sensitive or resistant to ara-C. B) miR24-3p levels were observed to be higher in cell lines sensitive to ara-C as compared to ara-C resistant cell lines.

Author Contributions: J.K.L. and N.S.B. were involved in designing the study; N.S.B., J.K.L., A.H.E., X.C. and S.P. performed statistical analysis. All authors contributed to manuscript writing. All authors read and approved the final manuscript.

References

1. Galmarini, C.M.; Clarke, M.L.; Jordheim, L.; Santos, C.L.; Cros, E.; Mackey, J.R.; Dumontet, C. Resistance to gemcitabine in a human follicular lymphoma cell line is due to partial deletion of the deoxycytidine kinase gene. *BMC Pharmacol.* **2004**, *4*, 8. [CrossRef] [PubMed]
2. Galmarini, C.M.; Thomas, X.; Calvo, F.; Rousselot, P.; Rabilloud, M.; El Jaffari, A.; Cros, E.; Dumontet, C. In vivo mechanisms of resistance to cytarabine in acute myeloid leukaemia. *Br. J. Haematol.* **2002**, *117*, 860–868. [CrossRef] [PubMed]
3. Lotfi, K.; Juliusson, G.; Albertioni, F. Pharmacological basis for cladribine resistance. *Leuk. Lymphoma* **2003**, *44*, 1705–1712. [CrossRef]
4. Mansson, E.; Flordal, E.; Liliemark, J.; Spasokoukotskaja, T.; Elford, H.; Lagercrantz, S.; Eriksson, S.; Albertioni, F. Down-regulation of deoxycytidine kinase in human leukemic cell lines resistant to cladribine and clofarabine and increased ribonucleotide reductase activity contributes to fludarabine resistance. *Biochem. Pharmacol.* **2003**, *65*, 237–247. [CrossRef]

5. Kent, O.A.; Mendell, J.T. A small piece in the cancer puzzle: MicroRNAs as tumor suppressors and oncogenes. *Oncogene* **2006**, *25*, 6188–6196. [CrossRef]
6. Rieger, J.K.; Reutter, S.; Hofmann, U.; Schwab, M.; Zanger, U.M. Inflammation-associated microRNA-130b down-regulates cytochrome P450 activities and directly targets CYP2C9. *Drug Metab. Dispos.* **2015**, *43*, 884–888. [CrossRef]
7. Pan, Y.Z.; Morris, M.E.; Yu, A.M. MicroRNA-328 negatively regulates the expression of breast cancer resistance protein (BCRP/ABCG2) in human cancer cells. *Mol. Pharmacol.* **2009**, *75*, 1374–1379. [CrossRef]
8. Mishra, P.J.; Humeniuk, R.; Mishra, P.J.; Longo-Sorbello, G.S.; Banerjee, D.; Bertino, J.R. A miR-24 microRNA binding-site polymorphism in dihydrofolate reductase gene leads to methotrexate resistance. *Proc. Natl. Acad. Sci. USA* **2007**, *104*, 13513–13518. [CrossRef] [PubMed]
9. Livak, K.J.; Schmittgen, T.D. Analysis of relative gene expression data using real-time quantitative PCR and the $2^{-\Delta\Delta C}{}_T$ Method. *Methods* **2001**, *25*, 402–408. [CrossRef] [PubMed]
10. Cancer Genome Atlas Research Network. Genomic and epigenomic landscapes of adult de novo acute myeloid leukemia. *N. Engl. J. Med.* **2013**, *368*, 2059–2074. [CrossRef] [PubMed]
11. Kruger, J.; Rehmsmeier, M. RNAhybrid: microRNA target prediction easy, fast and flexible. *Nucleic Acids Res.* **2006**, *34*, W451–W454. [CrossRef] [PubMed]
12. Kutmon, M.; Kelder, T.; Mandaviya, P.; Evelo, C.T.; Coort, S.L. CyTargetLinker: A cytoscape app to integrate regulatory interactions in network analysis. *PLoS ONE* **2013**, *8*, e82160. [CrossRef]
13. Bhise, N.S.; Chauhan, L.; Shin, M.; Cao, X.; Pounds, S.; Lamba, V.; Lamba, J.K. MicroRNA-mRNA Pairs Associated with outcome in AML: From in vitro cell-based studies to AML patients. *Front. Pharmacol.* **2015**, *6*, 324. [CrossRef] [PubMed]
14. Wallace, J.A.; O'Connell, R.M. MicroRNAs and acute myeloid leukemia: Therapeutic implications and emerging concepts. *Blood* **2017**, *130*, 1290–1301. [CrossRef]
15. Dumontet, C.; Fabianowska-Majewska, K.; Mantincic, D.; Callet Bauchu, E.; Tigaud, I.; Gandhi, V.; Lepoivre, M.; Peters, G.J.; Rolland, M.O.; Wyczechowska, D.; et al. Common resistance mechanisms to deoxynucleoside analogues in variants of the human erythroleukaemic line K562. *Br. J. Haematol.* **1999**, *106*, 78–85. [CrossRef]
16. Bhalla, K.; Nayak, R.; Grant, S. Isolation and characterization of a deoxycytidine kinase-deficient human promyelocytic leukemic cell line highly resistant to 1-β-D-arabinofuranosylcytosine. *Cancer Res.* **1984**, *44*, 5029–5037.
17. Verhoef, V.; Sarup, J.; Fridland, A. Identification of the mechanism of activation of 9-β-D-arabinofuranosyladenine in human lymphoid cells using mutants deficient in nucleoside kinases. *Cancer Res.* **1981**, *41*, 4478–4483.
18. Galmarini, C.M.; Thomas, X.; Calvo, F.; Rousselot, P.; El Jafaari, A.; Cros, E.; Dumontet, C. Potential mechanisms of resistance to cytarabine in AML patients. *Leuk. Res.* **2002**, *26*, 621–629. [CrossRef]
19. Garofalo, M.; Jeon, Y.J.; Nuovo, G.J.; Middleton, J.; Secchiero, P.; Joshi, P.; Alder, H.; Nazaryan, N.; di Leva, G. Correction: MiR-34a/c-dependent PDGFR-α/β downregulation inhibits tumorigenesis and enhances TRAIL-induced apoptosis in lung cancer. *PLoS ONE* **2015**, *10*, e0131729. [CrossRef]
20. Hong, J.H.; Roh, K.S.; Suh, S.S.; Lee, S.; Sung, S.W.; Park, J.K.; Byun, J.H.; Kang, J.H. The expression of microRNA-34a is inversely correlated with c-MET and CDK6 and has a prognostic significance in lung adenocarcinoma patients. *Tumour Biol.* **2015**, *36*, 9327–9337. [CrossRef]
21. Lu, G.; Sun, Y.; An, S.; Xin, S.; Ren, X.; Zhang, D.; Wu, P.; Liao, W.; Ding, Y.; Liang, L. MicroRNA-34a targets FMNL2 and E2F5 and suppresses the progression of colorectal cancer. *Exp. Mol. Pathol.* **2015**, *99*, 173–179. [CrossRef] [PubMed]
22. Qiao, P.; Li, G.; Bi, W.; Yang, L.; Yao, L.; Wu, D. microRNA-34a inhibits epithelial mesenchymal transition in human cholangiocarcinoma by targeting Smad4 through transforming growth factor-beta/Smad pathway. *BMC Cancer* **2015**, *15*, 469. [CrossRef]
23. Wang, X.; Li, J.; Dong, K.; Lin, F.; Long, M.; Ouyang, Y.; Wei, J.; Chen, X.; Weng, Y.; He, T.; et al. Tumor suppressor miR-34a targets PD-L1 and functions as a potential immunotherapeutic target in acute myeloid leukemia. *Cell. Signal.* **2015**, *27*, 443–452. [CrossRef]
24. Capizzi, R.L.; White, J.C.; Powell, B.L.; Perrino, F. Effect of dose on the pharmacokinetic and pharmacodynamic effects of cytarabine. *Semin. Hematol.* **1991**, *28* (Suppl. 4), 54–69. [PubMed]

25. Fridland, A.; Verhoef, V. Mechanism for ara-CTP catabolism in human leukemic cells and effect of deaminase inhibitors on this process. *Semin. Oncol.* **1987**, *14* (Suppl. 1), 262–268. [PubMed]
26. Liliemark, J.O.; Plunkett, W. Regulation of 1-β-D-arabinofuranosylcytosine 5′-triphosphate accumulation in human leukemia cells by deoxycytidine 5′-triphosphate. *Cancer Res.* **1986**, *46*, 1079–1083.
27. Gilbert, J.A.; Salavaggione, O.E.; Ji, Y.; Pelleymounter, L.L.; Eckloff, B.W.; Wieben, E.D.; Ames, M.M.; Weinshilboum, R.M. Gemcitabine pharmacogenomics: Cytidine deaminase and deoxycytidylate deaminase gene resequencing and functional genomics. *Clin. Cancer Res.* **2006**, *12*, 1794–1803. [CrossRef] [PubMed]
28. Xu, L.; Chen, Z.; Xue, F.; Chen, W.; Ma, R.; Cheng, S.; Cui, P. MicroRNA-24 inhibits growth, induces apoptosis, and reverses radioresistance in laryngeal squamous cell carcinoma by targeting X-linked inhibitor of apoptosis protein. *Cancer Cell Int.* **2015**, *15*, 61. [CrossRef] [PubMed]
29. Lu, K.; Wang, J.; Song, Y.; Zhao, S.; Liu, H.; Tang, D.; Pan, B.; Zhao, H.; Zhang, Q. miRNA-24-3p promotes cell proliferation and inhibits apoptosis in human breast cancer by targeting p27Kip1. *Oncol. Rep.* **2015**, *34*, 995–1002. [CrossRef] [PubMed]
30. Manvati, S.; Mangalhara, K.C.; Kalaiarasan, P.; Srivastava, N.; Bamezai, R.N. miR-24-2 regulates genes in survival pathway and demonstrates potential in reducing cellular viability in combination with docetaxel. *Gene* **2015**, *567*, 217–224. [CrossRef]
31. Zhao, G.; Liu, L.; Zhao, T.; Jin, S.; Jiang, S.; Cao, S.; Han, J.; Xin, Y.; Dong, Q.; Liu, X.; et al. Upregulation of miR-24 promotes cell proliferation by targeting NAIF1 in non-small cell lung cancer. *Tumour Biol.* **2015**, *36*, 3693–3701. [CrossRef] [PubMed]
32. Organista-Nava, J.; Gomez-Gomez, Y.; Illades-Aguiar, B.; del Carmen Alarcon-Romero, L.; Saavedra-Herrera, M.V.; Rivera-Ramirez, A.B.; Garzón-Barrientos, V.H.; Leyva-Vázquez, M.A. High miR-24 expression is associated with risk of relapse and poor survival in acute leukemia. *Oncol. Rep.* **2015**, *33*, 1639–1649. [CrossRef]
33. Gao, Y.; Liu, Y.; Du, L.; Li, J.; Qu, A.; Zhang, X.; Wang, L.; Wang, C. Down-regulation of miR-24-3p in colorectal cancer is associated with malignant behavior. *Med. Oncol.* **2015**, *32*, 362. [CrossRef]
34. Pan, B.; Chen, Y.; Song, H.; Xu, Y.; Wang, R.; Chen, L. Mir-24-3p downregulation contributes to VP16-DDP resistance in small-cell lung cancer by targeting *ATG4A*. *Oncotarget* **2015**, *6*, 317–331. [CrossRef] [PubMed]

5

Diagnostic and Therapeutic Strategies for Fluoropyrimidine Treatment of Patients Carrying Multiple *DPYD* Variants

Carin A. T. C. Lunenburg [1], Linda M. Henricks [2,3], André B. P. van Kuilenburg [4], Ron H. J. Mathijssen [5], Jan H. M. Schellens [2,3], Hans Gelderblom [1], Henk-Jan Guchelaar [6] and Jesse J. Swen [6,*]

1 Department of Medical Oncology, Leiden University Medical Center, 2333 ZA Leiden, The Netherlands; c.a.t.c.lunenburg@lumc.nl (C.A.T.C.L.); a.j.gelderblom@lumc.nl (H.G.)
2 Department of Clinical Pharmacology, Division of Medical Oncology, The Netherlands Cancer Institute, 1066 CX Amsterdam, The Netherlands; l.henricks@nki.nl (L.M.H.); j.schellens@gmail.com (J.H.M.S.)
3 Division of Pharmacology, The Netherlands Cancer Institute, 1066 CX Amsterdam, The Netherlands
4 Department of Clinical Chemistry, Amsterdam University Medical Centre, 1105 AZ Amsterdam, The Netherlands; a.b.vankuilenburg@amc.uva.nl
5 Department of Medical Oncology, Erasmus MC Cancer Institute, 3015 GD Rotterdam, The Netherlands; a.mathijssen@erasmusmc.nl
6 Department of Clinical Pharmacy & Toxicology, Leiden University Medical Center, 2333 ZA Leiden, The Netherlands; h.j.guchelaar@lumc.nl
* Correspondence: j.j.swen@lumc.nl

Abstract: *DPYD* genotyping prior to fluoropyrimidine treatment is increasingly implemented in clinical care. Without phasing information (i.e., allelic location of variants), current genotype-based dosing guidelines cannot be applied to patients carrying multiple *DPYD* variants. The primary aim of this study is to examine diagnostic and therapeutic strategies for fluoropyrimidine treatment of patients carrying multiple *DPYD* variants. A case series of patients carrying multiple *DPYD* variants is presented. Different genotyping techniques were used to determine phasing information. Phenotyping was performed by dihydropyrimidine dehydrogenase (DPD) enzyme activity measurements. Publicly available databases were queried to explore the frequency and phasing of variants of patients carrying multiple *DPYD* variants. Four out of seven patients carrying multiple *DPYD* variants received a full dose of fluoropyrimidines and experienced severe toxicity. Phasing information could be retrieved for four patients. In three patients, variants were located on two different alleles, i.e., in *trans*. Recommended dose reductions based on the phased genotype differed from the phenotype-derived dose reductions in three out of four cases. Data from publicly available databases show that the frequency of patients carrying multiple *DPYD* variants is low (< 0.2%), but higher than the frequency of the commonly tested *DPYD**13 variant (0.1%). Patients carrying multiple *DPYD* variants are at high risk of developing severe toxicity. Additional analyses are required to determine the correct dose of fluoropyrimidine treatment. In patients carrying multiple *DPYD* variants, we recommend that a DPD phenotyping assay be carried out to determine a safe starting dose.

Keywords: pharmacogenomics; pharmacogenetics; genotype; phenotype; alleles; precision medicine

1. Introduction

Fluoropyrimidines (including 5-fluorouracil (5-FU) and capecitabine) are the cornerstone of treatment for various types of cancer and are used by millions of patients worldwide each year [1–3]. However, up to one-third of treated patients experience severe toxicity (Common Terminology Criteria for Adverse Events (CTC-AE) grade ≥ 3), such as diarrhea, hand–foot syndrome, or mucositis upon treatment with fluoropyrimidines [4,5]. These adverse events can lead to mortality in approximately 1% of patients who experience severe toxicity [4,6]. Dihydropyrimidine dehydrogenase (DPD) is the key enzyme in the metabolism of 5-FU and its decreased activity is strongly associated with toxicity [7,8]. Variants in *DPYD*, the gene encoding DPD, can lead to decreased DPD enzyme activity [9–12]. Prospective *DPYD* genotyping of four main *DPYD* variants followed by dose reductions in patients carrying any of these four *DPYD* variants is safe, cost-effective, and feasible in clinical practice [13–15]. These *DPYD* variants are *DPYD**2A (rs3918290, c.1905+1G>A, IVS14+1G>A); *DPYD**13 (rs55886062, c.1679T>G, I560S); c.1236G>A/HapB3 (rs56038477, E412E); and c.2846A>T (rs67376798, D949V). For these four variants, convincing evidence has been provided warranting implementation in clinical practice [4,5,12,15–17].

An increasing number of hospitals apply prospective *DPYD* genotyping when treating patients with fluoropyrimidines [18]. Individual dosing guidelines for the abovementioned four *DPYD* variants are provided by the Dutch Pharmacogenetics Working Group (DPWG) and the Clinical Pharmacogenetics Implementation Consortium (CPIC) [19,20]. Dosing guidelines are based on the expected remaining DPD enzyme activity and can be applied to patients who are heterozygous carriers of a single *DPYD* variant. For homozygous *DPYD* variant allele carriers (two identical variants) and compound heterozygous *DPYD* variant allele carriers (two or more different variants), dosing guidelines are not yet available (or treatment with an alternative drug is advised), although safe treatment with low-dose fluoropyrimidines in these homozygous *DPYD* patients was demonstrated by a recent case series [21].

Patients who carry multiple variants (compound heterozygous) can carry the variants on a single allele (in *cis*) or on different alleles (in *trans*). In the first case, one functionally active allele remains, whereas in the latter case, both alleles are affected, which may result in a proportionally decreased enzyme activity (Figure 1). With currently used genotyping techniques, the allelic location of variants (phasing) cannot be determined. This uncertainty hampers adequate interpretation of the pharmacogenetic test result in compound heterozygous patients and makes it impossible to give an appropriate dose recommendation based on the genotype alone. Since it is likely that in the future, even more *DPYD* variants will be tested, the probability of finding compound heterozygous *DPYD* variant allele carriers will increase. The aims of this study are to examine diagnostic and therapeutic strategies for fluoropyrimidine treatment of patients carrying multiple *DPYD* variants and the frequency and phasing of variants of compound heterozygous *DPYD* patients in publicly available databases.

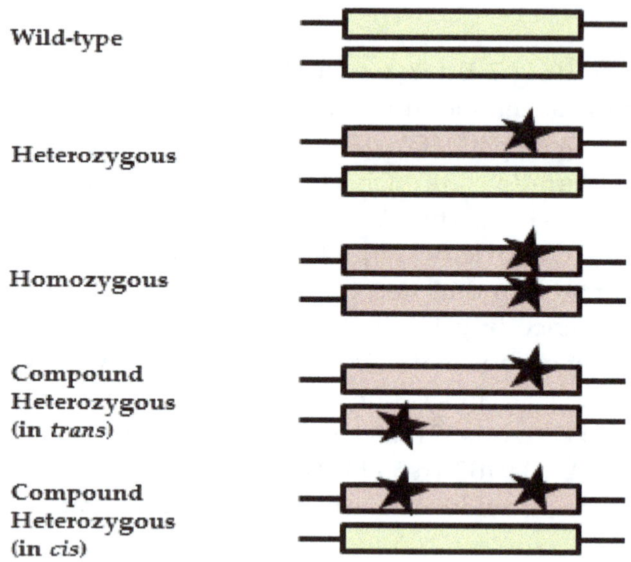

Figure 1. Illustration of zygosity and clinical interpretations. Black stars represent variants; boxes represent alleles. A wild-type patient carries no variants, resulting in normal-activity alleles (green). A heterozygous patient carries one variant, resulting in one reduced or inactive allele (red) and one active allele (green). A partly reduced enzyme activity is expected, since there is still one active allele left. For homozygous patients, both variants result in a reduced or inactive allele (red). Depending on the effect of the variants on the protein, a reduced or absent enzyme activity is expected. Compound heterozygous patients can carry variants on different alleles (in *trans*) or on one allele (in *cis*), resulting in differences in enzyme function, either like that of a heterozygous patient or a homozygous patient.

2. Materials and Methods

In this study, we present seven compounds heterozygous *DPYD* variant allele carriers as clinical cases. In addition, we have performed in silico research in publicly available databases.

2.1. Patients

Data and DNA from patient cases carrying multiple *DPYD* variants were collected. Patients were identified either after development of severe toxicity from fluoropyrimidine-containing therapy, by additional retrospective genotyping in a clinical trial (clinicaltrials.gov identifier NCT00838370, [13]), or prior to treatment in routine clinical care. The study was reviewed and approved by the institutional review board of the Leiden University Medical Centre (LUMC, G18.015). Patient data from the electronic medical records was handled following the codes of proper use and proper conduct in the self-regulatory codes of conduct [22]. Toxicity to fluoropyrimidine-containing therapy was graded by the treating physicians using the National Cancer Institute CTC-AE version 4.03 [23], and severe fluoropyrimidine-induced toxicity was defined as CTC-AE grade ≥ 3. In some cases, additional patient material to determine the phasing of the *DPYD* variants was collected. In these cases, additional patient consent was obtained.

2.2. Dihydropyrimidine Dehydrogenase Enzyme Activity Measurements

For all patients, DPD enzyme activity was determined. This could be either prior to treatment or retrospectively after the occurrence of severe toxicity. DPD enzyme activity measurement in peripheral blood mononuclear cells (PBMCs) [24,25] was used as a reference to assess DPD activity, and has been used previously to determine dosages in *DPYD* variant-carrying patients [21,26]. A validated method [27] was used, containing radiolabeled thymine as a substrate and consisting of high-performance liquid chromatography (HPLC) with online radioisotope detection using liquid scintillation counting. Normal values for healthy volunteers are 9.9 ± 2.8 nmol/(mg$\times$h), for DPD-deficient patients are 4.8 ± 1.7 nmol/(mg×h), and reference values range from 5.9 to 14 nmol/(mg×h) [28]. Dose reductions based on DPD enzyme activity were performed in a one-to-one ratio, as was previously described by Henricks et al. [21]. Thereafter, toxicity-guided dosing was used.

2.3. *Molecular Methods for Estimation of Phasing*

In regard to the size of the *DPYD* gene, the location of the variants, and the material available (DNA, RNA) from the patients, three molecular methods to determine the phasing of the variants could be used in this study. In four patients, we could execute one or more of these methods. These methods are explained and illustrated in the supplementary material (Figure S1). Details on these techniques have been published elsewhere [29–31].

2.4. *Frequencies of Compound Heterozygous DPYD Carriers*

To investigate the incidence of compound heterozygous *DPYD* variant allele carriers (of the four genotyped *DPYD* variants), large databases were queried [32,33]. The incidence was calculated using minor allele frequencies (MAFs) of each variant identified in the databases separately. Since the determined variants are not in the same haplotype, it was assumed that the inheritance of these individual *DPYD* variants is independent. All genotypes from the databases were calculated to be in Hardy–Weinberg equilibrium, except for *DPYD**2A and c.1236G>A for the Exome Aggregation Consortium (ExAC, http://exac.broadinstitute.org/) [32] and Genome Aggregation Database (gnomAD, http://gnomad.broadinstitute.org/) [33] due to a slight overrepresentation of homozygous cases. The calculated frequencies were compared to frequencies from databases in which phasing could be determined.

Exome Aggregation Consortium and Genome Aggregation Database

Both the ExAC [32] and gnomAD [33] databases collect exome sequencing data and aggregate the data for public use. The ExAC dataset (v0.3.1) contains sequenced data of 60,706 unrelated individuals. The gnomAD dataset (v2.0) contains sequenced data of 123,136 exomes and 15,496 genomes from unrelated individuals. In ExAC, 2791 *DPYD* variants, and in gnomAD, 2190 *DPYD* variants were found. MAFs of *DPYD* variants from these databases reflect those of the population due to the large group size in the databases. Since both ExAC and gnomAD do not contain individual matched or phased data, it is not possible to search for compound heterozygous patients in these databases.

2.5. *Phasing in Compound Heterozygous DPYD Carriers*

Three databases were used to identify compound heterozygous *DPYD* variant allele carriers and determine the phasing, i.e., allelic location, of variants.

2.5.1. Genome of the Netherlands Datasets

The Genome of the Netherlands (GoNL, http://www.nlgenome.nl/) trio datasets contain information of related fathers, mothers, and children, and phasing information is therefore available. Datasets were previously processed and phased using trio-aware variant calling [34]. After the exclusion of children, phased variant call format (VCF) files for 496 subjects (fathers and mothers) were obtained from the GoNL repository. The toolset Bedtools (https://bedtools.readthedocs.io/en/latest/, v2) was used to extract all variants found in the *DPYD* locus (chr1:97,543,300–98,386,615). Next, for all individuals, the carrier status of *DPYD**2A, *DPYD**13, c.1236G>A, and c.2846A>T was examined. Individuals who carry at least one of the four actionable *DPYD* variants were identified, and using a custom Python [35] script, the phasing of variants was assessed for individuals with multiple variants.

2.5.2. 1000 Genomes Database

The 1000 Genomes Project (http://www.internationalgenome.org/) is the largest publicly available catalogue of human variation and genotyped phased data. It originally ran from 2008 until 2015, and thereafter it was maintained and expanded by the International Genome Sample Resource (IGSR) [36]. On 27 October 2016, phased data of the *DPYD* gene (chr1: 97,543,300–98,386,615) was downloaded from the 1000 Genomes ftp server (phase 3; GRCh37; chr1: 97,543,300–98,386,615) using Tabix (v1.1) [37]. The statistical program R (v3.2.5) [38] was used to select the genotypes at four *DPYD* risk alleles in unrelated individuals of Caucasian descent.

2.5.3. Exome Trios Leiden University Medical Centre Database

This diagnostic database of the clinical genetics department of LUMC contains 433 complete exome trios (father, mother, and child). The exome was enriched by the Agilent sureselect v5 kit and sequenced using various Illumina (San Diego, CA, USA) sequencers (Hiseq 2000, 2500, 4000, Nextseq). Carrier status of the abovementioned *DPYD* variants was established by querying the trio VCF files. We also investigated all samples with sufficient coverage of this region to obtain a reliable frequency estimate. In the case of trios, only parents were taken into account.

3. Results

3.1. Patient Cases and Clinical Implications

Details of the demographics and clinical characteristics of the seven cases are described in the supplementary material (patient cases). All patients received treatment with fluoropyrimidines and were identified as compound heterozygous *DPYD* variant allele carriers either prior to the start of treatment or retrospectively. Table 1 shows an overview of the cases. Table 2 shows all genotype and phenotype results. With additional genetic testing, phasing could be determined in four out of seven patients. In three patients, the variants were located in *trans*, and one patient carried the variants in *cis*. With the phasing information available, it is possible to calculate a dose recommendation using publicly available pharmacogenetic dosing guidelines [19,20]. For example, patient 1 carried *DPYD**2A and c.1236G>A in *trans*. The gene activity values range from inactive (0) to fully active (1). *DPYD**2A and c.1236G>A/HapB3 have values of 0 and 0.5, respectively. As this patient carries the variants in *trans*, each allele contains one variant and no fully functional allele remains. Therefore, the cumulated gene activity score (GAS) is 0.5. The GAS can be used to determine dose recommendations according to the genotype, as was previously described [12]. The GAS ranges from 0 to 2, and a score of 0.5 corresponds to a dose recommendation of 25%. The DPD enzyme activity of patient 1 was 0.9 nmol/(mg×h). This was divided by the mean of the reference value (9.9), which results in a theoretical DPD activity of 9%. For each patient for whom phasing details were known, the GAS was determined and compared to the theoretical DPD activity. Dose recommendations according to the GAS (genotype) and theoretical DPD activity (phenotype) were divergent in almost all cases, as shown in Table 2.

3.2. Preventing Toxicity

Three of the seven case patients were identified as carriers of one or more *DPYD* variants prior to the start of therapy. For one patient, the DPD enzyme activity was determined prior to the start of therapy. Based on their genotype or phenotype, these three patients received initially reduced fluoropyrimidine dosages of 50%. They experienced limited and reversible toxicity (CTC-AE grades 0–2). The dose of one patient was increased to 70% in the second treatment cycle, after which CTC-AE grade 3 toxicity occurred.

Four of the seven case patients received a full dose, since their genotype was unknown prior to the start of therapy. These patients all experienced severe toxicity (CTC-AE grades 3–5), and three of them were admitted to the hospital for 7–14 days. An overview of cases, including the toxicity, is shown in Table 3.

3.3. *Frequencies of Compound Heterozygous DPYD Carriers without Phasing Information*

The ExAC and gnomAD databases revealed an average MAF for *DPYD**2A, *DPYD**13, c.1236G>A, and c.2846A>T of 0.55%, 0.03%, 1.43%, and 0.27%, respectively. MAFs for ExAC and gnomAD separately are summarized in Table 4. The probability of identifying a compound heterozygous *DPYD* patient for two variants according to these databases was $\leq$ 0.008%, as was calculated using frequencies of combinations of *DPYD* variants. Results for each combination of *DPYD* variants are shown in Table 5. With several million fluoropyrimidine users each year, thousands of patients worldwide are compound heterozygous for a subset of these four *DPYD* variants.

3.4. *Frequencies of Compound Heterozygous DPYD Carriers with Phasing Information*

In the GoNL database, genetic data from 496 subjects (fathers and mothers only) was reviewed. One subject was found who carried two *DPYD* variants. This subject was a carrier of the *DPYD* c.1236G>A and *DPYD* c.2846A>T variants, both of which were located on a single allele (in *cis*). Based upon the data in GoNL, the probability of having compound heterozygosity of the four *DPYD* variants is <0.2%.

In the 1000 Genomes database, data of 2513 individuals were available. After the selection of unique, unrelated individuals, 407 individuals remained. One subject was found who carried two *DPYD* variants. This subject was a carrier of *DPYD* c.1236G>A and *DPYD* c.2846A>T, both of which were located on different alleles (in *trans*). Based upon the data in 1000 Genomes, the probability of having compound heterozygosity of the four *DPYD* variants is <0.3%.

In the LUMC clinical genetics database (exome trios LUMC), the analysis was restricted to the children, since this would allow phasing. None of the 433 children carried more than one *DPYD* variant, thus compound heterozygosity in this database is <0.2%.

Despite the low frequency, compound heterozygous patients were identified in all databases except the LUMC clinical genetics database. However, the low frequency did not allow to determine the probability of in *cis* or in *trans* phasing of variants in a patient.

Table 1. Characteristics of patient cases. Shown per patient are primary tumor, treatment, capecitabine dose, executed assays (genotype, dihydropyrimidine dehydrogenase (DPD) enzyme activity, and additional assays) information. Additional assays are droplet digital PCR, PacBio sequencing (Menlo Park, CA, USA), or an in-house developed technique. For the executed assays, it is shown whether these were executed prior to treatment (P) or retrospectively (R). *Abbreviations:* BC: breast cancer; CRC: colorectal cancer; CAP: capecitabine; RT: radiotherapy; OX: oxaliplatin; BEV: bevacizumab; bid: *bis in die*/twice a day.

Patient #	Primary Tumor	Treatment	Capecitabine Dose	Executed Assays
1	BC	CAP	1000 mg/m^2/bid	Genotyping (R), DPD activity (R), in-house technique (R), droplet digital PCR (R)
2	BC	CAP	800 mg bid (50%)	Genotyping (P), DPD activity (R), in-house technique (R)
3	CRC	CAP + OX	900 mg bid (50%) [1]	Genotyping (P), DPD activity (P), PacBio (R)
4	BC	CAP	1500 mg bid	Genotyping (R), DPD activity (R [2])
5	CRC	CAP + RT	800 mg bid (50%)	Genotyping (P + R [3]), DPD activity (R [4]), PacBio (R)
6	CRC	CAP + OX	1000 mg/m^2/bid	Genotyping (R), DPD activity (R)
7	CRC	CAP + OX + BEV	1000 mg/m^2/bid	Genotyping (R), DPD activity (R)

[1] Increased to 70% in the second cycle; [2] during hospital admission; [3] *DPYD**2A was prospectively identified, c.2846A>T was retrospectively identified; [4] during treatment.

Table 2. Dose advice for compound heterozygous *DPYD* variant allele carriers. Shown per patient are *DPYD* variants, phasing of the *DPYD* variants, GAS, retrospective DPWG dosing advice based on phasing, DPD enzyme activity, and percentage of DPD enzyme activity considered for dose advice. According to the DPWG guidelines [19], a gene activity score can be given to compound heterozygous patients when phasing is known. Fully functional/reduced functionality = gene activity score of 1.5; fully functional/inactive = gene activity score of 1; reduced functionality/reduced functionality = gene activity score of 1; reduced functionality/inactive = gene activity score of 0.5; inactive/inactive = gene activity score of 0. *Abbreviations:* DPD: dihydropyrimidine dehydrogenase; GAS: gene activity score; DPWG: Dutch Pharmacogenetic Working Group; X: could not be determined.

Patient #	*DPYD* Variants	Phasing	GAS [12]	DPWG Dose Advice (% of Regular Dose)	DPD Activity (nmol/(mg×h))	Percentage of DPD Activity [1]
1	*DPYD**2A + c.1236G>A	in *trans*	0.5	25%	0.9	9%
2	*DPYD**2A + c.2846A>T	in *trans*	0.5	25%	6.0	60%
3	c.1236G>A + c.2846A>T	in *trans*	1	50%	4.5	45%
4	*DPYD**2A + c.2846A>T	unknown	X	X	0.11	1%
5	*DPYD**2A + c.2846A>T	in *cis*	1	50%	7.2	72%
6	*DPYD**2A + c.1236G>A	unknown	X	X	3.8	38%
7	*DPYD**2A + c.1236G>A	unknown	X	X	1.6	16%

[1] The reference DPD activity ranges from 5.9–14 nmol/(mg×h) [28], and therefore the percentage of DPD activity can be calculated using the average of the reference (9.9 nmol/(mg×h). This percentage could be used as a percentage of the regular dose.

Table 3. Toxicity profiles of compound heterozygous *DPYD* variant allele carriers. Shown per patient are *DPYD* variants, fluoropyrimidine dose as a percentage of the regular dose, and experienced toxicity with this dose. All patients retrospectively identified as *DPYD* variants carrier received full doses and experienced severe (CTC-AE $\geq$ 3) toxicity. All patients prospectively identified as *DPYD* variant(s) carrier received dose reductions and experienced a maximum of CTC-AE grade 2 toxicity with the initial dose. *Abbreviations:* CTC-AE: Common Terminology Criteria for Adverse Events v4.03.

Patient #	*DPYD* variants	Dose (% of Regular Dose)	Toxicity (Maximal CTC Grade)
1	*DPYD**2A + c.1236G>A	100%	4
2	*DPYD**2A + c.2846A>T	50%	1–2
3	c.1236G>A + c.2846A>T	50% → 70%	0 (on 50% dose) → 3 (on 70% dose)
4	*DPYD**2A + c.2846A>T	100%	5
5	*DPYD**2A + c.2846A>T	50%	0
6	*DPYD**2A + c.1236G>A	100%	4
7	*DPYD**2A + c.1236G>A	100%	3

Table 4. MAF per database. Three databases (GoNL, 1000 Genomes, and exome trios LUMC) containing phased data were checked for four *DPYD* variants. Two large online databases (ExAC and gnomAD) were checked to identify the MAFs of the individual *DPYD* variants. For each *DPYD* variant, the genotype distribution and MAF are shown. *Abbreviations:* MAF: minor allele frequency; HW: homozygous wild-type; HE: heterozygous carrier; HM: homozygous carrier; GoNL: Genome of the Netherlands; ExAC: Exome Aggregation Consortium; gnomAD: Genome Aggregation Database.

Variants / Databases	*DPYD**2A (rs3918290)		*DPYD**13 (rs55886062)		c.1236G>A (rs56038477)		c.2846A>T (rs67376798)	
	HW/HE/HM	MAF	HW/HE/HM	MAF	HW/HE/HM	MAF	HW/HE/HM	MAF
GoNL	489/7/0	0.7%	494/2/0	0.2%	475/21/0	2.1%	490/6/0	0.6%
1000 Genomes	405/2/0	0.2%	406/1/0	0.1%	389/18/0	2.2%	403/4/0	0.5%
Exome Trios LUMC	946/15/0	0.8%	946/0/0	0.00%	946/46/0	2.3%	946/2/0	0.1%
ExAC	60,627/624/5	0.5%	60,320/42/0	0.03%	60,652/1808/27	1.5%	60,687/317/1	0.3%
gnomAD	138,489/1586/10	0.6%	138,166/83/0	0.03%	138,407/3841/39	1.4%	138,478/792/1	0.3%

Table 5. Calculated frequencies for compound heterozygous *DPYD* patients. Using the average MAFs of the ExAC and gnomAD databases (for *DPYD**2A, *DPYD**13, c.1236G>A, and c.2846A>T, these are 0.55%, 0.03%, 1.43%, and 0.27%, respectively), possible combinations for two out of four currently genotyped *DPYD* variants are shown. *Abbreviations:* MAF: minor allele frequency; ExAC: Exome Aggregation Consortium; gnomAD: Genome Aggregation Database.

Combination of *DPYD* Variants	Calculated Frequency
*DPYD**2A + *DPYD**13	0.0002%
*DPYD**2A + c.1236G>A	0.008%
*DPYD**2A + c.2846A>T	0.001%
*DPYD**13 + c.1236G>A	0.0005%
*DPYD**13 + c.2846A>T	0.0001%
c.1236G>A + c.2846A>T	0.004%

4. Discussion

Prospective genotyping of *DPYD* variants followed by individual dose adjustments is increasingly applied as the standard of care for patients starting fluoropyrimidine therapy. Standard dose reductions from CPIC and DPWG guidelines cannot be applied in patients who carry more than one *DPYD* variant, as the phasing of the variants is unknown. Despite the low population frequency of < 0.2%, the absolute number of identified compound heterozygous patients will increase as the number of genotyped patients increases and the panel of tested variants is expanded. To the best of our knowledge, this is the first study that describes a case series of compound heterozygous *DPYD* variant allele carriers and investigates diagnostic and therapeutic strategies for these patients.

Our study shows the clinical need for further information on the genotype, as four patients were identified as compound heterozygous carriers retrospectively and all of them experienced severe toxicity. These compound heterozygous *DPYD* variant allele carriers have an increased risk of developing severe fluoropyrimidine-induced toxicity if dosages are not adequately adjusted. Previously, compound heterozygous patients have been described with severe or even lethal side effects after fluoropyrimidine treatment [39,40]. Three patients in this study were prospectively identified as compound heterozygous carriers, received initial dose reductions, and developed only mild toxicities.

Out of the four patients for whom we were able to retrieve phasing information, three were in *trans* and one was in *cis* orientation. Data from publicly available databases also showed that both in *cis* and in *trans* orientations exist. However, the recently updated CPIC guidelines on *DPYD* assumes in *trans* phasing for compound heterozygous patients [20]. The DPWG guidelines do not mention phasing; however, the dosing recommendations of the DPWG use the GAS, a score based on the activity of individual alleles [19]. This implies the need for phasing information. The assumption of in *trans* phasing could result in the underdosing of patients with variants phased in *cis*, and thus exemplifies the need for the determination of the phasing of variants.

In this study, we looked at different diagnostic strategies to determine the phasing of *DPYD* variants in compound heterozygous patients. In four patients, the phasing of *DPYD* variants could be determined using one of three different molecular methods. These methods are in the early phases of development, not routinely available, quite expensive, and not always conclusive. For two of these techniques, patient RNA is used, which degrades quickly after the blood draw unless specifically designed blood tubes are used. Compound heterozygous patients are rare, yet here we describe seven patients heterozygous for multiple *DPYD* variants. A limitation of our study is that most patients were identified retrospectively and in different institutions. Because of this, not enough of or not the right material was available for analysis, thus not all genotyping techniques could be executed in each patient. For two samples, tests failed or produced inconclusive results. For this reason, a formal comparison of their suitability to identify phasing was not possible. However, of the three explored molecular methods, PacBio sequencing seems most promising. While phasing improved the prediction of DPD enzyme activity, patients with identical combinations of *DPYD* variants and identical phasing showed considerable differences in DPD enzyme activity, which could potentially limit the added value of the determination of the phasing of *DPYD* variants. However, larger numbers of compound heterozygous *DPYD* variant allele carriers would be necessary to draw a firm conclusion.

The measurement of DPD enzyme activity in PBMCs was used as a reference to assess DPD activity. The method is well-established, commonly available, and shows limited intra- and interpatient variability [27]. However, recently, differences in intrapatient variability in DPD enzyme activity related to circadian rhythm were shown [41], which can result in the under- or overestimation of DPD enzyme activity. In this study, we present one patient with extremely low DPD enzyme activity, which could possibly be influenced by the presence of severe neutropenia, as DPD activity is normally measured in mononuclear cells. Therefore, DPD enzyme activity can differ depending on the clinical condition of the patient and should thus be measured prior to treatment.

A major question is whether genotyping or phenotyping is the best method to determine DPD activity to guide fluoropyrimidine dosing in patients carrying multiple *DPYD* variants. Despite the low population frequency, we present seven patients carrying multiple *DPYD* variants, of which three received initially reduced fluoropyrimidine dosages. However, based on these data, it is not possible to determine if a dose recommendation based on phased genetic information or DPD enzyme activity measured in PBMCs is safer. In three out of four cases, differences were observed between the theoretically calculated DPD activity using genotyping or phenotyping. These differences would result in different dosing recommendations. For example, there is a considerable interpatient variability in DPD enzyme activity in carriers of the *DPYD* variant c.1236G>A/HapB3 [12]. Due to this variability, genetic dose recommendations are categorized (e.g., 25 or 50%) on the average of the phenotypes. This categorization could explain the observed dosing differences derived from genotyping and phenotyping. Other variants of *DPYD* currently not routinely tested for or variants in other genes, e.g., *MIR27A* [42], might also be involved in reducing DPD activity or explaining fluoropyrimidine-induced toxicity. DPD enzyme activity measurements are well-established, and additional molecular methods to resolve phasing are still in early phases of development. Therefore, in our opinion, the current therapeutic strategy for compound heterozygous *DPYD* variant allele carriers should be to determine initial dose reductions based on a DPD phenotyping test, for example, by measuring enzyme activity in PBMCs. Dosing could be adjusted by the treating physician in subsequent cycles based on observed severe toxicity (or lack thereof).

5. Conclusions

In conclusion, patients carrying multiple *DPYD* variants are at high risk of developing severe toxicity. Additional analyses are required to determine the correct dose of fluoropyrimidine treatment. In patients carrying multiple *DPYD* variants, we recommend that a DPD phenotyping assay be carried out to determine a safe starting dose. The dose could be titrated in subsequent cycles based on observed toxicity.

Author Contributions: Conceptualization, C.A.T.C.L., H.G., H.-J.G. and J.J.S.; Data curation, C.A.T.C.L., L.M.H. and A.B.P.v.K.; Formal analysis, C.A.T.C.L., H.-J.G. and J.J.S.; Methodology, C.A.T.C.L., H.-J.G. and J.J.S.; Supervision, H.G., H.-J.G. and J.J.S.; Writing—original draft, C.A.T.C.L.; Writing—review & editing, L.M.H., A.B.P.v.K., R.H.J.M., J.H.M.S., H.G., H.-J.G. and J.J.S.

Acknowledgments: The authors thank S.Y. Anvar, G.W.E. Santen, E.B. van den Akker and H. Mei for assistance with the databases; R.H.A.M. Vossen, E.J. de Meijer and R.J.H.M van der Straaten for execution of the molecular methods for estimation of phasing; and F.M. de Man for the collection of patient material and clinical data.

References

1. *Scrip's Cancer Chemotherapy Report*; Scrip world pharmaceutical news; PJB Publications Ltd.: London, UK, 2002.
2. Walko, C.M.; Lindley, C. Capecitabine: A review. *Clin. Ther.* **2005**, *27*, 23–44. [CrossRef] [PubMed]
3. Malet-Martino, M.; Martino, R. Clinical studies of three oral prodrugs of 5-fluorouracil (capecitabine, UFT, S-1): A review. *Oncologist* **2002**, *7*, 288–323. [CrossRef] [PubMed]
4. Rosmarin, D.; Palles, C.; Pagnamenta, A.; Kaur, K.; Pita, G.; Martin, M.; Domingo, E.; Jones, A.; Howarth, K.; Freeman-Mills, L.; et al. A candidate gene study of capecitabine-related toxicity in colorectal cancer identifies new toxicity variants at *DPYD* and a putative role for *ENOSF1* rather than *TYMS*. *Gut* **2015**, *64*, 111–120. [CrossRef]
5. Terrazzino, S.; Cargnin, S.; Del Re, M.; Danesi, R.; Canonico, P.L.; Genazzani, A.A. *DPYD* IVS14+1G>A and 2846A>T genotyping for the prediction of severe fluoropyrimidine-related toxicity: A meta-analysis. *Pharmacogenomics* **2013**, *14*, 1255–1272. [CrossRef]
6. Saltz, L.B.; Niedzwiecki, D.; Hollis, D.; Goldberg, R.M.; Hantel, A.; Thomas, J.P.; Fields, A.L.; Mayer, R.J. Irinotecan fluorouracil plus leucovorin is not superior to fluorouracil plus leucovorin alone as adjuvant treatment for stage III colon cancer: Results of CALGB 89803. *J. Clin. Oncol.* **2007**, *25*, 3456–3461. [CrossRef] [PubMed]
7. Van Kuilenburg, A.B. Dihydropyrimidine dehydrogenase and the efficacy and toxicity of 5-fluorouracil. *Eur. J. Cancer* **2004**, *40*, 939–950. [CrossRef] [PubMed]
8. Gonzalez, F.J.; Fernandez-Salguero, P. Diagnostic analysis, clinical importance and molecular basis of dihydropyrimidine dehydrogenase deficiency. *Trends Pharmacol. Sci.* **1995**, *16*, 325–327. [CrossRef]
9. Van Kuilenburg, A.B.; Meijer, J.; Maurer, D.; Dobritzsch, D.; Meinsma, R.; Los, M.; Knegt, L.C.; Zoetekouw, L.; Jansen, R.L.; Dezentje, V.; et al. Severe fluoropyrimidine toxicity due to novel and rare *DPYD* missense mutations, deletion and genomic amplification affecting DPD activity and mRNA splicing. *Biochim. Biophys. Acta* **2017**, *1863*, 721–730. [CrossRef]
10. Meulendijks, D.; Henricks, L.M.; van Kuilenburg, A.B.; Jacobs, B.A.; Aliev, A.; Rozeman, L.; Meijer, J.; Beijnen, J.H.; de Graaf, H.; Cats, A.; et al. Patients homozygous for *DPYD* c.1129-5923C>G/haplotype B3 have partial DPD deficiency and require a dose reduction when treated with fluoropyrimidines. *Cancer Chemother. Pharmacol.* **2016**, *78*, 875–880. [CrossRef]
11. Offer, S.M.; Fossum, C.C.; Wegner, N.J.; Stuflesser, A.J.; Butterfield, G.L.; Diasio, R.B. Comparative functional analysis of *DPYD* variants of potential clinical relevance to dihydropyrimidine dehydrogenase activity. *Cancer Res.* **2014**, *74*, 2545–2554. [CrossRef]
12. Henricks, L.M.; Lunenburg, C.A.; Meulendijks, D.; Gelderblom, H.; Cats, A.; Swen, J.J.; Schellens, J.H.; Guchelaar, H.J. Translating *DPYD* genotype into DPD phenotype: Using the *DPYD* gene activity score. *Pharmacogenomics* **2015**, *16*, 1277–1286. [CrossRef] [PubMed]
13. Deenen, M.J.; Meulendijks, D.; Cats, A.; Sechterberger, M.K.; Severens, J.L.; Boot, H.; Smits, P.H.; Rosing, H.; Mandigers, C.M.; Soesan, M.; et al. Upfront genotyping of *DPYD**2A to individualize fluoropyrimidine therapy: A safety and cost analysis. *J. Clin. Oncol.* **2016**, *34*, 227–234. [CrossRef] [PubMed]
14. Lunenburg, C.A.; van Staveren, M.C.; Gelderblom, H.; Guchelaar, H.J.; Swen, J.J. Evaluation of clinical implementation of prospective *DPYD* genotyping in 5-fluorouracil- or capecitabine-treated patients. *Pharmacogenomics* **2016**, *17*, 721–729. [CrossRef] [PubMed]
15. Henricks, L.M.; Lunenburg, C.; de Man, F.M.; Meulendijks, D.; Frederix, G.W.J.; Kienhuis, E.; Creemers, G.J.; Baars, A.; Dezentje, V.O.; Imholz, A.L.T.; et al. *DPYD* genotype-guided dose individualisation of fluoropyrimidine therapy in patients with cancer: A prospective safety analysis. *Lancet Oncol.* **2018**, *19*, 1459–1467. [CrossRef]
16. Lunenburg, C.A.; Henricks, L.M.; Guchelaar, H.J.; Swen, J.J.; Deenen, M.J.; Schellens, J.H.; Gelderblom, H. Prospective *DPYD* genotyping to reduce the risk of fluoropyrimidine-induced severe toxicity: Ready for prime time. *Eur. J. Cancer* **2016**, *54*, 40–48. [CrossRef] [PubMed]
17. Meulendijks, D.; Henricks, L.M.; Sonke, G.S.; Deenen, M.J.; Froehlich, T.K.; Amstutz, U.; Largiader, C.R.; Jennings, B.A.; Marinaki, A.M.; Sanderson, J.D.; et al. Clinical relevance of *DPYD* variants c.1679T>G, c.1236G>A/HapB3, and c.1601G>A as predictors of severe fluoropyrimidine-associated toxicity: A systematic review and meta-analysis of individual patient data. *Lancet Oncol.* **2015**, *16*, 1639–1650. [CrossRef]

18. Result Survey Screening for DPD Deficiency. *Medische Oncologie*. October 2016. Available online: https://www.nvmo.org/magazine/ (accessed on 1 November 2016).
19. KNMP. Royal Dutch Society for the Advancement of Pharmacy. Fluorouracil/Capecitabine DPD Gene Activity Score and Guidelines. Available online: https://kennisbank.knmp.nl/article/farmacogenetica/2552-4893-4894.html (accessed on 5 May 2017).
20. Amstutz, U.; Henricks, L.M.; Offer, S.M.; Barbarino, J.; Schellens, J.H.M.; Swen, J.J.; Klein, T.E.; McLeod, H.L.; Caudle, K.E.; Diasio, R.B.; et al. Clinical pharmacogenetics implementation consortium (CPIC) guideline for dihydropyrimidine dehydrogenase genotype and fluoropyrimidine dosing: 2017 update. *Clin. Pharmacol. Ther.* **2018**, *103*, 210–216. [CrossRef]
21. Henricks, L.M.; Kienhuis, E.; de Man, F.M.; van der Veldt, A.A.M.; Hamberg, P.; van Kuilenburg, A.B.P.; van Schaik, R.H.N.; Lunenburg, C.A.T.C.; Guchelaar, H.J.; Schellens, J.H.M.; et al. Treatment algorithm for homozygous or compound heterozygous *DPYD* variant allele carriers with low dose capecitabine. *JCO Precis. Oncol.* **2017**, *1*, 1–10, Published online October 6. [CrossRef]
22. Federa. Available online: federa.org (accessed on 9 September 2017).
23. National Cancer Institute: Common Terminology Criteria for Adverse Events v4.03. Available online: https://evs.nci.nih.gov/ftp1/CTCAE/CTCAE_4.03_2010-06-14_QuickReference_8.5x11.pdf (accessed on 9 September 2017).
24. Meulendijks, D.; Cats, A.; Beijnen, J.H.; Schellens, J.H. Improving safety of fluoropyrimidine chemotherapy by individualizing treatment based on dihydropyrimidine dehydrogenase activity—Ready for clinical practice? *Cancer Treat. Rev.* **2016**, *50*, 23–34. [CrossRef]
25. Van Staveren, M.C.; van Kuilenburg, A.B.; Guchelaar, H.J.; Meijer, J.; Punt, C.J.; de Jong, R.S.; Gelderblom, H.; Maring, J.G. Evaluation of an oral uracil loading test to identify DPD-deficient patients using a limited sampling strategy. *Br. J. Clin. Pharmacol.* **2016**, *81*, 553–561. [CrossRef]
26. Henricks, L.M.; Siemerink, E.J.M.; Rosing, H.; Meijer, J.; Goorden, S.M.I.; Polstra, A.M.; Zoetekouw, L.; Cats, A.; Schellens, J.H.M.; van Kuilenburg, A.B.P. Capecitabine-based treatment of a patient with a novel *DPYD* genotype and complete dihydropyrimidine dehydrogenase deficiency. *Int. J. Cancer* **2018**, *142*, 424–430. [CrossRef]
27. Van Kuilenburg, A.B.; Van Lenthe, H.; Tromp, A.; Veltman, P.C.; Van Gennip, A.H. Pitfalls in the diagnosis of patients with a partial dihydropyrimidine dehydrogenase deficiency. *Clin. Chem.* **2000**, *46*, 9–17. [PubMed]
28. Van Kuilenburg, A.B.; Meinsma, R.; Zoetekouw, L.; Van Gennip, A.H. Increased risk of grade IV neutropenia after administration of 5-fluorouracil due to a dihydropyrimidine dehydrogenase deficiency: High prevalence of the IVS14+1g>a mutation. *Int. J. Cancer* **2002**, *101*, 253–258. [CrossRef]
29. Regan, J.F.; Kamitaki, N.; Legler, T.; Cooper, S.; Klitgord, N.; Karlin-Neumann, G.; Wong, C.; Hodges, S.; Koehler, R.; Tzonev, S.; et al. A rapid molecular approach for chromosomal phasing. *PLoS ONE* **2015**, *10*, e0118270. [CrossRef] [PubMed]
30. Buermans, H.P.; Vossen, R.H.; Anvar, S.Y.; Allard, W.G.; Guchelaar, H.J.; White, S.J.; den Dunnen, J.T.; Swen, J.J.; van der Straaten, T. flexible and scalable full-length CYP2D6 long amplicon PacBio sequencing. *Hum. Mutat.* **2017**, *38*, 310–316. [CrossRef]
31. Van der Straaten, T.; Swen, J.; Baak-Pablo, R.; Guchelaar, H.J. Use of plasmid-derived external quality control samples in pharmacogenetic testing. *Pharmacogenomics* **2008**, *9*, 1261–1266. [CrossRef] [PubMed]
32. ExAC. Exome Aggregation Consortium. ExAC Browser (Beta). Available online: http://exac.broadinstitute.org/ (accessed on 13 December 2017).
33. gnomAD. genome Aggregation Database. gnomAD browser (Beta). Available online: http://gnomad.broadinstitute.org/ (accessed on 14 July 2017).
34. Francioli, L.; Menelaou, A.; Pulit, S.; van Dijk, F.; Palamara, P.; Elbers, C.; Neerincx, P.; Ye, K.; Guryev, V.; Kloosterman, W.; et al. Genome of The Netherlands Consortium. Whole-genome sequence variation, population structure and demographic history of the Dutch population. *Nat. Genet.* **2014**, *46*, 818–825. [CrossRef] [PubMed]
35. Python. Python Software Foundation©. Available online: https://www.python.org/ (accessed on 9 September 2017).
36. IGSR. The International Genome Sample Resource. Available online: http://www.internationalgenome.org/ (accessed on 29 June 2017).

37. Li, H. Tabix: Fast retrieval of sequence features from generic TAB-delimited files. *Bioinformatics* **2011**, *27*, 718–719. [CrossRef] [PubMed]
38. R Core Team. R: A Language and Environment for Statistical Computing 2018. Available online: https://www.R-project.org. (accessed on 9 September 2017).
39. Toffoli, G.; Giodini, L.; Buonadonna, A.; Berretta, M.; De, P.A.; Scalone, S.; Miolo, G.; Mini, E.; Nobili, S.; Lonardi, S.; et al. Clinical validity of a *DPYD*-based pharmacogenetic test to predict severe toxicity to fluoropyrimidines. *Int. J. Cancer* **2015**, *137*, 2971–2980. [CrossRef] [PubMed]
40. Johnson, M.R.; Wang, K.; Diasio, R.B. Profound dihydropyrimidine dehydrogenase deficiency resulting from a novel compound heterozygote genotype. *Clin. Cancer Res.* **2002**, *8*, 768–774.
41. Jacobs, B.A.; Deenen, M.J.; Pluim, D.; van Hasselt, J.G.; Krahenbuhl, M.D.; van Geel, R.M.; de Vries, N.; Rosing, H.; Meulendijks, D.; Burylo, A.M.; et al. Pronounced between-subject and circadian variability in thymidylate synthase and dihydropyrimidine dehydrogenase enzyme activity in human volunteers. *Br. J. Clin. Pharmacol.* **2016**, *82*, 706–716. [CrossRef] [PubMed]
42. Meulendijks, D.; Henricks, L.M.; Amstutz, U.; Froehlich, T.K.; Largiader, C.R.; Beijnen, J.H.; de Boer, A.; Deenen, M.J.; Cats, A.; Schellens, J.H. Rs895819 in *MIR27A* improves the predictive value of *DPYD* variants to identify patients at risk of severe fluoropyrimidine-associated toxicity. *Int. J. Cancer* **2016**, *138*, 2752–2761. [CrossRef] [PubMed]

6

Focal Recurrent Copy Number Alterations Characterize Disease Relapse in High Grade Serous Ovarian Cancer Patients with Good Clinical Prognosis

Matteo Dugo [1,*,†], Andrea Devecchi [1,†], Loris De Cecco [1], Erika Cecchin [2], Delia Mezzanzanica [3], Marialuisa Sensi [1] and Marina Bagnoli [3,*]

1 Platform of Integrated Biology, Department of Applied Research and Technological Development, Fondazione IRCCS Istituto Nazionale dei Tumori, 20133 Milan, Italy
2 Experimental and Clinical Pharmacology Unit, Centro di Riferimento Oncologico, IRCCS National Cancer Institute, 33081 Aviano, Pordenone, Italy
3 Molecular Therapy Unit, Department of Research, Fondazione IRCCS Istituto Nazionale dei Tumori, 20133 Milan, Italy
* Correspondence: matteo.dugo@istitutotumori.mi.it (M.D.); marina.bagnoli@istitutotumori.mi.it (M.B.)
† Equally contributing authors.

Abstract: High grade serous ovarian cancer (HGSOC) retains high molecular heterogeneity and genomic instability, which currently limit the treatment opportunities. HGSOC patients receiving complete cytoreduction (R0) at primary surgery and platinum-based therapy may unevenly experience early disease relapse, in spite of their clinically favorable prognosis. To identify distinctive traits of the genomic landscape guiding tumor progression, we focused on the R0 patients of The Cancer Genome Atlas (TCGA) ovarian serous cystadenocarcinoma (TCGA-OV) dataset and classified them according to their time to relapse (TTR) from surgery. We included in the study two groups of R0-TCGA patients experiencing substantially different outcome: Resistant (R; TTR $\leq$ 12 months; n = 11) and frankly Sensitive (fS; TTR $\geq$ 24 months; n = 16). We performed an integrated clinical, RNA-Sequencing, exome and somatic copy number alteration (sCNA) data analysis. No significant differences in mutational landscape were detected, although the lack of BRCA-related mutational signature characterized the R group. Focal sCNA analysis showed a higher frequency of amplification in R group and deletions in fS group respectively, involving cytobands not commonly detected by recurrent sCNA analysis. Functional analysis of focal sCNA with a concordantly altered gene expression identified in R group a gain in Notch, and interferon signaling and fatty acid metabolism. We are aware of the constraints related to the low number of OC cases analyzed. It is worth noting, however, that the sCNA identified in this exploratory analysis and characterizing Pt-resistance are novel, deserving validation in a wider cohort of patients achieving complete surgical debulking.

Keywords: ovarian cancer; platinum resistance; focal copy number alterations; whole exome sequencing

---

1. Introduction

High grade serous ovarian cancer (HGSOC) is the most common and lethal epithelial ovarian cancer (EOC) subtype, causing 70–80% of ovarian cancer deaths worldwide [1]. Due to the lack of specific symptoms it is generally diagnosed at advanced stages when it has diffusely metastasized into the peritoneal cavity. Standard treatment includes aggressive primary debulking surgery (PDS) followed by platinum (Pt)-based therapy; but, despite the improvement of surgical approaches and drug development, survival rate has changed little in the last decades [2].

Pt-based therapy remains the cornerstone treatment type and, currently, *BRCA1/2* mutation status is the only biomarker that allows up-front identification of patients with Pt-sensitive or resistant disease [3]. As a consequence, around 30% of patients undergoing Pt-based chemotherapy do not respond to treatment. Also, around 80% of those patients achieving complete response will relapse with a median progression-free survival of 18 months, developing a disease that progressively becomes Pt-resistant, a largely incurable state [2,3].

The opportunity to effectively treat and control HGSOC progression is limited by tumor heterogeneity and genomic instability. HGSOC following p53 mutation undergo multiple sequential mutational processes that shape a complex genome, strongly dominated by somatic copy number aberrations (sCNA). As a result, HGSOC like other CNA driven tumors, as esophageal cancer, non-small-cell lung cancer and triple negative breast cancer, have a low frequency of recurrent oncogenic mutations and a few recurrent sCNA [4]. These multiple mutational forces acting on HGSOC cause difficulties in the identification of targetable genetic lesion(s).

At present, no residual tumor (R0) after PDS is the most important prognostic factor for survival in advanced stage disease [2]. Analyzing clinical data of The Cancer Genome Atlas (TCGA) ovarian serous cystadenocarcinoma (TCGA-OV) we observed that in the group of patients experiencing early relapse were included also those who received optimal clinical treatment (Pt-based therapy and no residual disease after PDS) supporting the notion that intrinsic characteristic(s) of the tumor play a major role in the lack of responsiveness.

The aim of the present pilot study is to decipher the genomic landscape characterizing the highly selected cohort of HGSOC patients who experienced an early relapse, in spite of their expected favorable outcome as assessed by clinical parameters.

2. Materials and Methods

2.1. Data Source and Samples Selection

Mutational and copy number data of TCGA-OV samples were downloaded from the Broad Institute Firehose web portal (https://gdac.broadinstitute.org/) with data version 2016_01_28. Clinical data were obtained from the ovarian cancer landmark paper [5]. RNA-Seq raw counts data were obtained from the Genomic Data Commons data portal (https://portal.gdc.cancer.gov/) with accession date 12th March 2019.

For genomic analyses we selected patients with: (i) no residual disease (R0) after PDS; (ii) whole-exome sequencing data available; (iii) sCNA data available; (iv) a follow-up time $\geq$ 12 months. Forty-eight patients having these characteristics were then classified according to their time to relapse (TTR). Since the time of end-of-treatment was not recorded, the disease-free interval was calculated from the date of surgery. Patients were categorized on the basis of disease-free period length and we identified two subgroups having very different TTR: the refractory/resistant (R) group with TTR $\leq$ 12 months (n = 11), and the frankly Sensitive (fS) groups with TTR $\geq$ 24 months (n = 16). These 27 patients (5.9% of the entire TCGA-OV cohort) constitute the TCGA-OV27 cohort, analyzed in the present study. All analyses described in the following sections were performed in the R environment version 3.5.2.

2.2. RNA-Seq Data Analysis

RNA-Seq data were available for 23 patients (9 R and 14 fS) of the TCGA-OV27 dataset. Raw read counts were normalized using the Trimmed Mean of M-values (TMM) method [6], implemented in the edgeR Bioconductor package [7]. TMM estimates a scaling factor used to reduce technical bias between samples due to differences in library size. Normalized data were then filtered removing genes with at least 1 count per million reads in less than 5% of samples. The final dataset included

23391 unique genes. Differential expression between R and fS was performed using the limma/voom pipeline [8]. p-values were corrected for multiple testing using the Benjamini–Hochberg false discovery rate (FDR) method. Ensembl gene IDs were associated to HUGO gene symbols using the GENCODE v22 annotation. Gene Set Enrichment Analysis [9] between R and fS was performed using the Fast Gene Set Enrichment Analysis (fgsea) package ranking genes according to the t-statistic obtained with limma. Gene sets of the "Hallmark" collection from the Molecular Signatures Database (MSigDB, http://software.broadinstitute.org/gsea/msigdb/) were tested. Gene sets with an FDR < 0.05 were considered significant.

2.3. Mutational Data Analysis

Mutation Annotation Format (MAF) files used to store somatic variants detected were summarized, analyzed, annotated, and visualized using the maftools Bioconductor package [10]. Only variants assumed to have high or moderate (disruptive) impact in the protein, probably causing protein truncation, loss of function or triggering nonsense mediated decay were included in the analysis of most frequently mutated genes. For the calculation of tumor mutational load we considered both high/moderate impact mutation and all somatic mutations.

The DeconstructSigs package [11] was used to perform the mutational signature analysis. This tool evaluates the contribution of 30 signatures reported in COSMIC (https://cancer.sanger.ac.uk/cosmic/signatures) [12] to the mutational profile of each sample. Mutational signatures were calculated considering all somatic mutations in a given sample. The obtained signature scores were then analyzed in association with sensitivity class using Wilcoxon rank-sum test. Samples were grouped according to the top-5 most contributing mutational signatures using unsupervised hierarchical clustering performed with Euclidean distance and Ward linkage.

To identify mutations associated to sensitivity class we used the clinicalEnrichment function of *maftools* package [10] that performs Fisher's exact tests to identify mutated genes associated with the class of interest. Analysis at the level of oncogenic pathways described in Sanchez-Vega et al. [13] was performed using the *OncogenicPathways* function of *maftools*. For each sample we classified each pathway as mutated if at least one of its genes carried a mutation. We then associated mutated pathways to sensitivity class using Fisher's exact test. The same analysis was repeated using the "Hallmark" gene sets from MSigDB.

2.4. sCNA Data Analysis

Genomic Identification of Significant Targets in Cancer (GISTIC) [14] algorithm was used to analyze sCNA data.

Segmented copy number data were analyzed using GISTIC [14] to identify significantly recurrent sCNA in the whole TCGA-OV27 cohort, independently of sensitivity class. GISTIC output was parsed using the maftools package [10]. In addition to the regions recurrently affected by sCNA, GISTIC provides a gene-level copy number status for all genes of the genome in each sample (all_thresholded.by_genes.txt output file). Thus, we tested the association with sensitivity class both for recurrently amplified or deleted regions (GISTIC FDR < 0.1) and for each single gene. For these analyses amplifications and deletions were analyzed separately. For amplifications, a region was assigned a value of 1 if amplified or 0 if the region was not altered or deleted. The same criterion was applied to deletions. The binary amplification and deletion data were then analyzed in relation to sensitivity class using Fisher's exact test. p-values were corrected for multiple testing using the Benjamini-Hochberg FDR method.

Per sample genomic instability was calculated according to: (i) The number of segments in the segmented copy number data; (ii) the total number of genes with a copy number alteration; (iii) the sum of deleted or amplified genes. Association between genomic instability and sensitivity class was assessed by Wilcoxon rank-sum test.

2.5. Statistical Power and Sample Size Calculation

The statistical power for Fisher's exact test applied to the TCGA-OV27 cohort for mutational and sCNA data analyses was calculated using the power2x2 function of the exact2x2 R package. From TCGA-OV27 data we observed that the genes mostly associated to the phenotype of interest were altered (mutated, amplified or deleted) in 27% and 94% of R and fS patients, respectively. Considering these proportions and hypothesizing to test 20,000 genes, the present study has a statistical power of 2.4% of detecting at least one significant finding at an FDR threshold of 5%. To achieve a power of 80% at the same FDR threshold at least 31 patients per group are required. This sample size was calculated using the ss2x2 function of the R-package.

2.6. Integrated sCNA and RNA-Seq Functional Analysis

Functional analysis was carried out on a subset of genes that showed coherent copy number status and differential expression in R compared to fS patients. Over-representation of molecular and cellular functions in the list of selected genes was carried out using: (i) Reactome canonical pathways gene sets from the C2 collection of MSigDB (http://software.broadinstitute.org/gsea/msigdb/annotate.jsp) to map the genes in known functional pathways; (ii) Ingenuity® Pathway Analysis (IPA®, Qiagen; Bioinformatics, Redwood City, CA, USA; http://www.qiagen.com/ingenuity) to derive predictions about the activation status. Enrichments with an FDR < 0.05 were considered statistically significant.

3. Results

From TCGA-OV dataset we selected patients with no residual disease (R0) after PDS with WES and sCNA data available and with a follow-up time ≥ 12 months.

Then, considering that the subgroup of R0 patients is expected to have a good prognosis, for the pilot analysis we further refined the cohort selecting Resistant (R, n = 11) with an unfavorable outcome and frankly Sensitive (fS, n = 16) patients. Overall 27 patients, the TCGA-OV27 cohort, were included in the study and their associated clinical data are summarized in Table 1.

Table 1. Clinical characteristics of The Cancer Genome Atlas (TCGA) ovarian serous cystadenocarcinoma (TCGA-OV) 27 cohort.

	Total (n = 27)	R (n = 11)	Fs (n = 16)
		Stage	
III	23	9	14
IV	4	2	2
		Grading	
G2	3	0	3
G3	23	10	13
NA	1	1	0
		Relapse	
yes	18	11	7
no	9	0	9

R = Resistant; fS = frankly Sensitive.

Transcriptomic analysis of TCGA-OV27 cohort did not reveal differentially expressed genes between R and fS patients at an FDR < 0.05. However, when we considered a nominal p-value < 0.05 and a fold-change of 2, 210 and 214 genes were down- and up-regulated respectively, in R patients. Comparison of the two groups using GSEA highlighted 29 hallmark gene sets significantly enriched in one of the two groups at an FDR < 0.05. (Figure S1). In particular, 1 gene set related to oxidative phosphorylation was positively enriched in fS patients while the remaining 28 gene sets were positively enriched in the R group. Overall, gene sets positively enriched in R patients are supporting of a more aggressive phenotype for this subset of tumors but did not highlighted specific mechanisms possibly associated with Pt-resistance.

3.1. *Mutational Landscape of TCGA-OV27 Cohort*

To identify genomic features associated with early relapse we then analyzed mutational data of the selected cohort. Consistent with genome landscape studies of the whole TCGA-OV cohort and most recent studies on ovarian cancer [15,16], p53 is mutated in 89% of TCGA-OV27 patients (Figure 1). Among the prevalent mutated genes we found, as expected, *CDK12*, *NF1*, and *RB1*, together with *CSMD1*, *NOTCH4*, and *TMEM132D* genes, which seem to be a specific trait of this cohort. Considering genes mutated in at least three patients we did not observe any significantly unbalanced distribution of these predominantly mutated genes within R/fS classes (Figure 1A).

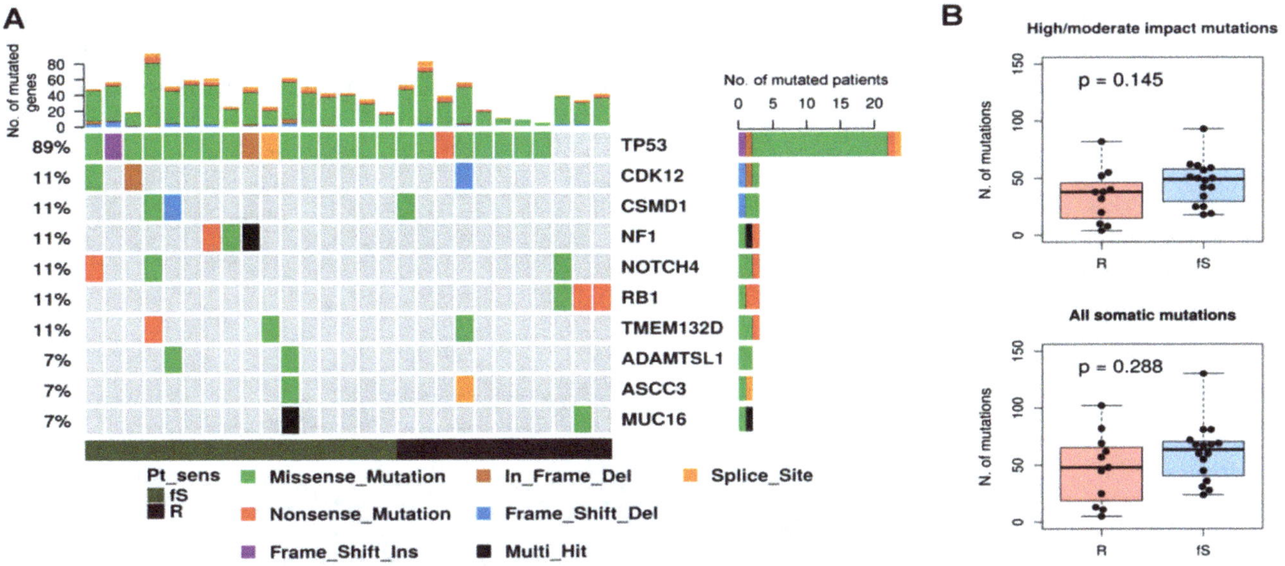

Figure 1. Mutational spectrum of TCGA-OV27 samples. (**A**) Oncoplot of the top-10 most frequently mutated genes in cytoreduction (R0) patients of the TCGA-OV27 dataset, grouped according to sensitivity class. Each column represents a sample and each row a different gene. Colored squares show mutated genes, while grey squares show no mutated genes. Different type of mutations are colored according to the variant type as indicated in the legend at the bottom. Genes annotated as "Multi_Hit" have more than one mutation in the same sample. The barplot at the top shows the number of mutated genes for each patient colored according to the mutation type. The barplot on the right reports the number of mutated patients for each gene, colored according to the mutation type. (**B**) Boxplot showing the tumor mutational load of R and fS samples, calculated both considering only mutations with high/moderate impact (upper panel) or all somatic mutations (lower panel). *P*-value was calculated by Wilcoxon rank-sum test.

We compared the tumor mutational load in the two sensitivity classes considering either only mutations with high/moderate impact (Figure 1B upper panel) or all somatic mutations (Figure 1B lower panel); even if fS patients tend to have a slightly higher number of mutations, we did not detect significant differences between the two classes.

Overall, we identified in at least one sample 1115 variants with high/moderate impact affecting 1005 unique genes. To reduce the high inter-patient heterogeneity of mutational data we grouped genes into pathways and compared pathways mutated in R or fS patients. For this analysis we considered 50 gene sets from the 'Hallmark' collection of MSigDB database that summarize well-defined biological states or processes and ten canonical oncogenic pathways [13]. We called a pathway mutated if at least one of its genes was mutated. According to our analysis, none of the pathways tested was found to be significantly associated to sensitivity class, even at a less stringent nominal p-value < 0.05 (Tables S1 and S2).

3.2. *Mutational Signatures of TCGA-OV27 Cohort*

Basing on the relative frequency of somatic base substitution events, 30 distinct mutational signatures, reflecting distinct mutational process associated with specific biological status and/or altered functions have been described (COSMIC; https://cancer.sanger.ac.uk/cosmic/signatures) [12]. These mutational signatures were analyzed in the TCGA-OV27 cohort considering all somatic variants independently of their functional consequences. A hierarchical clustering based on the scores of the five most represented mutational signatures identified two major clusters mainly driven by different contribution of Signature 1 (related to endogenous mutational processes) and Signature 3 (related to defective homologous repair of double-strand DNA break). Even if the association between these clusters and sensitivity was not significant (Fisher's exact test p-value $= 0.054$), we observed a clear trend of enrichment of R patients in the cluster driven by Signature 1 and an enrichment of fS patients in the cluster driven by Signature 3 (Figure 2). The comparison of each signature's score between the two classes is reported in Table S3 and a nominal p-value < 0.05 (Wilcoxon rank-sum test) was observed for Signature 3 only.

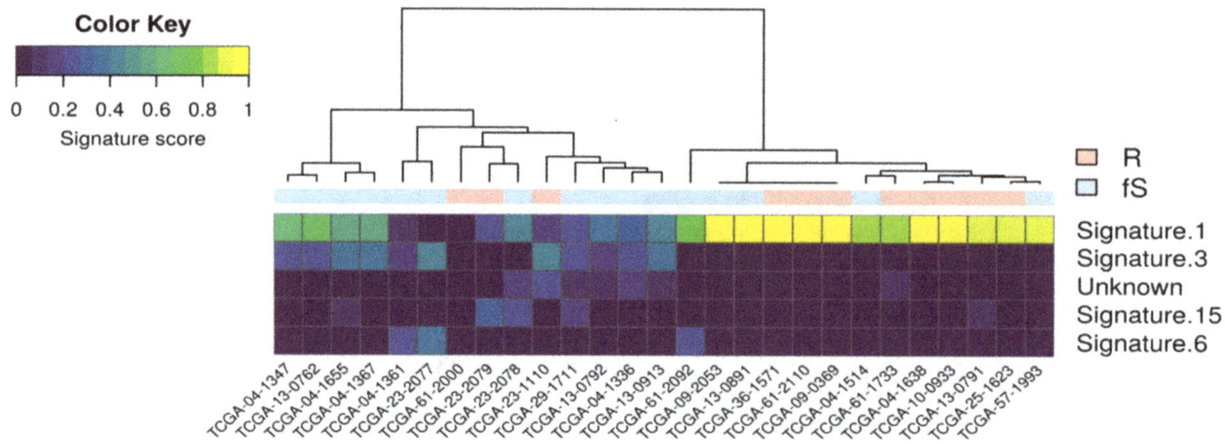

Figure 2. Mutational signatures in TCGA-OV27 cohort. Heatmap showing the contribution of the top-5 most represented COSMIC signatures in the mutational profiles of TCGA-OV27 samples.

3.3. *Genomic Instability and sCNA Landscape of TCGA-OV27 Cohort*

On the basis of recent studies defining sCNA as the prevalent genomic alteration affecting HGSOC [17], we assessed whether R or fS patients of our selected cohort could be distinguished by specific sCNA.

We used sCNA data to obtain a measure of genomic instability for each patient, using different approaches all based on the GISTIC algorithm. We firstly considered the number of regions with different copy number (number of segments; Figure 3A), with the assumption that a higher number of segments should describe a more fragmented (instable) genome. We next considered within each sample either the total number of genes affected by sCNA (Figure 3B) or, separately, the total number of amplified or deleted genes (Figure 3C,D). Overall, we observed a trend for higher sCNA in fS compared to R patients. This trend was significant when we considered the number of genes affected by aberrations in general (Wilcoxon rank-sum test p-value $= 0.03$) and this difference was mainly driven by deletions (Wilcoxon rank-sum test p-value $= 0.034$).

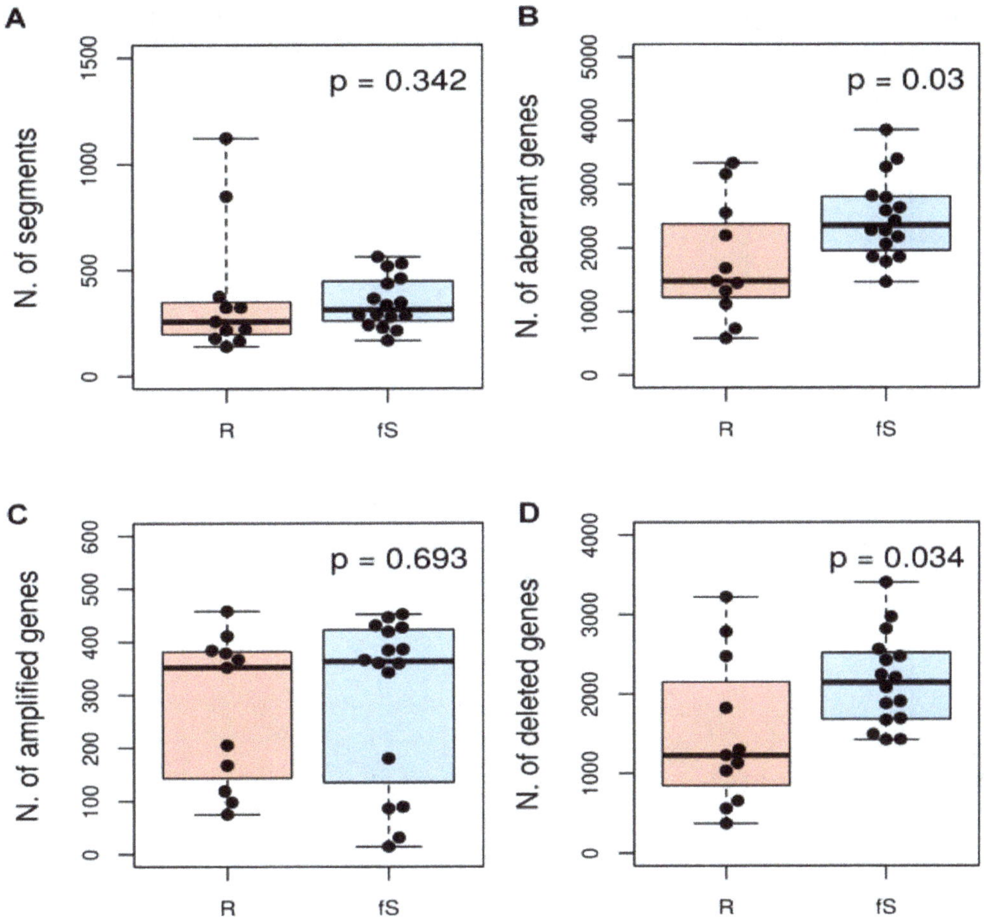

Figure 3. Association between genomic instability and sensitivity class in TCGA-OV27 dataset. As measure of genomic instability for each sample we considered: (**A**) the number of segments that represents the number of regions with different copy number levels within a genome; (**B**) the total number of amplified or deleted genes; the total number of amplified genes only (**C**) or deleted genes only (**D**). *P*-values are according to Wilcoxon rank-sum test.

To identify recurrent sCNA we applied GISTIC to copy number data of the TCGA-OV27 cohort. We identified 10 regions significantly amplified and 12 regions significantly deleted across samples (Figure 4A). All sCNA events, as well as detail in category, chromosome location genes in the region and cytobands are in Table S4.

The frequency plot distribution of sCNA detected in the TCGA-OV27 cohort (Figure 4B), shows that 3q26.2 gain, 17q11.2, 19p13.3, and 4q34.3 loss were the most frequently altered regions (>80% of patients). The frequency of samples positive for the recurrently amplified or deleted regions in the two subgroups (R and fS) of patients is showed in Figure S2. However, when we compared the frequency of the recurrent sCNA identified by GISTIC between the two sensitivity classes, no significant association to Pt-sensitivity was observed (Table S5).

We repeated the analysis of sCNA at the gene-level, considering 23110 amplified or deleted genes. Due to the low number of samples available for each class, no significant findings were detected after multiple-testing correction, while we detected 1270 genes more frequently altered at a nominal p-value < 0.05 (Fisher's exact test) in R or fS patients (166 amplified and 1104 genes deleted, Table S6). Considering the explorative nature of this pilot study, we further explored the genes list being aware of the limitations associated with analysis of small group of patients and the high risk of detecting false positive hits (see Materials and Methods, Section 2.5 for power calculation of the present study). Among these genes we observed that amplifications were more frequently detected in R rather than in fS group (median percentage of patients with amplified genes: 57% in R vs 12% in fS; Range: 36–82% in

R group, 0–37% in fS group). On the other side deletions were more frequently detected in fS patients (median percentage of patients with deleted genes: 15% in R vs 62% in fS group; Range: 0–63% in R group, 19–87% in fS group).

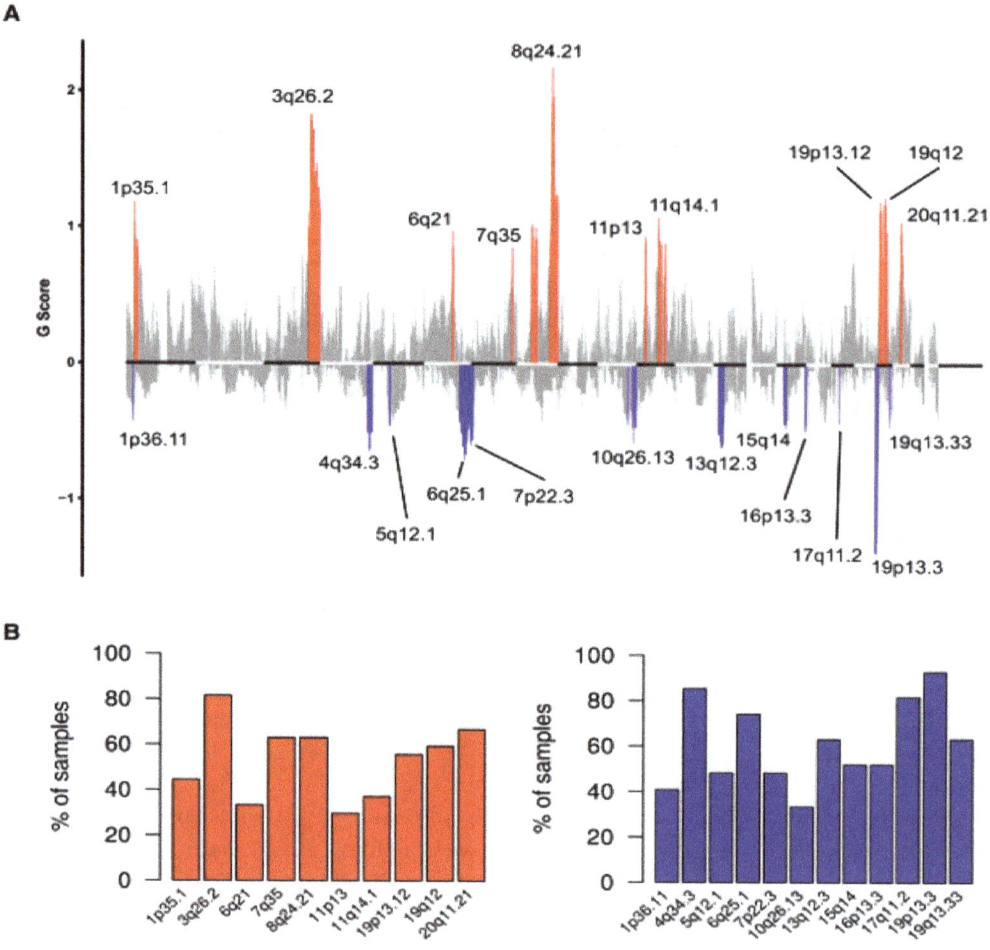

Figure 4. Recurrent somatic copy number alterations (sCNA) in R0 patients of TCGA-OV27 cohort. (**A**) Plot of G scores (defined as the amplitude of the copy number multiplied by its frequency across samples) calculated by Genomic Identification of Significant Targets in Cancer (GISTIC) for genomic regions recurrently amplified (red) or deleted (blue) in the TCGA-OV27 dataset, at an FDR < 0.1. (**B**) Barplot showing the frequency of samples positive for the recurrently amplified (left) or deleted (right) regions identified by GISTIC.

3.4. Association between sCNA and Altered Gene/Pathways Expression in Pt-Sensitivity Classes

We investigated the relationships between sCNA, alteration of genes' expression and relevant functional pathways possibly affected by these alterations.

The complete decision tree for gene selection is shown in Figure 5A. We first removed genes that were not assessed by RNA-Seq from the list of 1270 genes significantly amplified or deleted in R or fS patients. We next filtered this list according to the observed relative frequency of amplification or deletion for each sensitivity class. Finally, we removed genes whose log2 fold change (FC) was not compatible with its copy number status (e.g., a gene preferentially amplified but down-regulated in R group) and among the concordant genes we selected those with a log2 FC of at least 0.5 between R and fS patients. The final gene list included 128 genes (Table S7), consisting of 16 genes preferentially amplified and up-regulated in R group and 112 genes more frequently deleted and down-regulated in fS patients. The relative frequency of associated altered cytobands is reported in Figure 5B. Interestingly, these cytobands were not included among the significantly recurrent aberrant regions identified by GISTIC.

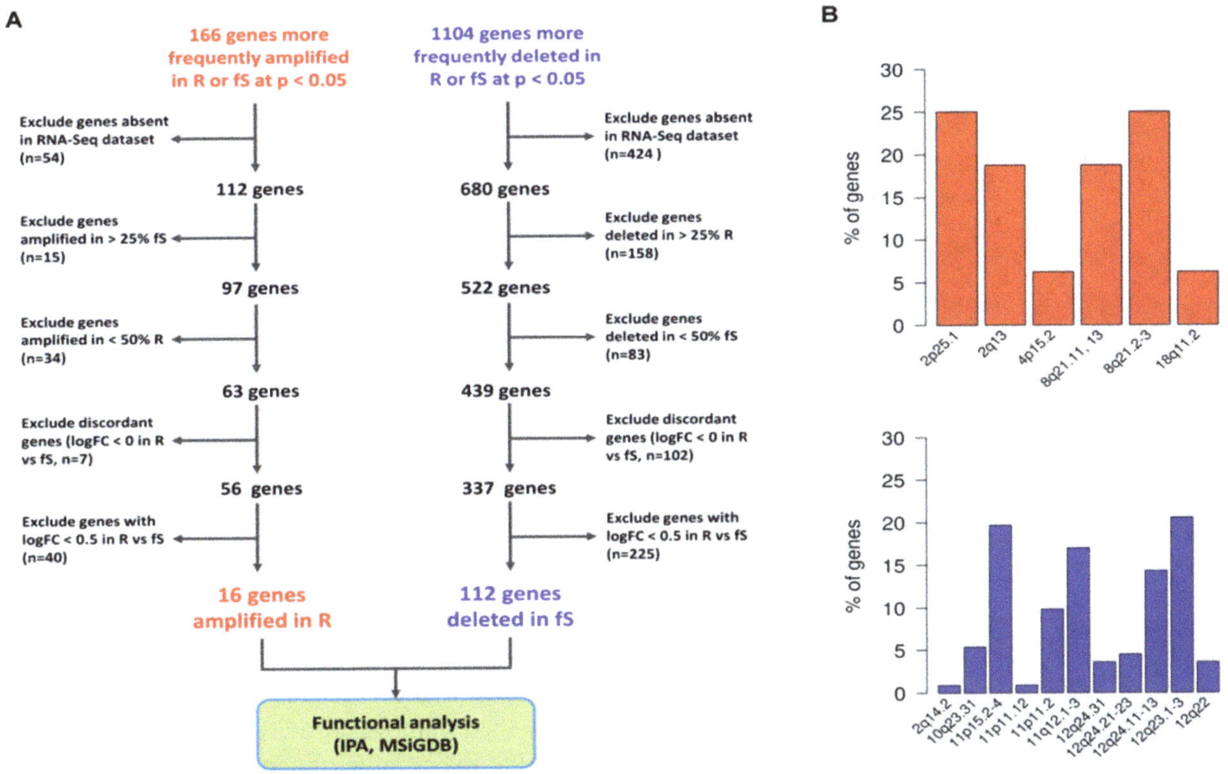

Figure 5. Association between sCNA and altered gene expression in Pt-sensitivity classes. (**A**) Selection of significant focal sCNA with concordant alteration of gene expression. Gene expression was assessed by RNA-sequencing (RNASeq) data, and for each altered gene, the logFC expression ratio of R vs fS patients was calculated. The workflow guiding selection of both amplified and deleted genes with concordant expression is shown. (**B**) Cytobands associated with significant sCNA and altered gene expression. In the plot are reported the cytobands affected by significant amplification (upper panel, red bars) and deletions (lower panel, blue bars). For each type of alteration, the relative frequency of each cytoband affected is shown.

To map the 128 altered genes into known functional pathways we firstly assessed over-representation of Reactome canonical pathways included in the C2 gene set collection of MSiGDB. Seven gene sets, related to interferon (IFN) and cytokine signaling, fatty acid and lipid metabolism, were found significantly over-represented (FDR < 0.05) and 23 out of the 128 genes overlapped with at least one of them (Figure 6).

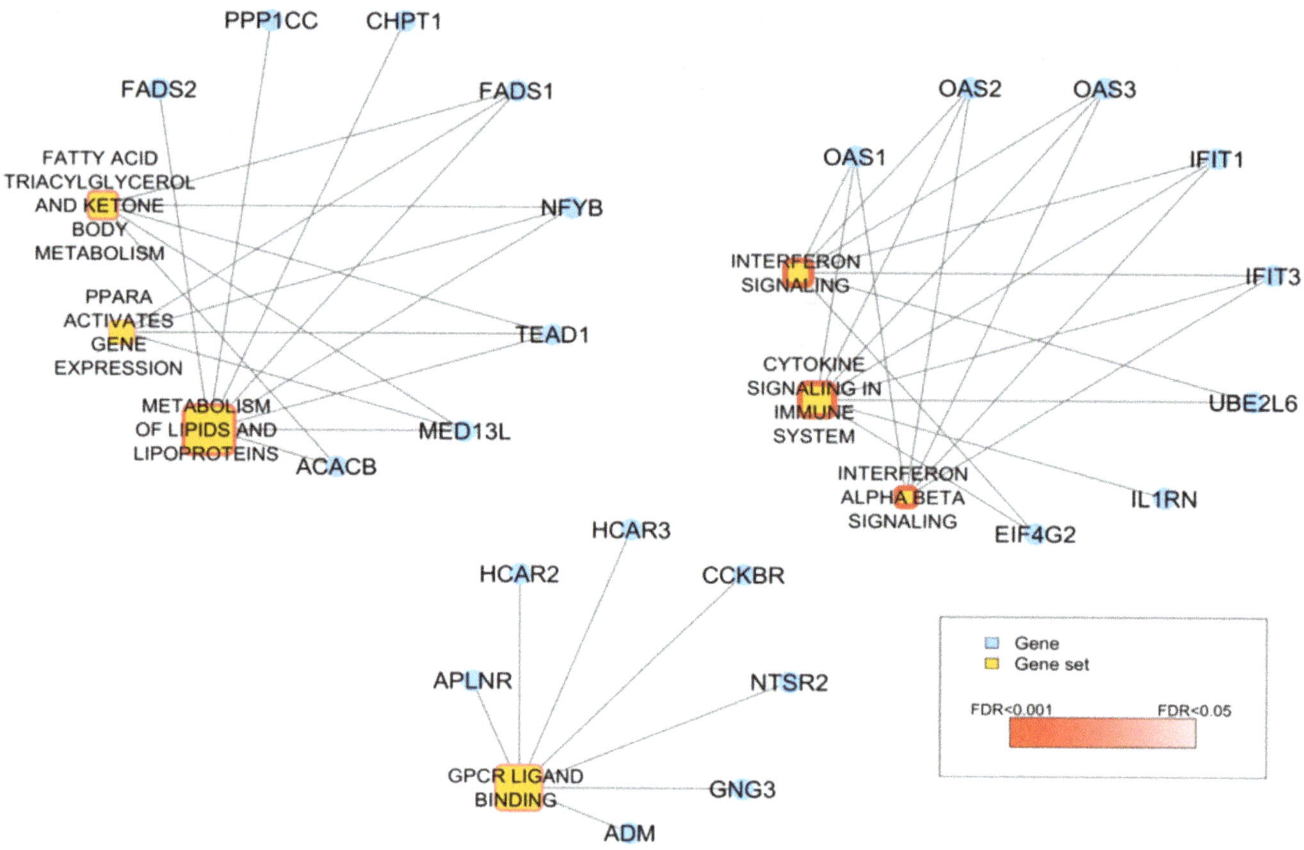

Figure 6. Over-representation analysis of the 128 genes with concordant sCNA and expression. Network showing the 7 Reactome gene sets significantly over-represented in the list of 128 genes. Yellow nodes represent gene sets and the size of the node is proportional to the number of genes catalogued in the gene set. The significance of the over-representation is represented by a dark-to-light red color scale. Blue nodes represent genes and are connected to a gene set if they are among its gene members.

Then, to examine biological relationship and investigate functional effects related to sCNA of these 128 genes, we run Ingenuity Pathway Analysis. Canonical pathways analysis confirmed a significant modulation in IFN signaling, mostly related to *IFIT* and *OAS2* genes deletion, and fatty acid metabolism dependent on alterations in desaturase genes (FADS1 and FADS2). We also observed significant modulation of G-alpha proteins signaling pathways (Table 2). The most significant Regulatory Networks affected by the altered gene expression are listed in Table 3.

Table 2. Canonical Pathways identified by Ingenuity® Pathway Analysis (IPA).

Ingenuity Canonical Pathways	-Log(*p*-Value)	Genes
Interferon signaling	2.87	*OAS1, IFIT1, IFIT3*
Oleate biosynthesis II (animals)	2.8	*FADS1, FADS2*
Graft-versus-host Disease signaling	2.62	*IL1RN, IL36RN, FAS*
Gαs signaling	2.4	*CNGB3, GNG3, HCAR3, HCAR2*
γ-linolenate biosynthesis II (animals)	2.33	FADS1, FADS2
Gαi signaling	2.15	*APLNR, GNG3, HCAR2, CHRM4*

Table 3. Top regulatory networks identified by IPA. Genes detected in the TCGA-OV27 cohort are shown in bold.

Top Diseases and Functions	Molecules in Network	Score	Focus Molecules
Dermatological diseases and conditions, Organismal injury and abnormalities, immunological disease	**ACTA2, ADM, APLNR**, Akt, **CCKBR, CD6**, ERK, ERK1/2, **FAS, GLI2, HCAR2, IFIT1, IFIT3, IL1RN, ILK,** Interferon alpha, Jnk, **MAPK8IP1**, Mek, NFkB (complex), **OAS1, OAS2, OAS3**, P38 MAPK, PI3K (family), **PPP1CC**, Raf, SH2B3, **SLC15A3, SLC43A3,** TCR, **TRIM22, UBE2L6, UNG, WEE1**	44	24
Gastrointestinal disease, organismal injury and abnormalities, cell death and survival	**ADM, AHNAK,** ATG7, C3, CFTR, CLDN7, CST5, CTSS, **DENND5**A, DUSP10, **FADS1, FADS2**, HAS1, **HCAR3**, HLA-B, IFNGR1, IL13, IL1B, **IL36RN**, LBP, MAFF, **MS4A4A**, NFKBIE, **NRIP3, PQLC3, SEL1L3, SLC43A3,** SMARCA4, **STK33, STMN2, SYT7**, TNF, TP63, **TUB, WWP1**	27	17
Gene expression, cell cycle, cellular growth and proliferation	ACAD10, BAG1, CBS/CBSL, CCNB2, **CDK17, CORO1C**, CTR9, **DCHS1**, ESR1, **FGD6, GREB1**, HAUS8, HDAC1, HLTF, LTB, **NEDD1, NFYB**, NR1D1, **NR2C1**, NR3C1, NUPR1, PLK1, PRMT6, **SCUBE2,** SMARCE1, SMYD2, SMYD3, SP1, **TBX3, TEAD1**, TFAP2C, TNFAIP6, **TRAFD1,** YWHAG, estrogen receptor	19	13
Cellular development, cellular growth and proliferation, cell cycle	CCND1, CDCA2, CDK5, CHD7, **CMKLR1,** Ctbp, **DRAM1, E2F5**, ERBB2, **GCN1, HCAR1, HEY1,** JAG1, LINC-ROR, **LIPF**, MAFB, **MED13L**, NOTCH2, NOTCH4, **NUAK1,** NUMB, OIP5-AS1, PCLAF, PPARGC1A, RFC1, **RMST**, RUNX3, SLC16A1, SMTN, SOX2, SUV39H1, **TMEM119, TMPO**, TP53, let-7a-5p	17	12
Gene expression, cell signaling, cellular development	26s Proteasome, **ACACB, ACTA2**, AR, **ASCL1, ATP6V0D2,** BAG1, CD55, CDK5, CDKN1C, **CHRM4, CHST1**, CKAP4, DAB2, DLL4, FSH, GBP1, H2AFY, HES1, **HRK**, IER3, **LYVE1**, Lh, MED12, MTOR, NOTCH1, PGR, PRKD1, PRKD2, SMARCE1, **SMTNL1, SSH1**, TOP1, **TP53I11**, YWHAB	17	12
DNA replication, recombination, and repair, cell morphology, cellular function and maintenance	ACTG1, **CHPT1**, CLOCK, DDX11, DDX5, **DTX4, EIF4G2**, EP300, **FEN1**, GATA1, **HBB**, HNRNPC, HNRNPD, HNRNPU, HUS1, MAX, MYB, **OAS3**, OTUB1, **PARPBP,** PCLAF, PCNA, RAD51, RAD9A, RFC1, RHOA, Rnr, SATB1, **TMEM241**, TP53BP1, **TRPV4, USP44, UTP20**, XRN2, YBX1	15	11

The top-scoring Network (Dermatological Diseases and Conditions, Organismal Injury and Abnormalities, Immunological Disease) whose graphical representation is reported in Figure 7, shows a number of molecular relationships centered on interferon, in accordance with previously described pathway analysis. Interestingly, among the top regulatory networks we also identified a number of networks whose functions are mainly related to cell growth and proliferation and cell development. Accordingly, Cellular Development, Cell Morphology, Cellular Growth and Proliferation were the most significantly modulated Molecular Cell Function (Table S8), while Invasion, Migration and Cell Movement were the only Disease and Functions significantly predicted to be increased in R patients (Table S9).

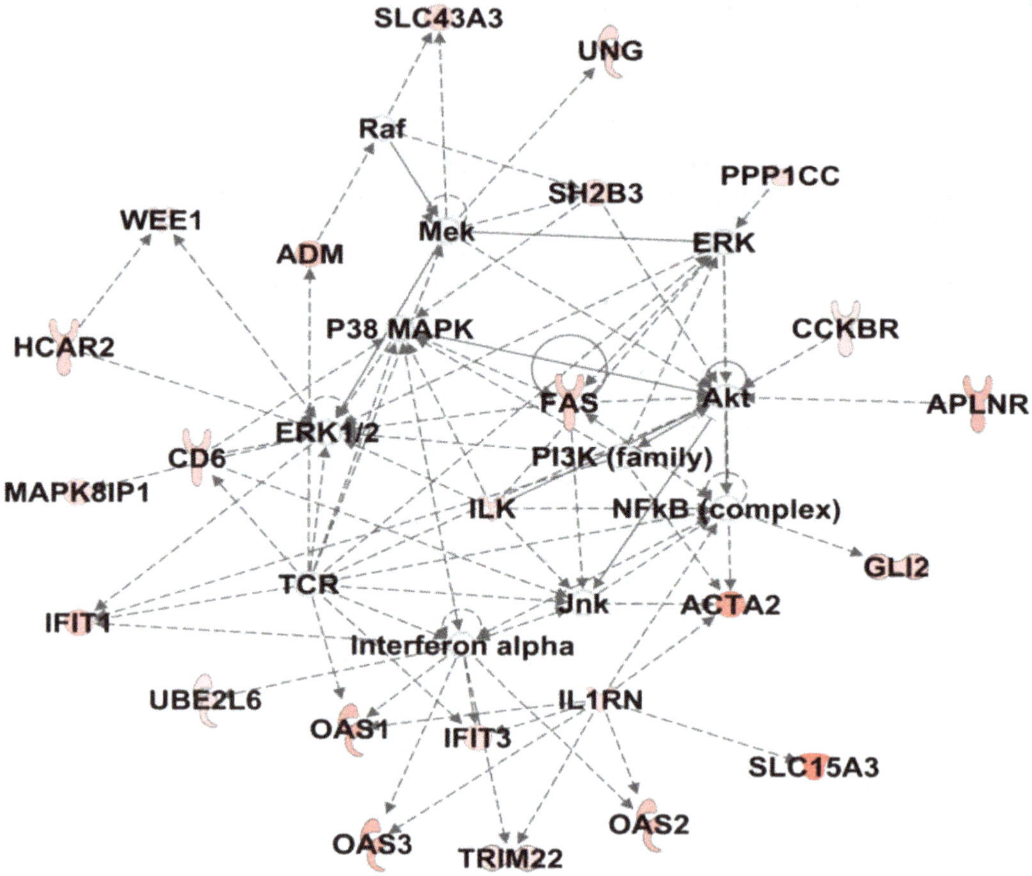

Figure 7. IPA analysis of the 128 significantly altered genes. The top-scoring regulatory network built from Core Analysis and named Dermatological Diseases and Conditions, Organismal Injury and Abnormalities, Immunological Disease is shown. Colored nodes are the genes of the dataset participating to the network.

4. Discussion

The relationship between post-operative residual tumor burden and clinical outcome is consolidated for ovarian cancer [2,18]. Consequently, the concept of optimal cytoreduction is evolving along time and, although the metric for optimal debulking is still defined as tumor nodules not greater than 1 cm, the literature and meta-data analysis clearly show that R0 patients, those with no residual tumor after primary surgery, have the best overall outcome. Nevertheless, some of those R0 patients with an expected favorable clinical outcome still experience early disease relapse, due to intrinsic molecular characteristics of their tumors. We focused our attention on this small, poorly characterized subgroup of patients with an unexpectedly unfavorable prognosis (R patients; PFS < 12 months from surgery). To possibly identify molecular traits associated with Pt-resistant disease in R0 patients we analyzed their genomic portrait in comparison to those of R0 patients with good prognosis (fS patients; PFS > 24 months from surgery).

The approach to compare the gene expression of two series of patients with marked opposite outcomes, with the assumption that this selection may enhance discovering relevant molecular pathways associated to sensitivity to pt- or cetuximab/pt-based treatment was previously applied with some success to small cohorts of gastric [19] and head and neck cancers [20]. Comparison of transcriptomes in the two R0 HGSOC Pt-sensitivity classes, showed in R patients modifications that could be commonly referred to an increased aggressiveness of tumors but were not directly suggestive of specific actionable alterations. Similarly, the mutational profile of the R0 cohort did not substantially differ from the overall TCGA study population, where, apart the prevalent p53 mutation, few other genes were commonly mutated and in a small fraction of patients, thus confirming the high mutational heterogeneity of this tumor type. Also, none of these prevalently mutated genes was significantly associated with Pt-sensitivity classes. Interestingly, from the overall analysis of the somatic mutational status we did not observe any enrichment for *BRCA1/2* mutations in the fS group and not all fS patients were characterized by mutational Signature 3 related to defective Homologous Repair of double-strand DNA breaks. These findings are substantially in agreement with recent data obtained on long term survivor ovarian cancer patients [15] where the authors propose that the BRCA-associated signature alone could not be prognostic of Pt-sensitivity in HGSOC. Nevertheless, the analysis of genomic instability in our R0 cohort disclosed a higher number of sCNA in fS patients as compared to R ones. Since genomic instability can be attributed to defects in HR pathway [21] these data are in accordance with the observed enrichment of fS patient in the cluster characterized by mutational Signature 3 and overall support their Pt-sensitivity. This trend appeared to be mainly driven by deletions rather than amplification, in accordance with data obtained from focal (gene-level) sCNA analysis, which described deletions as the prominent event distinctive of the fS group. At the same time these observations confirm that the maintenance of potential oncogenic pro-survival functions is a requirement for Pt-resistance and, concordantly, their inactivation might be an opportunity to overcome Pt-resistance. Noteworthy, the sCNA profile of the R0, fS patients of the TCGA-OV27 cohort appeared to be different from the HR-deficient TCGA-OV cohort [5], possibly because of the specific molecular setting of R0 tumors, which have been shown to be intrinsically different from those ovarian tumors more massively diffused in the peritoneal cavity and less-likely to be completely removed at primary surgery [22].

sCNA are known drivers of HGSOC development and progression [17]. Interestingly, in a recent paper studying the spatial and temporal heterogeneity of HGSOC [23], the authors suggest that in this tumor type the relapsed disease is mostly related to the emergence of pre-existing rather than de-novo clones and observe that sCNA maintain a low level of intra-patient heterogeneity. Therefore, sCNA analysis promises to be an effective strategy to identify cancer-causing genes, which could be used for treatment decisions. Accordingly, Cyclin E (*CCNE1*) amplification is a known trait in ovarian cancers with intact HR. It occurs in around 20% of all HGSOC and since it is mutually exclusive with *BRCA1/2* mutation [24], patients harboring *CCNE1* amplification will not benefit from *PARP*i treatment and will likely be less responsive to Pt treatment [5,17]. Nevertheless, these finding provided the rationale for the development of therapeutic approach that specifically exploit the tumor dependence upon *CCNE1* amplification, for instance by targeting *CDK2* and *AKT* activities [25].

CCNE1 locates on chr19q12 cytoband, which we identified to be amplified in the whole TCGA-OV27 cohort. However, possibly due to the small number of samples analyzed, we did not identify any significant enrichment of 19q12 amplification in the R subgroup of patients and, concordantly, we did not have any evidence about significant enrichment of *CCNE1* amplification in the same subgroup when we performed the analysis at gene-level. Of note, none of the cytobands identified as significantly altered in both R and fS class of R0 patients at gene level is comprised in the recurrent chromosomal aberrations identified and only 5 genes (*FAS, HEY1, SH2B3, TBX3, USP44*) were included in the COSMIC (Catalogue of Somatic Mutations in Cancer) Cancer Gene Census list, suggesting that new information can be acquired with this approach.

Among these newly identified genes, we found *HEY1*, to be amplified in the R group. Interestingly, *HEY1* is a downstream mediator of Notch-dependent signals [26], it has a putative role as oncogene (COSMIC) and its expression was recently associated with an EMT phenotype, increased invasion and cell migration as well as Pt resistance in head and neck cancers [27]. These observations are in agreement with IPA describing a predicted increase in functions (cell growth and proliferation and cell development) overall suggestive of a stemness program. Also, Notch1 signaling pathway has been described to contribute to chemoresistance in ovarian cancer [28], it is a key for maintenance of cancer stem cell in ovarian cancer [29] and the development of new treatment strategies targeting these pathways to control stem-cell replication is a current active field of research.

Pt-resistance is recognized to be a multifactorial event and the search for determinants (genes) guiding response to Pt treatments still continues to be a key issue in ovarian cancer translational research. In this context, it has been proven the involvement of aberrant DNA methylation and modification of histone marks [17,30] in the development of Pt-resistance and a number of synthetically lethal approaches are under investigation, with cell cycle check points (CHK1, Wee1, DNA-PK) and related cyclins inhibitors being among the most promising (see [31,32] for an overview).

To our knowledge, this is the first study of R0 HGSOC that specifically investigates sensitivity to Pt-based therapy by transcriptomics and genomics analyses and biology behind. We are aware that our study has to be considered explorative. The major limit rests in the small number of samples included in the TCGA-OV27 cohort, which account for about 6% of the entire TCGA-OV cohort. This limitation is inherently related to the reduced number of ovarian cancer patients having these clinical characteristics and with full molecular data available. The statistical power of our analyses is constrained to 2.4% by the sample size of the TCGA-OV27 cohort, which should triplicate to endow a statistical significance. Our results should be interpreted with caution. Nevertheless, the overall data presented here, based on tumors with marked opposite treatment outcomes, are suggestive of a specific Pt-resistance molecular trait driven by sCNA, and these observations deserve to be further explored in wider cohort of patients with selected clinical characteristics. If verified and upon appropriate independent validation, it could possibly drive toward the development of a new tool based on the sCNA pattern, which may help clinicians in defining sensitivity to Pt treatment.

Supplementary Materials:
Figure S1: Enrichment plots of hallmark gene sets significantly enriched at an FDR < 0.01. Gene sets were tested against the list of genes ranked according to their differential expression significance and fold change, from the most up-regulated to the most down-regulated in R versus fS. The Gene Ranks column shows the location of the genes of each gene set along the pre-ranked gene list. NES: normalized enrichment score; padj: adjusted p-value (FDR). Figure S2: Barplot showing for each sensitivity class the frequency of samples positive for the recurrently amplified (left panel) or deleted (right panel) regions identified by GISTIC. Table S1. Association between mutated hallmark gene sets and sensitivity class. P-value by Fisher's exact test. FDR: false discovery rate. Table S2. Association between mutated oncogenic pathways and sensitivity class. P-value by Fisher's exact test. FDR: false discovery rate. Table S3. Association between mutational signatures scores of the top-5 most represented COSMIC signatures and sensitivity class. P-value by Wilcoxon rank-sum test. FDR: false discovery rate. Table S4. Recurrently amplified or deleted regions in the TCGA-OV27 dataset identified by GISTIC. Table S5. Association of recurrently amplified or deleted regions identified by GISTIC and sensitivity class. P-value by Fisher's exact test. FDR: false discovery rate. Table S6. Association of copy number status at the gene level and sensitivity class. P-value by Fisher's exact test. Table S7. List of the 128 genes selected after integration of sCNA and RNA-Seq data. Table S8. IPA on 128 genes list. Molecular cell functions significantly modulated Table S9. Prediction of Disease and Function activation state by IPA on 128 genes list.

Author Contributions: Conceptualization: M.D.; M.S. and M.B.; Formal Analysis: M.D., A.D. and M.B.; Data Curation, M.D., A.D. and L.D.C.; Writing—Original Draft Preparation, M.B, M.D., A.D.; Writing—Review and Editing. M.S., D.M., E.C., M.D. and M.B.; Supervision: D.M., M.S. All authors read and approved the final manuscript.

Acknowledgments: We thank Silvana Canevari (Fondazione IRCCS Istituto Nazionale dei Tumori Milano, Italy) for fruitful discussion and critical reading of the manuscript.

References

1. Siegel, R.L.; Miller, K.D.; Jemal, A. Cancer statistics, 2019. *CA Cancer J. Clin.* **2019**, *69*, 7–34. [CrossRef] [PubMed]
2. Jayson, G.C.; Kohn, E.C.; Kitchener, H.C.; Ledermann, J.A. Ovarian cancer. *Lancet* **2014**, *384*, 1376–1388. [CrossRef]

3. Lheureux, S.; Gourley, C.; Vergote, I.; Oza, A.M. Epithelial ovarian cancer. *Lancet* **2019**, *393*, 1240–1253. [CrossRef]
4. Ciriello, G.; Miller, M.L.; Aksoy, B.A.; Senbabaoglu, Y.; Schultz, N.; Sander, C. Emerging landscape of oncogenic signatures across human cancers. *Nat. Genet.* **2013**, *45*, 1127–1133. [CrossRef] [PubMed]
5. Cancer Genome Atlas Research Network. Integrated genomic analyses of ovarian carcinoma. *Nature* **2011**, *474*, 609–615. [CrossRef]
6. Robinson, M.D.; Oshlack, A. A scaling normalization method for differential expression analysis of RNA-seq data. *Genome Biol.* **2010**, *11*, R25. [CrossRef] [PubMed]
7. Robinson, M.D.; McCarthy, D.J.; Smyth, G.K. edgeR: A Bioconductor package for differential expression analysis of digital gene expression data. *Bioinformatics* **2010**, *26*, 139–140. [CrossRef]
8. Law, C.W.; Chen, Y.; Shi, W.; Smyth, G.K. voom: Precision weights unlock linear model analysis tools for RNA-seq read counts. *Genome Biol.* **2014**, *15*, R29. [CrossRef]
9. Subramanian, A.; Tamayo, P.; Mootha, V.K.; Mukherjee, S.; Ebert, B.L.; Gillette, M.A.; Paulovich, A.; Pomeroy, S.L.; Golub, T.R.; Lander, E.S.; et al. Gene set enrichment analysis: A knowledge-based approach for interpreting genome-wide expression profiles. *Proc. Natl. Acad. Sci. USA* **2005**, *102*, 17745–17750. [CrossRef]
10. Mayakonda, A.; Lin, D.C.; Assenov, Y.; Plass, C.; Koeffler, H.P. Maftools: Efficient and comprehensive analysis of somatic variants in cancer. *Genome Res.* **2018**, *28*, 1747–1756. [CrossRef]
11. Rosenthal, R.; McGranahan, N.; Herrero, J.; Taylor, B.S.; Swanton, C. DeconstructSigs: Delineating mutational processes in single tumors distinguishes DNA repair deficiencies and patterns of carcinoma evolution. *Genome Biol.* **2016**, *17*, 31. [CrossRef] [PubMed]
12. Alexandrov, L.B.; Nik-Zainal, S.; Wedge, D.C.; Aparicio, S.A.; Behjati, S.; Biankin, A.V.; Bignell, G.R.; Bolli, N.; Borg, A.; Borresen-Dale, A.L.; et al. Signatures of mutational processes in human cancer. *Nature* **2013**, *500*, 415–421. [CrossRef] [PubMed]
13. Sanchez-Vega, F.; Mina, M.; Armenia, J.; Chatila, W.K.; Luna, A.; La, K.C.; Dimitriadoy, S.; Liu, D.L.; Kantheti, H.S.; Saghafinia, S.; et al. Oncogenic signaling pathways in The Cancer Genome Atlas. *Cell* **2018**, *173*, 321–337. [CrossRef] [PubMed]
14. Mermel, C.H.; Schumacher, S.E.; Hill, B.; Meyerson, M.L.; Beroukhim, R.; Getz, G. GISTIC2.0 facilitates sensitive and confident localization of the targets of focal somatic copy-number alteration in human cancers. *Genome Biol.* **2011**, *12*, R41. [CrossRef] [PubMed]
15. Yang, S.Y.C.; Lheureux, S.; Karakasis, K.; Burnier, J.V.; Bruce, J.P.; Clouthier, D.L.; Danesh, A.; Quevedo, R.; Dowar, M.; Hanna, Y.; et al. Landscape of genomic alterations in high-grade serous ovarian cancer from exceptional long- and short-term survivors. *Genome Med.* **2018**, *10*, 81. [CrossRef] [PubMed]
16. Macintyre, G.; Goranova, T.E.; De, S.D.; Ennis, D.; Piskorz, A.M.; Eldridge, M.; Sie, D.; Lewsley, L.A.; Hanif, A.; Wilson, C.; et al. Copy number signatures and mutational processes in ovarian carcinoma. *Nat. Genet.* **2018**, *50*, 1262–1270. [CrossRef]
17. Patch, A.M.; Christie, E.L.; Etemadmoghadam, D.; Garsed, D.W.; George, J.; Fereday, S.; Nones, K.; Cowin, P.; Alsop, K.; Bailey, P.J.; et al. Whole-genome characterization of chemoresistant ovarian cancer. *Nature* **2015**, *521*, 489–494. [CrossRef]
18. Nick, A.M.; Coleman, R.L.; Ramirez, P.T.; Sood, A.K. A framework for a personalized surgical approach to ovarian cancer. *Nat. Rev. Clin. Oncol.* **2015**, *12*, 239–245. [CrossRef] [PubMed]
19. Lo, N.C.; Monteverde, M.; Riba, M.; Lattanzio, L.; Tonissi, F.; Garrone, O.; Heouaine, A.; Gallo, F.; Ceppi, M.; Borghi, F.; et al. Expression profiling and long lasting responses to chemotherapy in metastatic gastric cancer. *Int. J. Oncol.* **2010**, *37*, 1219–1228.
20. Bossi, P.; Bergamini, C.; Siano, M.; Cossu, R.M.; Sponghini, A.P.; Favales, F.; Giannoccaro, M.; Marchesi, E.; Cortelazzi, B.; Perrone, F.; et al. Functional genomics uncover the biology behind the responsiveness of head and neck squamous cell cancer patients to cetuximab. *Clin. Cancer Res.* **2016**, *22*, 3961–3970. [CrossRef]
21. Negrini, S.; Gorgoulis, V.G.; Halazonetis, T.D. Genomic instability—An evolving hallmark of cancer. *Nat. Rev. Mol. Cell Biol.* **2010**, *11*, 220–228. [CrossRef] [PubMed]
22. Riester, M.; Wei, W.; Waldron, L.; Culhane, A.C.; Trippa, L.; Oliva, E.; Kim, S.H.; Michor, F.; Huttenhower, C.; Parmigiani, G.; et al. Risk prediction for late-stage ovarian cancer by meta-analysis of 1525 patient samples. *J. Natl. Cancer Inst.* **2014**, *106*. [CrossRef] [PubMed]

23. Ballabio, S.; Craparotta, I.; Paracchini, L.; Mannarino, L.; Corso, S.; Pezzotta, M.G.; Vescio, M.; Fruscio, R.; Romualdi, C.; Dainese, E.; et al. Multisite analysis of high-grade serous epithelial ovarian cancers identifies genomic regions of focal and recurrent copy number alteration in 3q26.2 and 8q24.3. *Int. J. Cancer* **2019**. [CrossRef] [PubMed]
24. Etemadmoghadam, D.; Weir, B.A.; Au-Yeung, G.; Alsop, K.; Mitchell, G.; George, J.; Davis, S.; D'Andrea, A.D.; Simpson, K.; Hahn, W.C.; et al. Synthetic lethality between *CCNE1* amplification and loss of *BRCA1*. *Proc. Natl. Acad. Sci. USA* **2013**, *110*, 19489–19494. [CrossRef] [PubMed]
25. Au-Yeung, G.; Lang, F.; Azar, W.J.; Mitchell, C.; Jarman, K.E.; Lackovic, K.; Aziz, D.; Cullinane, C.; Pearson, R.B.; Mileshkin, L.; et al. Selective targeting of Cyclin E1-amplified high-grade serous ovarian cancer by cyclin-dependent kinase 2 and AKT inhibition. *Clin. Cancer Res.* **2017**, *23*, 1862–1874. [CrossRef]
26. Belandia, B.; Powell, S.M.; Garcia-Pedrero, J.M.; Walker, M.M.; Bevan, C.L.; Parker, M.G. Hey1, a mediator of notch signaling, is an androgen receptor corepressor. *Mol. Cell Biol.* **2005**, *25*, 1425–1436. [CrossRef]
27. Fukusumi, T.; Guo, T.W.; Sakai, A.; Ando, M.; Ren, S.; Haft, S.; Liu, C.; Amornphimoltham, P.; Gutkind, J.S.; Califano, J.A. The NOTCH4-HEY1 pathway induces epithelial-mesenchymal transition in head and neck squamous cell carcinoma. *Clin. Cancer Res.* **2018**, *24*, 619–633. [CrossRef]
28. Chen, C.; Wang, X.; Huang, S.; Wang, L.; Han, L.; Yu, S. Prognostic roles of Notch receptor mRNA expression in human ovarian cancer. *Oncotarget* **2017**, *8*, 32731–32740. [CrossRef]
29. Venkatesh, V.; Nataraj, R.; Thangaraj, G.S.; Karthikeyan, M.; Gnanasekaran, A.; Kaginelli, S.B.; Kuppanna, G.; Kallappa, C.G.; Basalingappa, K.M. Targeting Notch signalling pathway of cancer stem cells. *Stem Cell Investig.* **2018**, *5*, 5. [CrossRef]
30. Fang, F.; Cardenas, H.; Huang, H.; Jiang, G.; Perkins, S.M.; Zhang, C.; Keer, H.N.; Liu, Y.; Nephew, K.P.; Matei, D. Genomic and epigenomic signatures in ovarian cancer associated with resensitization to platinum drugs. *Cancer Res.* **2018**, *78*, 631–644. [CrossRef]
31. Brown, J.S.; O'Carrigan, B.; Jackson, S.P.; Yap, T.A. Targeting DNA repair in cancer: Beyond PARP inhibitors. *Cancer Discov.* **2017**, *7*, 20–37. [CrossRef] [PubMed]
32. Gourley, C.; Balmana, J.; Ledermann, J.A.; Serra, V.; Dent, R.; Loibl, S.; Pujade-Lauraine, E.; Boulton, S.J. Moving from poly (ADP-Ribose) polymerase inhibition to targeting DNA repair and DNA damage response in cancer therapy. *J. Clin. Oncol.* **2019**. [CrossRef] [PubMed]

7

FARMAPRICE: A Pharmacogenetic Clinical Decision Support System for Precise and Cost-Effective Therapy

Rossana Roncato [1], Lisa Dal Cin [1], Silvia Mezzalira [1], Francesco Comello [1], Elena De Mattia [1], Alessia Bignucolo [1], Lorenzo Giollo [2], Simone D'Errico [2], Antonio Gulotta [2], Luca Emili [3], Vincenzo Carbone [3], Michela Guardascione [1], Luisa Foltran [4], Giuseppe Toffoli [1,*] and Erika Cecchin [1,*]

1 Clinical and Experimental Pharmacology, Centro di Riferimento Oncologico di Aviano (CRO) IRCCS, 33081 Aviano, Italy; rroncato@cro.it (R.R.); lisa.dalcin@cro.it (L.D.C.); silvia.mezzalira@cro.it (S.M.); francesco.comello@cro.it (F.C.); edemattia@cro.it (E.D.M.); alessia.bignucolo@cro.it (A.B.); michela.guardascione@cro.it (M.G.)

2 GPI, Società per Azioni (SpA), 38123 Trento, Italy; lorenzo.giollo@gpi.it (L.G.); simone.derrico@gpi.it (S.D.); antonio.gulotta@gpi.it (A.G.)

3 InSilicoTrials Technologies società a responsabilità limitata (s.r.l.), 34148 Trieste, Italy; luca.emili@insilicotrials.com (L.E.); vincenzo.carbone@insilicotrials.com (V.C.)

4 Department of Medical Oncology, Centro di Riferimento Oncologico di Aviano (CRO), IRCSS, 33081 Aviano, Italy; luisa.foltran@cro.it

* Correspondence: gtoffoli@cro.it (G.T.); ececchin@cro.it (E.C.)

Abstract: Pharmacogenetic (PGx) guidelines for the precise dosing and selection of drugs remain poorly implemented in current clinical practice. Among the barriers to the implementation process is the lack of clinical decision support system (CDSS) tools to aid health providers in managing PGx information in the clinical context. The present study aimed to describe the first Italian endeavor to develop a PGx CDSS, called FARMAPRICE. FARMAPRICE prototype was conceived for integration of patient molecular data into the clinical prescription process in the Italian Centro di Riferimento Oncologico (CRO)-Aviano Hospital. It was developed through a coordinated partnership between two high-tech companies active in the computerization of the Italian healthcare system. Introducing FARMAPRICE into the clinical setting can aid physicians in prescribing the most efficacious and cost-effective pharmacological therapy available.

Keywords: CDSS; pharmacogenetics; implementation

---

1. Introduction

The response to drugs is highly variable among individuals. Indeed, genetic variants are estimated to affect between 20–95% of the response variability, depending on the drug [1]. Germline genetic variants can influence drug Adsorption, Distribution, Metabolism, and Elimination (ADME) and they can be responsible for reduced drug efficacy or increased toxicity. Patients might benefit from using pharmacogenetics (PGx) to inform treatment decisions regarding drug selection and dosing. The PGx approach has the potential of improving drug efficacy and/or avoiding unwanted side effects; these improvements could lead to better treatment adherence and outcomes [2]. An inherently personalized approach to medicine could provide non-negligible offsets to Healthcare system costs [3,4].

PGx guidelines for drug dosing have become available for a wide range of medications associated with gene-drug interactions that could potentially be clinically actionable. To date, over 160 medications, ranging from heart disease medications to psychiatric drugs, currently have PGx labeling registered with the US Food and Drug Administration (FDA) [5]. The publicly available online knowledge base, PharmGKB [6], is an interactive tool that collects PGx recommendations. It includes PGx-based drug dosing guidelines established by the Clinical Pharmacogenetics Implementation Consortium (CPIC), the Royal Dutch Association for the Advancement of Pharmacy—Pharmacogenetics Working Group (DPWG), the Canadian Pharmacogenomics Network for Drug Safety (CPNDS) and other professional societies.

PGx tests have been used in the past, but mainly as a reactive approach to an aberrant clinical outcome in individual patients. Physicians typically ordered PGx tests on an "as needed" basis, after the occurrence of unexpected severe toxicity or a lack of response. Currently, the use of PGx as a tool for evidence-based medication management is gaining acceptance among many healthcare providers. PGx tests can be used to predict drug efficacy and side effects in individual patients. Consequently, PGx testing has moved to the pre-therapeutic setting, where the test is typically ordered at the first prescription of a drug that is associated with a PGx guideline.

Despite a recent survey, which showed that 97.6% of clinicians agreed that genetic variations might influence drug response, only 12.9% of clinicians had ordered a PGx test during the prior six months. In fact, translating PGx knowledge into clinical practice has been slow and hindered by many barriers that have prevented its large-scale implementation. Apart from the established statistical associations between PGxs and drug therapy outcomes (clinical validity), large scale implementation of PGx translation requires evidence of clinical-utility and cost-effectiveness. Moreover, that evidence will likely result in favorable reimbursement decisions from payers [7]. Additionally, to aid the implementation of PGx in clinical practice, we need to set up a straightforward workflow from the test prescription to the application of the guidelines, combined with appropriate training and education programs about the clinical use of PGx for healthcare practitioners [8].

The poor application of PGx in the clinical routine is related to the need for a "physician-friendly" electronic "educational resource" that aids clinicians in managing PGx results during routine clinical practice [9]. The implementation of a point-of-care electronic clinical decision support system (CDSS) is urgently needed to guide drug prescriptions in a community-based practice setting [10].

In recent years, a growing body of literature has been produced in developing and implementing PGx CDSSs for improving patient care. A PGx CDSS is a critical tool that can address some of the barriers to implementing PGx guidelines into the clinical routine. They are computer-based systems intended to improve medical decision-making at the point-of-care by supporting physicians in decisions regarding prescriptions. The CDSS infrastructure was designed to store the patient's genomic data and create filtered PGx information, such as pop-up alerts, to inform physicians and other healthcare providers when a gene-drug interaction is available for a specific patient [11]. Thus, this information technology (IT) tool can translate genetic information into practical therapeutic recommendations. It can be used to customize, as much as possible, pharmacological treatments, in terms of drug selection and dosing. The dynamic nature of PGx guidelines warrants long-term maintenance and continuous updating of the PGx CDSS, as new evidence becomes available. To that end, PGx CDSS tools must be fully scalable and sustainable in an automated way [12].

With the aim of providing clinicians with an IT infrastructure (CDSS) for the automated management of patient molecular data, which could be translated into specific prescription indications the FARMAPRICE partnership was created. The partnership comprises the Clinical and Experimental Pharmacology unit of the Centro di Riferimento Oncologico (CRO)-Aviano Hospital and two high-tech companies, InSilicoTrials Technologies, Trieste, Italy, and GPI company, Trento, Italy, which are active in developing solutions for the healthcare system. They put forth a coordinated effort to bring together scientific, clinical and technological expertise in the PGx field. In 2017, the FARMAPRICE partnership proposed a project that was financed by POR FESR 2014–2020, which aimed to promote innovation in the drug prescription process by implementing the preemptive PGx approach in Italy.

The present article aimed to describe the Italian project, FARMAPRICE, a CDSS designed for integration into the clinical prescription process in the Italian CRO-Aviano Hospital.

2. Materials and Methods

FARMAPRICE CDSS was designed to aid clinicians in prescribing the most efficacious and cost-effective pharmacological therapy available by providing support for prescribing drugs within available PGx guidelines. Prescribing physicians can interrogate the FARMAPRICE platform to get specific dosing recommendation. To that end, the FARMAPRICE platform queries two repositories: The first is the patient's complete genetic data; the second is the list of all PGx guidelines based on validated gene-drug interactions (Figure 1).

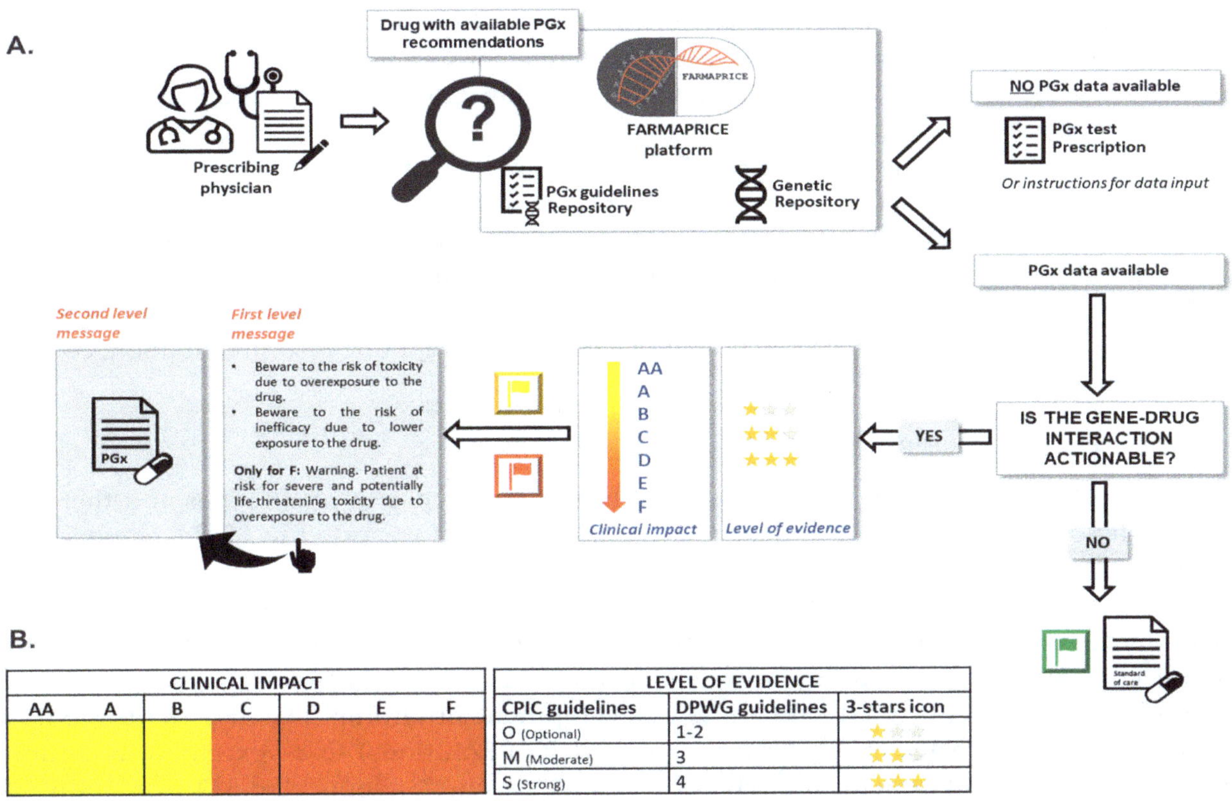

Figure 1. FARMAPRICE platform workflow. (**A**) The prescribing physician interrogates FARMAPRICE platform to discover if the drug to be prescribed presents validated gene-drug interactions and if that specific patient has a potentially clinically actionable genotype. In the negative case instructions are given for a pharmacogenetic (PGx) test prescription. In the affirmative case, a PGx-based recommendation integrated with its level of evidence and clinical impact will be provided. This will allow prescribers to weigh the strength of evidence available and to decide whether to follow the recommendation or not. A PGx-based recommendation will be first delivered as a "first level message" briefly describing the involved risk (inefficacy or toxicity) for that specific patient at standard dosage. A "second level message" (complete PGx-based drug selection or dosing recommendation) is displayed by clicking on "first level message". (**B**) Clinical impact of a specific gene-drug interaction is delivered with a different colors flag icon basing on Swen et al. [13]. Correspondence between rating from AA to F and the color code is here defined. Conversely, the level of evidence will be delivered as a three-star icon basing on both Clinical Pharmacogenetics Implementation Consortium (CPIC) and Royal Dutch Association for the Advancement of Pharmacy—Pharmacogenetics Working Group (DPWG) latest guidelines available for that gene-drug interaction as herein described.

The development of the project was divided into three phases: First, the selection of actionable gene-drug pairs to be integrated into the CDSS; second, the development of a CDSS prototype; and third, an evaluation of the IT platform prototype in a medical setting.

2.1. First Phase: The Selection of Actionable Gene-Drug Pairs to be Integrated into the CDSS

Between January and June 2018, the PGx team of the Experimental and Clinical Pharmacology Unit of CRO-Aviano elaborated a list of gene-drug interactions based on the most recent PGx guidelines [6].

In the first phase of the project, the PharmGKB website was consulted to obtain the most complete, up-to-date list of all available PGx guidelines. The PharmGKB summarizes guidelines from the two most widely recognized consortia, CPIC and DPWG. Although these consortia are currently working on harmonizing their clinical recommendations, controversial information might arise from different guidelines, which could generate uncertainty in treatment decisions. Within the FARMAPRICE development project, the PGx-based recommendations provided by the CPIC and DPWG consortia were merged into a unique therapeutic recommendation. In cases of discrepancies, the software provides prescribing physicians with the most restrictive/conservative recommendation, to ensure patient safety, and it adds the following statement: "Further modification of the therapy is advised, based on the patient's individual response".

Gene-drug pairs to be integrated were selected based on their actionability and on the availability of the drug in Italy. The genetic variants of these pharmacogenes were selected based on the most recent scientific publications and the level of evidence on the functional effect of the genetic variant on the encoded protein, according to the most updated CPIC guidelines [14]. These genetic variants were classified according to their functional impact. Then, they were combined to obtain all possible genotypes and diplotypes that could be linked to a specific therapeutic recommendation, consistent with published guidelines [15].

2.2. Second Phase: Development of the FARMAPRICE Prototype

A series of synoptic tables was created that linked genotypes to phenotypes and therapeutic recommendations for each selected drug. These tables were forwarded to IT developers for the configuration of the CDSS prototype. The IT tools for collecting medical-molecular data were configured together with corresponding protocols for the acquisition and integration of molecular data in a standardized form. To guarantee greater longevity, open source solutions were implemented: The application was developed using Protected Health Information (PHI) Technology, an open-source framework based on Eclipse IDE (Integrated Development Environment). It provides tools and components to design eHealth applications (named PHI Solutions) to be executed in a runtime environment independent from the underlying operating system. It adopts Model Driven Architecture (MDA) and Business Processes Management (BPM) tools combined with Service Oriented Architecture (SOA), completely based on the latest open standards (HL7, IHE, DICOM, XDS).

These elements assure the longest lifetime of the applications and back the whole diagnostic, therapeutic and processes. This choice guarantees a high level of interoperability, in view of potential integration into systems of production and in complex environments, such as hospital information systems, including the EHR [16].

2.3. Third Phase: FARMAPRICE User Experience

Ideally, the genetic reports and the service provided should be formatted and focused, based on feedback from clinicians. Maximizing the effectiveness of the alerts will aid in the integration of CDSSs and their adoption by practitioners [17]. The IT companies involved in FARMAPRICE development carried out a study to determine the software requirements for the most effective user experience on: (i) Platform usability, (ii) functional specifications and content requirements, (iii) information architecture, and (iv) Information design, interface design, and navigation.

Software requirements were gathered by the project partners to collect, analyze and document the System Requirements Specification. The approach adopted was not the usual waterfall model where software development follows a linear succession of steps to the final product. A prototypal approach was implemented, instead. The development of a prototype with a minimum set of functionalities made the formalization of the requirements easier and the adaptation to the users' real needs through consecutive approximation. The partners carried out a study to determine the best software Graphical User Interface (GUI) using the designing tools of the User Experience (UX). Users were separated into two classes of archetypical users (so called personas) who represent the needs of a larger group of users, i.e., "clinicians" and "researchers". The observation of these two classes was realized considering the environment in which a persona operates, which tools it uses, its background information, and the behavior working patterns. As a result, the study output gives back slightly different users' interactions with the software that will be considered in further implementations. The use of REST (Representational State Transfer) services ensures the separation between the application back-end and front-end. Process execution, information classes and the persistence management (permanent data storage) are then unlinked by the front-end that can be migrated to other frameworks (Angular JS, React etc.) with no impact on the application business logic.

The study outcome indicated the necessity of two different interfaces and two different sets of data access and access privileges, due to privacy concerns. About the latter, "clinicians" have data access to all the information (i.e., they can see all the data without modification of genomic data), while "researchers" have data access constraints to patient personal data, but have access privileges to modify all genetic information (i.e., they cannot see who the patient is, but can update/modify the data, the PGx guidelines, etc.). The "clinicians" GUI is oriented to the clinical aspects, similarly to an EHR presenting the evidence-based therapeutic recommendations, together with the actual clinical impact; the "researchers" GUI is designed for the collection, modification, integration of the background information.

3. Results

3.1. First Phase: The Selection of Actionable Gene-Drug Pairs to be Integrated into the CDSS

The selection process of gene-drug pairs based on both their actionability and availability of the drug in Italy resulted in the inclusion of 46 drugs in the final selection. FARMAPRICE drugs span several pharmacological classes, including anti-neoplastic agents, anti-viral agents, anti-coagulant agents, oral contraceptives, analgesics, anti-emetics, immunosuppressives, anti-epileptics, anti-arrhythmics, anti-gout drugs, anti-depressants (SSRI, TCA and other), psychostimulants, anti-psychotics, anti-hypertensive drugs, drugs for cystic fibrosis treatment, cholesterol-lowering drugs, and anti-fungals (Table 1). Among the pharmacogenes that impacted the outcome of the identified drugs, 14 were included in the final selection. This selection process identified 374 variants with documented impact on gene transcription.

Table 1. Drugs included in FARMAPRICE clinical decision support system (CDSS).

Drug Classification	Drugs
Analgesics	Codeine, Tramadol
Anti-arrhythmics	Propafenone, Flecainide
Anti-coagulant agents	Acenocoumarol, Phenprocoumon, Clopidrogel, Warfarin
Antidepressant	Venlafaxine
Antidepressant (SSRI)	Citalopram, Escitalopram, Sertraline, Paroxetine
Anti-depressants (TCA)	Amitriptyline, Clomipramine, Nortriptyline, Trimipramine
Anti-emetics	Ondasetron, Tropisetron
Anti-epileptics	Carbamazepine, Phenytoin, Oxacarbamazepine
Anti-fungals	Voriconazole
Anti-gout drugs	Allopurinol, Rasburicase

Table 1. *Cont.*

Drug Classification	Drugs
Anti-hypertensive drugs	Metoprolol
Anti-neoplastic agents	5-Fluorouracil, Capecitabine, Irinotecan, Tamoxifen, Tioguanine, Mercaptopurine, Azathioprine
Anti-psychotics	Aripiprazole, Haloperidol, Zuclopenthixol
Anti-viral agents	Abacavir, Atazanavir, Ribavirin, PEG-IFN
Cholesterol-lowering drugs	Atorvastatin, Simvastatin
Cystic fibrosis treatment	Ivacaftor
Immunosuppressives	Tacrolimus
Oral contraceptives	Hormonal contraceptives for systemic use
Psychostimulants	Atomoxetine

3.2. Second Phase: Development of the FARMAPRICE Prototype

FARMAPRICE was developed as an active PGx CDSS functional prototype integrated with PGx guidelines and patient genetic information in a web service platform. It was considered that the Italian health care system is currently lacking a common EHR platform among its different regions, thus resulting in a fragmented healthcare delivery system with limited EHR interoperability. Since sharing healthcare data among different providers is hampered, FARMAPRICE was conceived as a stand-alone system that could be eventually integrated into the EHR system. Specific requirements were then to guarantee a correct exchange of data, in particular the checking of data entry (in support of the researchers and the clinicians to eliminate any input errors), the certification of the prescription algorithm (avoiding the risk of incurring possible modifications), and the verification of the output data (to have indications for further improvement of the effectiveness of the guidelines underlying the system itself). Specifically, the solution has been designed as a web application, implemented using open-source components and technologies: The integration with an EHR can be reached through integration profiles that manage HL7 input/output messages. It is designed to be a module: It defines and enforce logical boundaries, it is pluggable with another module that expects its interface, and it is a single unit to be easily deployed, overcoming fragmentation issues.

The prototype is structured into four principal parts. The section "Patients" provides the prescribing physician access to the patient's genetic data (genetic data repository). Moreover, in this section, the prescriber can configure a new patient record and input the relevant genetic data. In the section "Prescription", the clinician can interrogate the system to obtain a specific recommendation for a selected patient that requires a new drug prescription. An alphabetically ordered drug list will pop-up. Once a new drug prescription is selected, the dosing recommendation will be provided, based on the patient's genetic profile. When relevant genetic data are missing, the system will request input of additional information to ensure the correct drug recommendation is provided. In addition, the user can track a patient's clinical history to obtain information about all the drugs previously prescribed through FARMAPRICE. Other sections (e.g., "File configuration" and "Drug configuration") are reserved for developers and researchers that update the FARMAPRICE CDSS with the latest PGx guidelines.

Due to the security risks associated with storing large quantities of personal data, specifically genetic data, the CDSS prototype was implemented on a "research and development" project setting, meaning that all the genetic data were handled anonymously. For future developments, an electronic register has been designed for the safe storage and management of acquired genetic data, and for qualitative-quantitative analysis, aiming to enlarge the register with new data deriving from other hospital structures present in the region. The OpenClinica technology (OpenClinica, LLC, Waltham, MA, USA), representing the first open source clinical trial software in the world for the management of clinical data (CDM) of Electronic Data Capture (EDC), was chosen for the underlying electronic database. The underlying technologies of the OpenClinica web application are: Java as a programming language, Spring Framework as an application framework and PostgreSQL as a report database.

The early modular design was prepared for integration with security technologies on the cloud, such as Microsoft Azure, to benefit from safety and compliance in the healthcare field with the latest standards of anonymization, security, and data maintenance as required by the European Medicine Agency (EMA) and the Food and Drug Administration (FDA) USA.

FARMAPRICE employs both types of alert messages typically used by CDSS: "Pre-test" and "Post-test" alerts. Pre-test alerts can be useful for reminding clinicians when a PGx test is necessary to ensure that a specific drug is safe for the patient. When prescribing a medication that is affected by a PGx guideline, the alert informs the clinician that the patient record lacks genotyping results. Conversely, a post-test alert appears when the PGx test results are available. This alert informs the prescribing physician that the patient has an actionable genotype and recommends a corresponding therapy [18]. This alert includes patient-specific dosing recommendations and highlights the strength of supporting evidence.

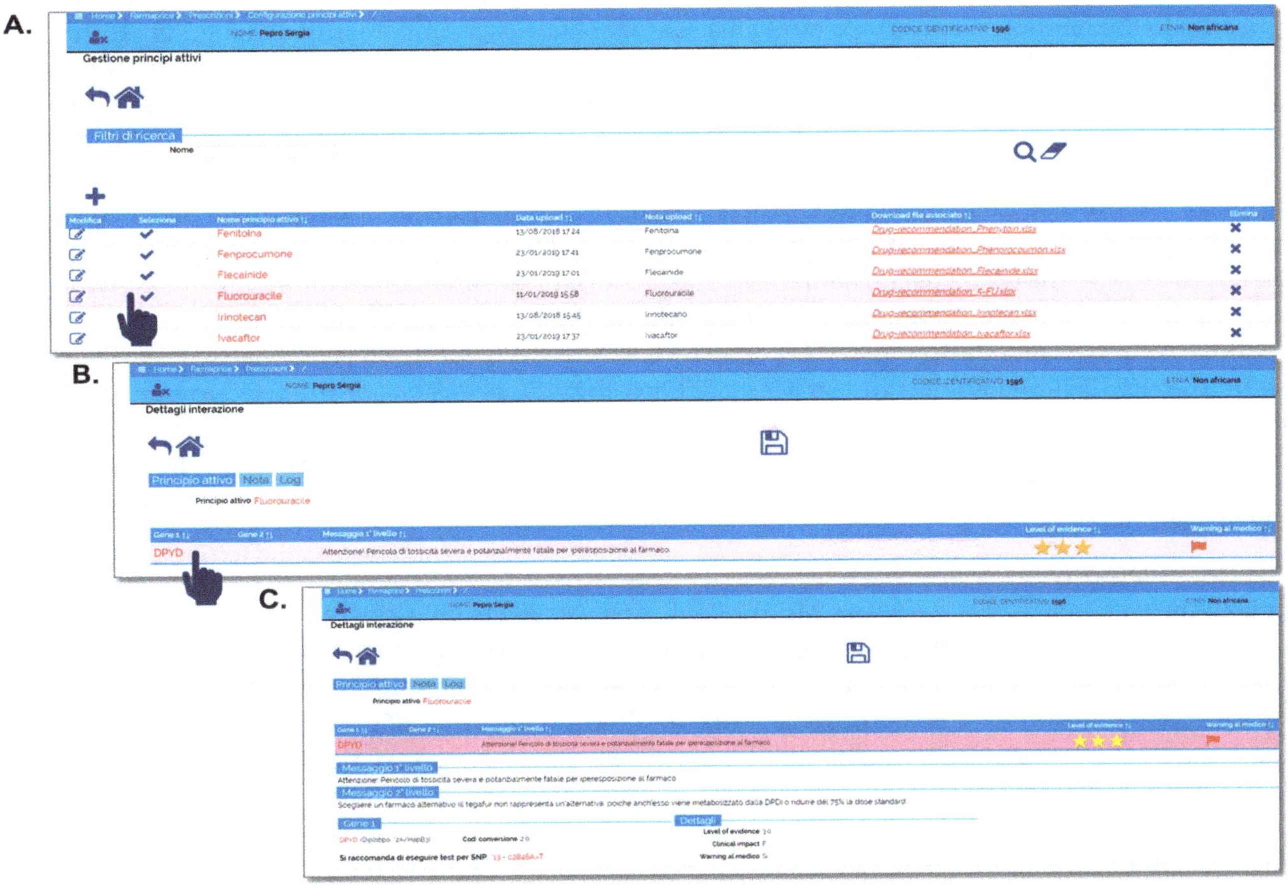

Figure 2. Demo prescription using FARMAPRICE tool. (**A**) the physician prescribes 5-fluorouracil to a patient who is DihydroPYrimidine-Dehydrogenase (*DPYD*) poor metabolizer. (**B**) This action triggers a pop-up with a first level message. (**C**) This in turn can trigger the real PGx-based recommendation of drug selection or dosage by clicking directly on the first level message.

Post-test alerts consist of two levels of messages. At the time a drug is ordered, a pop-up alert (first level message) appears when the patient has an actionable genotype listed in the PGx results repository. This first level message is a standardized text that describes the expected clinical effect of a specific genotype-drug interaction. This text was designed to be concise, and it includes the most important information needed for a prescription. Next to the first level text message, FARMAPRICE places stars and flags to indicate the *level of evidence* and the *clinical impact*, respectively, of the proposed dosing guideline. The *level of evidence* refers to the strength of the literature-based evidence that links the genotype to the phenotype. FARMAPRICE indicates the level of evidence with one to three stars to indicate the lowest to highest levels of evidence, respectively. The *clinical impact* is related to the clinical relevance of the potential adverse drug event. The clinical impact is indicated with colored flags: Yellow for low clinical impact (scored AA to C in the DPWG guidelines); red for high clinical impact (D to Fin the DPWG guidelines [13]); and green for no clinical impact. Thus, a green flag combined with the first level message, "no recommendation, start with the standard dosage", indicates that no actionable genotype-drug interaction is available. For red and yellow flags, the prescribing physician can click on the first-level message to activate a hypertext link that will redirect to a second-level message. This message gives a recommendation on drug dosing and alternate drug selection. This second level message contains a more extensive text explanation, with details on the recommended changes in drug dosing and selection (Figure 2).

3.3. Third Phase: FARMAPRICE User Experience

Once the prototype was ready, the graphical interface was accurately reviewed and modified according to the medical doctors feed-back. The software GUI was implemented using PHI Technology GUI Designer which provides web-based user interfaces created on the underlying processes. This capability to render a GUI model is owed to the modeling framework of Eclipse, combined with the templating framework and guarantee a framework based on the logical processes of the software user, to consider all the crucial information. Yet this does not ensure the intuitiveness of the UI: Icons symbolize common actions which are consistent for homogeneous groups of users (i.e., "clinicians" and "researchers"). The feedback provided by the users led to the selection of an alternative set of icons understandable to the CDSS users, namely "clinicians" and "researchers". Warning messages were also implemented to allow prescribers to better weigh the strength of evidence available and decide whether to follow the recommendation or not [2]. The FARMAPRICE prototype is currently in experimental use by the medical oncologists of the Medical Oncology Department of the CRO-Aviano Hospital. These physicians have agreed to provide feed-back on their user experience, which will inform the developers on ways to optimize the software graphical interface and its operative performance.

4. Discussion

The preemptive PGx approach is typically used only for single gene-drug pairs with a relevant clinical impact, as is the case for highly toxic drugs, such as capecitabine, 5-fluorouracil, or 6-mercaptopurine. Preferably, in the future, this type of preemptive testing will be integrated into clinical practice. In that context, patients could be screened for drug-related genes in anticipation of future prescription events, consistent with the lifetime value of PGx testing. Then, in decisions regarding prescriptions, PGx results will be considered an inherent patient characteristic, like age, weight, renal function, and allergy status. Indeed, physicians are in a front-line position to handle the potential volume of such information by reviewing, interpreting, and delivering PGx test results and providing follow-up to the patient. Moreover, in future, the PGx knowledge base is likely to increase with the discovery of new gene-drug interactions, as next generation sequencing (NGS) continues to advance. In this study we have presented the results of an Italian coordinated effort to develop a CDSS tool, FARMAPRICE, that could help the PGx implementation in the current clinical practice.

Many initiatives both in Europe and the United States are and have been trying to address this hurdle. The main research networks involved in the integration of genetic data into the EHR are the Electronic Medical Records and Genomics Network (eMERGE) and the Implementing Genomics in Practice (IGNITE) [19]. The eMERGE network was formed by a partnership between eMERGE and the Pharmacogenomics Research Network (PGRN), which involves ten US sites. One of its main goals is to integrate clinically validated PGx genotypes into the EHR and associated CDSSs and to assess the process and clinical outcomes of implementation [20]. A few medical institutions have pilot projects that have surpassed "reactive genotyping" to include "preemptive genotyping". For example, the Mayo Clinic, with the RIGHT project, the Icahn School of Medicine at Mount Sinai, with CLIPMERGE, and Vanderbilt University Medical Center (VUMC), with PREDICT. These projects aim to drive point-of-care CDSSs with the integration of clinically actionable PGx variants into the EHR [21–23].

The Mayo clinic Biobank enrolled 1013 participants within 3 years into the "Right Drug, Right Dose, Right Time" project. The study aimed at optimizing preemptive genotyping in patients with a high probability of initiating statin therapy during the study period. One result of that study was the integration of PGx results into the EHR and the development of a point-of-care CDSS, including: (i) Pre-test and post-test alerts; and (ii) a CDSS integrated with additional PGx educational support links to aid clinicians. In addition, the Mayo Clinic developed a long-term maintenance strategy, with a CDSS that could automatically update itself with newly discovered gene-drug interactions. Moreover, that CDSS could automatically send an email to the technical team when an unreadable result occurred [11,19,21,24,25].

A member of the eMERGE network, the CLIPMERGE PGx program at Mount Sinai Medical Center, developed an active CDSS that delivered post-PGx-test alerts to clinicians at the point-of-care. That project aimed to implement the use of PGx testing by integrating it in CDSS and EHR using a DNA biobank-derived cohort (*BioMe*). Initially, 1500 pilot participants were recruited and preemptively genotyped for known variants associated with the use of warfarin, clopidogrel, simvastatin, and several types of antidepressants [22,25,26].

As mentioned previously, another relevant network involved in the integration of patient genetic data into clinical care is the IGNITE network. This network includes six US sites, and of these, three deal with PGx implementation: The University of Florida's Personalized Medicine Program; Indiana University's INGENIOUS program; and Vanderbilt University's I3P program [27]. Other initial efforts that aim to implement PGx in clinical care include Cleveland Clinic's Personalized Medication Program, St. Jude Children's Research Hospital's PG4KDS program, the University of Chicago's 1200 Patient Project, and the University of Maryland's Personalized Anti-Platelet Pharmacogenetics Program [18,28–30]. In Europe the PREemptive Pharmacogenomic testing for prevention of Adverse drug Reactions (PREPARE) clinical trial was conducted within the European Ubiquitous Pharmacogenomics (U-PGx) project [26,31]. They selected a panel of 50 variants in 13 pharmacogenes. This project put together different implementation sites in different European countries, with widely varying health care systems. In this context a spectrum of complementary CDSS solutions was developed, with the unique implementation experience of a portable CDSS, the "Safety-Code card".

For many years, genotyping was limited by the single-gene approach. The recent introduction of genotyping array technologies in the clinical practice made it possible to simultaneously evaluate several relevant pharmacogenes [32]. This technological approach has led to high-quality and economically affordable results. Indeed, the genotyping method for preemptive testing that has been adopted by ongoing implementation programs is mainly based on the use of array genotyping platforms [33]. These platforms offer robust interpretations of the results, and they are well-suited to automation, where PGx results are automatically uploaded into a structured IT system. The most suitable genotyping approach should be selected from the currently available commercial and custom panels. This selection is guided by features of feasibility and cost-effectiveness, such as: The turnaround time from isolated DNA to genotype; the instrumental and technical equipment of the laboratory involved in generating the genotype; the potential number of samples per array; the cost of the array; and the content and potential flexibility of the array [34].

A CDSS can be designed as an active or passive system. In the passive (or asynchronous) CDSS, the information is available only when the clinician specifically requests it, and it is reported as a static warning note. In contrast, the active (or synchronous) CDSS processes information and interacts with clinical data by following rules and issuing alerts [12,24]. Indeed, FARMAPRICE can be interrogated by healthcare providers at the point-of-care by accessing the web-based platform to determine whether a specific drug has a potentially clinically actionable gene-drug interaction. Rules will predict phenotype-predicted genotype and interactive alerts will be triggered both when a high-risk drug is prescribed and when a specific PGx result should be obtained before prescribing the intended drug.

PGx CDSSs are typically developed as stand-alone systems that function autonomously as a web service or a mobile application, rather than being integrated into the existing local hospital infrastructure. However, because PGx results are relevant throughout a patient's life, ideally, they should be stored in a time-independent manner to ensure accessibility to future providers [12]. Currently, the long-term availability of PGx results at the point-of-care can only be guaranteed by a CDSS that is embedded into an Electronic Health Record (EHR) [35]. With this method, PGx results can be shared among different healthcare providers (pharmacists, general practitioners, specialists), and they can be used at different stages of the clinical workflow to guide clinical decision-making processes [19]. However, linking the EHR to the CDSS is challenging; thus, it is not yet a common practice. Caraballo et al pointed out that modern EHRs have not been designed for long-term storage of genetic data. Due to the lack of a specific repository, to date, PGx data have been stored in EHRs on either a "problem list" or an "allergy list", which provides time-independent documentation of possible gene-drug interactions. Other issues that make it challenging to incorporate PGx results into the EHR are the increasing amount of genetic data and the unstandardized formats of available data, which makes them difficult to share in a multi-center setting [19,24]. The Italian health care system is currently lacking a common EHR platform among its different regions. This lack has resulted in a fragmented healthcare delivery system with limited EHR interoperability. Thus, sharing healthcare data among different providers is hampered. Consequently, FARMAPRICE was conceived as a stand-alone system that could be eventually integrated into the EHR system.

Indeed, successful implementation of a CDSS is not only related to its clinical utility in terms of improving treatment safety and efficacy, but also to its perceived feasibility and usability by the prescribing physicians. When looking at the software requirements for the most effective user experience, clinicians considered that excess alerts (e.g., not relevant or repeated alerts, a phenomenon termed "alert fatigue") could put a strain on the clinician's workload, and this could have adverse effects on patient care [36]. In the evaluation of FARMAPRICE prototype, a user-friendly design was sought and designed to ensure that the interruptions would not overload busy clinicians [24]. The user experience is now in the experimental evaluation phase by prescribing physicians in the CRO-Aviano hospital.

It must be further considered that, in the first place, the use of this kind of tool is primarily related to the health practitioners personal motivation and of their awareness of the opportunity to use PGx in their everyday routine. Other implementation experiences have demonstrated that although physicians may perceive the benefit of using PGx, the lack of formal training about PGx, together with concerns regarding feasibility, clinical utility, and integration in the clinical workflow have been reported by physicians as the major barriers to a more routine use of PGx [8]. It must be not forgotten that education is a crucial step for implementing PGx into the clinic. Educational and training programs must be offered to health practitioners in an interprofessional context to drive interest and continuous learning about PGx, to allow a critical and conscious use of PGx in the clinical practice also with the aid of innovative IT tools, such as FARMAPRICE.

5. Conclusions

Patients and healthcare providers are important stakeholders in the implementation of PGx. Among the provider-perceived barriers to adopting this information are inadequate knowledge about PGx, the lack of clear guidelines for many drugs, and the absence of convincing cost-effectiveness data to support PGx clinical utility. In addition, an emerging barrier to the PGx clinical implementation process is the lack of user-friendly tools to integrate genetic information and their interpretation into the clinical prescription workflow.

Health-related ITs, such as the CDSS, are designed to support clinicians in the decision-making process; to address the growing information pool, which overloads clinicians; and to provide a platform for incorporating evidence-based knowledge into care delivery. An Italian consortium has been set up to create FARMAPRICE, a CDSS designed to be used in the clinical setting to facilitate the use of PGx in the drug prescription process in Italy. A prototype has been created and is ready to be presented to clinicians for use in their routine practice. It is likely that, in the next few years, pre-treatment patient genotyping will become a more common clinical practice, and FARMAPRICE will represent a user-friendly, stand-alone system that can be integrated into every clinical context to manage genetic data and optimize patient treatments.

Author Contributions: Conceptualization: E.C., G.T., L.G., and L.E.; methodology: E.C., R.R., L.D.C., S.M., and F.C.; software: V.C., and E.D.S.; validation: M.G., E.D.M., A.B., L.F., and F.C.; original manuscript draft preparation: E.C., R.R., L.D.C., S.M., F.C., and E.D.M.; funding acquisition: E.C., L.G., L.E.

References

1. Arwood, M.J.; Chumnumwat, S.; Cavallari, L.H.; Nutescu, E.A.; Duarte, J.D. Implementing Pharmacogenomics at Your Institution: Establishment and Overcoming Implementation Challenges. *Clin. Trans. Sci.* **2016**, *9*, 233–245. [CrossRef]
2. Mukerjee, G.; Huston, A.; Kabakchiev, B.; Piquette-Miller, M.; van Schaik, R.; Dorfman, R. User considerations in assessing pharmacogenomic tests and their clinical support tools. *Genom. Med.* **2018**, *3*, 26. [CrossRef]
3. Roncato, R.; Cecchin, E.; Montico, M.; De Mattia, E.; Giodini, L.; Buonadonna, A.; Solfrini, V.; Innocenti, F.; Toffoli, G. Cost Evaluation of Irinotecan-Related Toxicities Associated With the UGT1A1*28 Patient Genotype. *Clin. Pharmacol. Ther.* **2017**, *102*, 123–130. [CrossRef] [PubMed]
4. Toffoli, G.; Innocenti, F.; Polesel, J.; De Mattia, E.; Sartor, F.; Dalle Fratte, C.; Ecca, F.; Dreussi, E.; Palazzari, E.; Guardascione, M.; et al. The Genotype for DPYD Risk Variants in Patients With Colorectal Cancer and the Related Toxicity Management Costs in Clinical Practice. *Clin. Pharmacol. Ther.* **2019**, *105*, 994–1002. [CrossRef] [PubMed]
5. US Food and Drug Administration Home Page. Available online: https://www.fda.gov/ (accessed on 11 February 2019).
6. PharmGKB. Available online: https://www.pharmgkb.org/ (accessed on 14 February 2019).
7. Janssens, A.C.J.W.; Deverka, P.A. Useless until proven effective: The clinical utility of preemptive pharmacogenetic testing. *Clin. Pharmacol. Ther.* **2014**, *96*, 652–654. [CrossRef] [PubMed]
8. Borden, B.A.; Galecki, P.; Wellmann, R.; Danahey, K.; Lee, S.M.; Patrick-Miller, L.; Sorrentino, M.J.; Nanda, R.; Koyner, J.L.; Polonsky, T.S.; et al. Assessment of provider-perceived barriers to clinical use of pharmacogenomics during participation in an institutional implementation study. *Pharmacogenet. Genom.* **2019**, *29*, 31–38. [CrossRef] [PubMed]
9. Johansen Taber, K.A.; Dickinson, B.D. Pharmacogenomic knowledge gaps and educational resource needs among physicians in selected specialties. *Pharmgenom. Pers. Med.* **2014**, *7*, 145–162. [CrossRef] [PubMed]
10. Relling, M.V.; Evans, W.E. Pharmacogenomics in the clinic. *Nature* **2015**, *526*, 343–350. [CrossRef] [PubMed]
11. Hinderer, M.; Boeker, M.; Wagner, S.A.; Lablans, M.; Newe, S.; Hülsemann, J.L.; Neumaier, M.; Binder, H.; Renz, H.; Acker, T.; et al. Integrating clinical decision support systems for pharmacogenomic testing into clinical routine—A scoping review of designs of user-system interactions in recent system development. *BMC Med. Inform. Decis. Mak.* **2017**, *17*, 81. [CrossRef]
12. Hicks, J.K.; Dunnenberger, H.M.; Gumpper, K.F.; Haidar, C.E.; Hoffman, J.M. Integrating pharmacogenomics into electronic health records with clinical decision support. *Am. J. Health Syst. Pharm.* **2016**, *73*, 1967–1976. [CrossRef]
13. Swen, J.J.; Nijenhuis, M.; de Boer, A.; Grandia, L.; Maitland-van der Zee, A.H.; Mulder, H.; Rongen, G.A.P.J.M.; van Schaik, R.H.N.; Schalekamp, T.; Touw, D.J.; et al. Pharmacogenetics: From bench to byte—An update of guidelines. *Clin. Pharmacol. Ther.* **2011**, *89*, 662–673. [CrossRef] [PubMed]

14. Kalman, L.V.; Agúndez, J.; Appell, M.L.; Black, J.L.; Bell, G.C.; Boukouvala, S.; Bruckner, C.; Bruford, E.; Caudle, K.; Coulthard, S.A.; et al. Pharmacogenetic allele nomenclature: International workgroup recommendations for test result reporting. *Clin. Pharmacol. Ther.* **2016**, *99*, 172–185. [CrossRef] [PubMed]
15. Caudle, K.E.; Dunnenberger, H.M.; Freimuth, R.R.; Peterson, J.F.; Burlison, J.D.; Whirl-Carrillo, M.; Scott, S.A.; Rehm, H.L.; Williams, M.S.; Klein, T.E.; et al. Standardizing terms for clinical pharmacogenetic test results: Consensus terms from the Clinical Pharmacogenetics Implementation Consortium (CPIC). *Genet. Med.* **2017**, *19*, 215–223. [CrossRef] [PubMed]
16. PHI Technology White Paper. Available online: http://wiki.hl7.org/index.php?title=PHI_TECHNOLOGY_white_paper (accessed on 4 April 2019).
17. Lazaridis, K.N. PACE Forward-Making Pharmacogenomics Testing Available for Real-Life Clinical Utility. *Clin. Pharmacol. Ther.* **2019**, *105*, 42–44. [CrossRef] [PubMed]
18. Hicks, J.K.; Stowe, D.; Willner, M.A.; Wai, M.; Daly, T.; Gordon, S.M.; Lashner, B.A.; Parikh, S.; White, R.; Teng, K.; et al. Implementation of Clinical Pharmacogenomics within a Large Health System: From Electronic Health Record Decision Support to Consultation Services. *Pharmacotherapy* **2016**, *36*, 940–948. [CrossRef]
19. Caraballo, P.J.; Bielinski, S.J.; Sauver, J.S.; Weinshilboum, R.M. Electronic Medical Record-Integrated Pharmacogenomics and Related Clinical Decision Support Concepts. *Clin. Pharmacol. Ther.* **2017**, *102*, 254–264. [CrossRef] [PubMed]
20. Rasmussen-Torvik, L.J.; Stallings, S.C.; Gordon, A.S.; Almoguera, B.; Basford, M.A.; Bielinski, S.J.; Brautbar, A.; Brilliant, M.H.; Carrell, D.S.; Connolly, J.J.; et al. Design and anticipated outcomes of the eMERGE-PGx project: A multicenter pilot for preemptive pharmacogenomics in electronic health record systems. *Clin. Pharmacol. Ther.* **2014**, *96*, 482–489. [CrossRef]
21. Bielinski, S.J.; Olson, J.E.; Pathak, J.; Weinshilboum, R.M.; Wang, L.; Lyke, K.J.; Ryu, E.; Targonski, P.V.; Van Norstrand, M.D.; Hathcock, M.A.; et al. Preemptive genotyping for personalized medicine: Design of the right drug, right dose, right time-using genomic data to individualize treatment protocol. *Mayo Clin. Proc.* **2014**, *89*, 25–33. [CrossRef]
22. Gottesman, O.; Scott, S.A.; Ellis, S.B.; Overby, C.L.; Ludtke, A.; Hulot, J.-S.; Hall, J.; Chatani, K.; Myers, K.; Kannry, J.L.; et al. The CLIPMERGE PGx Program: Clinical implementation of personalized medicine through electronic health records and genomics-pharmacogenomics. *Clin. Pharmacol. Ther.* **2013**, *94*, 214–217. [CrossRef] [PubMed]
23. Pulley, J.M.; Denny, J.C.; Peterson, J.F.; Bernard, G.R.; Vnencak-Jones, C.L.; Ramirez, A.H.; Delaney, J.T.; Bowton, E.; Brothers, K.; Johnson, K.; et al. Operational implementation of prospective genotyping for personalized medicine: The design of the Vanderbilt PREDICT project. *Clin. Pharmacol. Ther.* **2012**, *92*, 87–95. [CrossRef] [PubMed]
24. Caraballo, P.J.; Hodge, L.S.; Bielinski, S.J.; Stewart, A.K.; Farrugia, G.; Schultz, C.G.; Rohrer-Vitek, C.R.; Olson, J.E.; St Sauver, J.L.; Roger, V.L.; et al. Multidisciplinary model to implement pharmacogenomics at the point of care. *Genet. Med.* **2017**, *19*, 421–429. [CrossRef] [PubMed]
25. Dunnenberger, H.M.; Crews, K.R.; Hoffman, J.M.; Caudle, K.E.; Broeckel, U.; Howard, S.C.; Hunkler, R.J.; Klein, T.E.; Evans, W.E.; Relling, M.V. Preemptive clinical pharmacogenetics implementation: Current programs in five US medical centers. *Annu. Rev. Pharmacol. Toxicol.* **2015**, *55*, 89–106. [CrossRef]
26. Van der Wouden, C.H.; Cambon-Thomsen, A.; Cecchin, E.; Cheung, K.C.; Dávila-Fajardo, C.L.; Deneer, V.H.; Dolžan, V.; Ingelman-Sundberg, M.; Jönsson, S.; Karlsson, M.O.; et al. Implementing Pharmacogenomics in Europe: Design and Implementation Strategy of the Ubiquitous Pharmacogenomics Consortium. *Clin. Pharmacol. Ther.* **2017**, *101*, 341–358. [CrossRef] [PubMed]
27. Weitzel, K.W.; Alexander, M.; Bernhardt, B.A.; Calman, N.; Carey, D.J.; Cavallari, L.H.; Field, J.R.; Hauser, D.; Junkins, H.A.; Levin, P.A.; et al. The IGNITE network: A model for genomic medicine implementation and research. *BMC Med. Genom.* **2016**, *9*, 1. [CrossRef]
28. Hoffman, J.M.; Haidar, C.E.; Wilkinson, M.R.; Crews, K.R.; Baker, D.K.; Kornegay, N.M.; Yang, W.; Pui, C.-H.; Reiss, U.M.; Gaur, A.H.; et al. PG4KDS: A Model for the Clinical Implementation of Pre-emptive Pharmacogenetics. *Am. J. Med. Genet. Semin. Med. Genet.* **2014**, *166C*, 45–55. [CrossRef]
29. O'Donnell, P.H.; Danahey, K.; Jacobs, M.; Wadhwa, N.R.; Yuen, S.; Bush, A.; Sacro, Y.; Sorrentino, M.J.; Siegler, M.; Harper, W.; et al. Adoption of a clinical pharmacogenomics implementation program during outpatient care—Initial results of the University of Chicago "1200 Patients Project". *Am. J. Med. Genet. Semin. Med. Genet.* **2014**, *166C*, 68–75. [CrossRef] [PubMed]

30. Shuldiner, A.R.; Palmer, K.; Pakyz, R.E.; Alestock, T.D.; Maloney, K.A.; O'Neill, C.; Bhatty, S.; Schub, J.; Overby, C.L.; Horenstein, R.B.; et al. Implementation of Pharmacogenetics: The University of Maryland Personalized Anti-Platelet Pharmacogenetics Program. *Am. J. Med. Genet. Semin. Med. Genet.* **2014**, *166C*, 76–84. [CrossRef]
31. Cecchin, E.; Roncato, R.; Guchelaar, H.J.; Toffoli, G. Ubiquitous Pharmacogenomics Consortium Ubiquitous Pharmacogenomics (U-PGx): The Time for Implementation is Now. An Horizon2020 Program to Drive Pharmacogenomics into Clinical Practice. *Curr. Pharm. Biotechnol.* **2017**, *18*, 204–209. [CrossRef] [PubMed]
32. Di Francia, R.; Frigeri, F.; Berretta, M.; Cecchin, E.; Orlando, C.; Pinto, A.; Pinzani, P. Decision criteria for rational selection of homogeneous genotyping platforms for pharmacogenomics testing in clinical diagnostics. *Clin. Chem. Lab. Med.* **2010**, *48*, 447–459. [CrossRef]
33. Dunnenberger, H.M.; Biszewski, M.; Bell, G.C.; Sereika, A.; May, H.; Johnson, S.G.; Hulick, P.J.; Khandekar, J. Implementation of a multidisciplinary pharmacogenomics clinic in a community health system. *Am. J. Health Syst. Pharm.* **2016**, *73*, 1956–1966. [CrossRef]
34. Johnson, J.; Burkley, B.; Langaee, T.; Clare-Salzler, M.; Klein, T.; Altman, R. Implementing Personalized Medicine: Development of a Cost-Effective Customized Pharmacogenetics Genotyping Array. *Clin. Pharmacol. Ther.* **2012**, *92*, 437–439. [CrossRef] [PubMed]
35. Swen, J.J.; Nijenhuis, M.; van Rhenen, M.; de Boer-Veger, N.J.; Buunk, A.-M.; Houwink, E.J.F.; Mulder, H.; Rongen, G.A.; van Schaik, R.H.N.; van der Weide, J.; et al. Pharmacogenetic Information in Clinical Guidelines: The European Perspective. *Clin. Pharmacol. Ther.* **2018**, *103*, 795–801. [CrossRef] [PubMed]
36. McCoy, A.B.; Thomas, E.J.; Krousel-Wood, M.; Sittig, D.F. Clinical decision support alert appropriateness: A review and proposal for improvement. *Ochsner. J.* **2014**, *14*, 195–202. [PubMed]

8

Impact of *CYP2C9* and *VKORC1* Polymorphisms on Warfarin Sensitivity and Responsiveness in Jordanian Cardiovascular Patients during the Initiation Therapy

Laith N. AL-Eitan [1,2,*], Ayah Y. Almasri [1] and Rame H. Khasawneh [3]

1 Department of Applied Biological Sciences, Jordan University of Science and Technology, Irbid 22110, Jordan; ayalmasri13@sci.just.edu.jo

2 Department of Biotechnology and Genetic Engineering, Jordan University of Science and Technology, Irbid 22110, Jordan

3 Department of Hematopathology, King Hussein Medical Center (KHMC), Jordan Royal Medical Services (RMS), Amman 11118, Jordan; rami.khasawneh@jaf.mil.jo

* Correspondence: lneitan@just.edu.jo

Abstract: Warfarin is an oral anticoagulant frequently used in the treatment of different cardiovascular diseases. Genetic polymorphisms in the *CYP2C9* and *VKORC1* genes have produced variants with altered catalytic properties. A total of 212 cardiovascular patients were genotyped for 17 Single Nucleotide Polymorphisms (SNPs) within the *CYP2C9* and *VKORC1* genes. This study confirmed a genetic association of the *CYP2C9**3 and *VKORC1* rs10871454, rs8050894, rs9934438, and rs17708472 SNPs with warfarin sensitivity. This study also found an association between *CYP2C9* and *VKORC1* genetic haplotype blocks and warfarin sensitivity. The initial warfarin dose was significantly related to the *CYP2C9**3 polymorphism and the four *VKORC1* SNPs ($p < 0.001$). There were significant associations between rs4086116 SNP and TAT haplotype within *CYP2C9* gene and rs17708472 SNP and CCGG haplotype within *VKORC1* gene and warfarin responsiveness. However, possessing a *VKORC1* variant allele was found to affect the international normalized ratio (INR) outcomes during initiation of warfarin therapy. In contrast, there was a loose association between the *CYP2C9* variant and INR measurements. These findings can enhance the current understanding of the great variability in response to warfarin treatment in Arabs.

Keywords: *CYP2C9*; *VKORC1*; warfarin; warfarin initiation phase of therapy; INR; pharmacogenetics study

1. Introduction

Warfarin is a commonly prescribed oral anticoagulant that is employed for the treatment of venous and arterial thromboembolic disorders and cardiac valve replacements [1]. However, interindividual genetic variation causes great variability in dosage requirements, making the latter a problematic issue for physicians. A higher or lower dose than needed could lead to bleeding and thrombotic risk, respectively [2,3]. Two-thirds of warfarin dose variation was due to environmental factors like age, body mass index, smoking status, gender, and diet, among others, while the remaining one-third is caused by genetic factors such as the *CYP2C9* and *VKORC1* genes [4–6].

Belonging to the cytochrome P450 superfamily, the *CYP2C9* gene is involved in the metabolism and clearance of S-warfarin, the latter of which is a racemic form of warfarin together with R-warfarin [7,8]. *CYP2C9* is located on the long arm of chromosome 10, and like other members of *CYP2C*, *CYP2C9* is highly polymorphic [9–11]. Although there are over 50 single nucleotide polymorphisms (SNPs) located in the regulatory and coding region of the *CYP2C9* sequence, the most studied *CYP2C9* polymorphisms are *CYP2C9**2 (R144C) and *CYP2C9**3 (I359L) [12,13]. It was found that individuals carrying the *CYP2C9* *2 *3 alleles reduced the elimination of S-warfarin and, therefore, plasma concentrations of the latter increased significantly compared to the wild-type allele and the individuals with these variant alleles need a lower warfarin maintenance dose [14].

Similarly, the *VKORC1* gene encodes the vitamin K epoxide reductase complex subunit 1 and it is a warfarin target [5]. The vitamin K epoxide reductase complex subunit 1 normally catalyzes the carboxylation reaction of the vitamin K-dependent protein glutamic acid residues in order to activate it, the latter of which are responsible for catalyzing the clotting factor pathway [15]. Several genetic studies conducted in different populations suggest that the G3673A (rs9923231), C6484T (rs9934438), and G9041A (rs7294) polymorphisms of the *VKORC1* gene are the most common and well-studied [7,16].

Analysis of *CYP2C9* and *VKORC1* gene polymorphisms revealed that they were responsible for 10% and 40% of warfarin dose requirement variance, respectively [17]. Combined with clinical data, both of the aforementioned genes can explain up to 60% of the warfarin variance [18,19]. More than 50 years ago, the dose of warfarin was determined by trial and error, with an initial dose (2–10 mg/day) dependent on the indication of warfarin and clinical factors, regardless of the effect of the genetic factor [20]. Patients are treated with warfarin in two stages, the first called the initiation phase of treatment, which is considered as the stage in which the initial international normalized ratio (INR) value of the patient is unstable and fluctuates up and down. With the second (maintenance) stage of the therapy, the patient is within the therapeutic INR for at least two consecutive visits [21]. However, pharmacogenetics for specific populations including Jordanian Arabs is necessary. Therefore, the objective of this study was to recognize genetic variations within the *CYP2C9* and *VKORC1* genes that are involved in warfarin sensitivity and responsiveness in Jordanian cardiovascular patients of Arab descent during initiation of treatment.

2. Materials and Methods

2.1. Patient Population and Study Design

The study population consisted of 212 unrelated warfarin intake patients selected from the Jordanian-Arab population, from the Anticoagulation Clinic at the Queen Alia Heart Institute (QAHI) in Amman, Jordan. Informed consent was obtained from all subjects. The study protocol was approved by the Human Ethics Committee at Jordan University of Science and Technology in Irbid, Jordan, and the Royal Medical Services in Amman, Jordan. Ethical approval code: 13/78/2014.

In this study, patients have cardiovascular diseases and are prescribed warfarin as an anticoagulant therapy. Inclusion criteria involved patients being 18 years or older and having received warfarin for at least three months. Patients who did not provide informed written consent, did not visit the anticoagulation clinic regularly, took *CYP2C9* inducers or inhibitors, or did not have a complete data set were excluded.

Initially, 350 patients were screened and, based on the aforementioned inclusion and exclusion criteria, 300 patients were approached to participate in this study (Figure 1). 80 patients were subsequently excluded because of inability to complete the treatment program or refusal. Of the remaining patients, 220 accepted to be part of this study, after which an additional eight patients were excluded from the final analysis because of a failure in genotyping. In total, whole sets of data were obtained from 212 patients with cardiovascular disease who were being treated with warfarin. Data was collected on demographic (age, gender, and body mass index) and lifestyle (smoking status and diet) characteristics as well as medical history (diseases and clinical features of warfarin therapy). Clinical features included the target INR, mean weekly warfarin doses required to reach the target INR, and the use of concomitant medication, all of which are required to be known in order to adjust warfarin doses. All data were blinded and obtained through semi-standardized interviews and medical records.

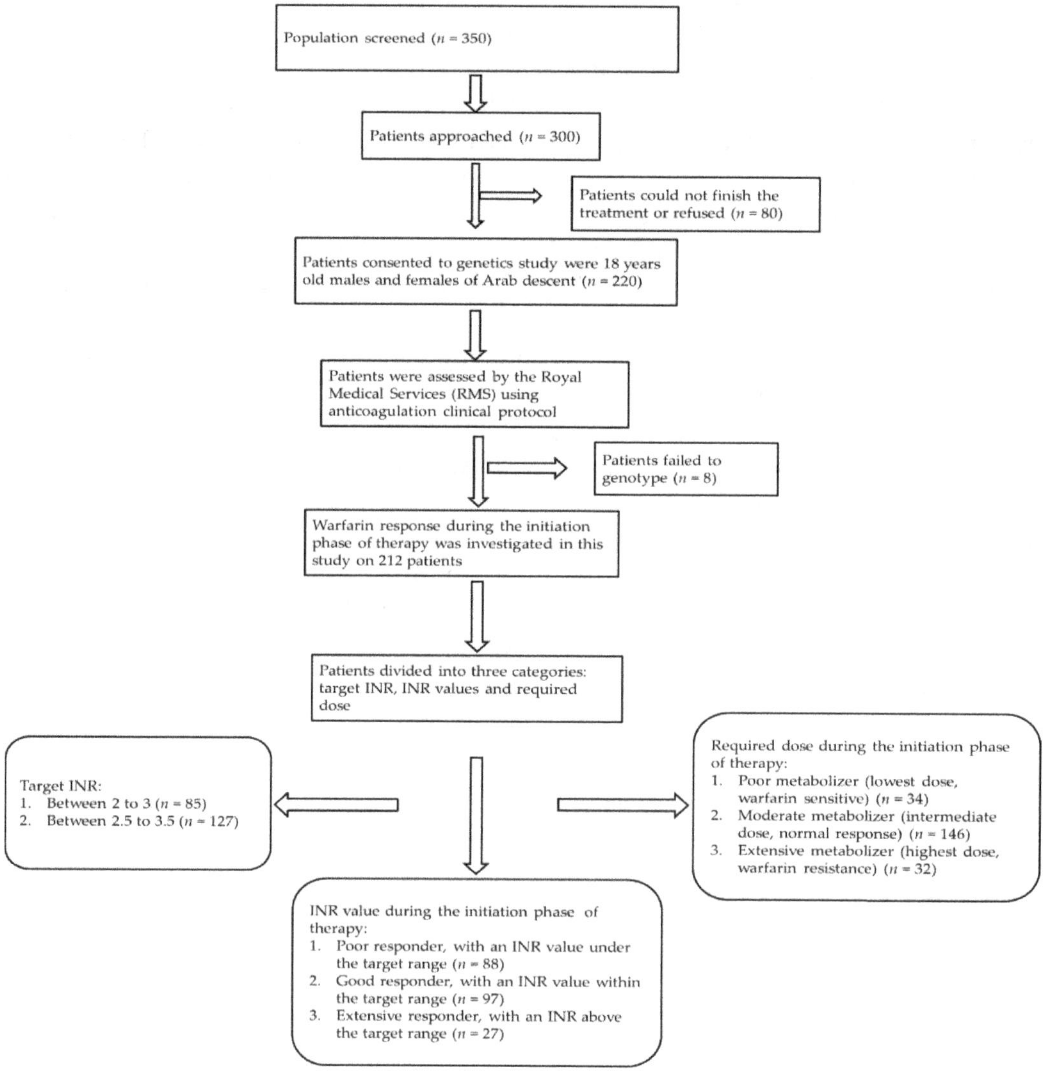

Figure 1. Flow chart depicting study design. INR: international normalized ratio.

All subjects in this study received warfarin anticoagulant therapy according to RMS anticoagulation protocol, which began with 2.5 to 10 mg nightly doses. INR monitoring is required at least once a week for the first three to four weeks after the initiation of therapy. After three consecutive visits, a patient with stable INR reaches the maintenance dose and is monitored for warfarin treatment administration by clinic protocol.

2.2. Outcome Measurement

Oral anticoagulant therapy was mandated by the prothrombin time (PT) that is, evaluated using an automated method over STAGO coagulometric unit in the QAHI laboratory. To calculate INR, there was a blood coagulation (clotting) test. INR monitoring for dose adjustments was determined by the physician and pharmacist. INR values between January 2014 and November 2015 were obtained from medical records, and these values were then used to divide the patients according to warfarin responsiveness into: (1) good responders, with an INR value within the target range; (2) poor responders, with an INR value under the target range; and (3) extensive responders, with an INR above the target range.

Further, based on their warfarin sensitivity, patients were divided into resistant, normal, or sensitive to warfarin as follows: (1) warfarin resistance (or Poor metabolizer), largest daily doses were required to keep a patient's INR within a therapeutic range (dose required > 49 mg/week); (2) warfarin normal patient (or Intermediate metabolizer), intermediate doses required (doses between 21–49 mg/week); and (3) warfarin sensitive patient (or Extensive metabolizer) lowest doses required (required dose <21 mg/week) [22].

2.3. SNP Selection, DNA Extraction, and Genotyping

In this study, 17 SNPs in the *CYP2C9* and *VKORC1* genes were selected from public databases and genotypes. Information about the aforementioned SNPs is shown in Table S1. Genomic DNA was extracted within one week of blood collection using the commercially available Wizard Genomic DNA Purification Kit (Promega Corporation, Madison, WI, USA) according to the manufacturer's instructions. After extraction, the DNA was diluted in 96-well plates using an automated robotic system to achieve concentrations of 20 ng/μL (50–500 μL). Concentrations were confirmed with the Nano-Drop ND-100 (Thermo Scientific, Wilmington, DE, USA). Genotyping was carried out by means of the MassARRAY®system (iPLEX GOLD) (Sequenom, San Diego, CA, USA), which was carried out at the Australian Genome Research Facility (AGRF) (Sequenom).

2.4. Statistical Analysis

Discrepancy and call rates were calculated using Microsoft Excel, and the deviation from Hardy Weinberg Equilibrium (HWE) was assessed using the Pearson X2 test. Minor allele frequencies (MAF) and HWE *p*-values for genotypic distribution were calculated via the Court lab-HW calculator. To test which of the chosen SNPs is associated with warfarin response, various statistical genetic association analyses were conducted, such as the chi-square, nonparametric correlation tests (Kruskal-Wallis and Tukey Pairwise comparison) and haplotype genetic analysis test. The Statistical Package for the Social Sciences (SPSS) version 21.0 and the SNPStat Web Tool (https://www.snpstats.net/start.htm) were used to perform all analyses.

3. Results

3.1. Study Group

The study group comprised of 212 unrelated Jordanian-Arabs patients treated with warfarin, with a mean age (±SD) of 56.03 (±17.68) years, a median age of 60, and an age range of 18 to 85 years. There were 34 poor responders (16%), 146 moderate responders (68.9%), and 32 extensive responders (15.1%). Table 1 summarizes the demographic, lifestyle, and medical characteristics of each of the three groups.

In total, 17 SNPs (100%) passed the quality control measures for throughput genotyping and were analyzed by the MassARRAY®system (iPLEX GOLD) with high accuracy and a 97% average success rate. The genotypic discrepancy average (±SD) rate over the 17 loci was only 0.06% (±0.0004%) out of the entire cohort (212 subjects). Genotypic and allelic frequencies are shown in Table S2.

For the 17 SNPs examined in this study, all were in accordance with the HWE. Ten polymorphisms (rs104894539, rs104894540, rs104894541, rs104894542, and rs61742245 in *VKORC1*, and rs28371685, rs28371686, rs72558191, rs9332131, and rs9332239 in *CYP2C9*) were non-polymorphic. In contrast, the seven remaining SNPs (rs10871454, rs8050894, rs9934438, and rs17708472 located in *VKORC1*, and rs1799853, rs4086116, and rs1057910 located in *CYP2C9*) were polymorphic and thus included in the study. The minor alleles and their frequencies for the successful genotyped SNPs are shown in Table S3.

3.2. *Effect of* CYP2C9 *and* VKORC1 *Polymorphisms on Warfarin Sensitivity during Initiation Phase of Therapy*

Regarding the association of *VKORC1* and *CYP2C9* SNPs with warfarin sensitivity among the three inclusion groups, significant differences in proportions among genotypes were observed at all tested *VKORC1* SNPs ($p < 0.001$) (Table 2). Significant differences were also observed between two SNPs of the *CYP2C9* gene (rs4086116 ($p = 0.012$) and rs1057910 ($p < 0.001$)), as shown in Table 2. Moreover, there was a significant association observed between *VKORC1* and *CYP2C9* haplotypes and warfarin sensitivity ($p < 0.0001$) (Table 3).

Table 1. Descriptive analysis of demographics and clinical characteristics of 212 cardiovascular patients treated with warfarin at the Queen Alia Heart Institute.

Category	Subcategory	Extensive Metabolizer	Good Metabolizers	Poor Metabolizers
Demographics	Patients (N, %)	(32/212) 15.1%	(146/212) 68.9%	(34/212) 16%
	Age [a] (years)	56.0 (17.68)	55.0 (14.64)	48.29 (15.09)
	BMI [a]	27.87 (3.72)	27.7 (4.85)	27.42 (3.45)
	Smoking (N, %)	31.25%	18.6%	41.2%
	Male	59.4%	51.4%	67.6%
	Female	40.6%	48.6%	32.4%
Concomitant Disease	Co morbidity	56.3%	68.5%	55.9%
	Hypertension	34.4%	42.5%	23.5%
	Diabetes mellitus	18.8%	21.9%	26.5%
	CHD [b]	28.1%	25.3%	29.4%
	Thyroid	0%	3.4%	2.9%
	Lipid	3.1%	6.8%	2.9%
Medication	Aspirin	62.5%	65.8%	76.5%
Indication of Treatment	MVR [c]	18.8%	10.3%	20.6%
	AVR [d]	6.3%	24.0%	20.6%
	AF [e]	34.4%	19.2%	20.6%
	DVR [f]	9.4%	15.8%	11.8%
	Others	9.4%	7.5%	0.0%
Target INR	2–3	43.8%	39.7%	38.2%
	2.5–3.5	56.3%	60.3%	61.8%
Mean weakly dose [a]		16.699 (2.79)	35.896 (7.39)	67.44 (42.48)
Mean INR [a]		2.82 (0.72)	2.38 (0.75)	2.44 (0.83)

[a] Mean Standard deviation in square brackets. [b] CHD: Chronic heart disease. [c] MVR:Mitral valve replacement. [d] AVR: Aortic valve replacement. [e] AF: Atrial Fibrillation. [f] DVR: Double valve replacement.

Table 2. Association of *VKORC1* and *CYP2C9* single nucleotide polymorphism (SNPs) with warfarin sensitivity during the initiation phase of therapy of 212 cardiovascular patients.

Gene	SNP ID	Genotype	Sensitive	Moderate	Resistance	*p*-Value *
VKORC1	rs10871454	CC	4.3%	57.4%	38.3%	<0.001
		CT	10.0%	76.4%	13.6%	
		TT	34.5%	63.6%	1.8%	
	rs8050894	CC	2.3%	60.5%	37.2%	<0.001
		CG	10.9%	74.5%	14.5%	
		GG	32.2%	64.4%	3.4%	
	rs9934438	CC	4.2%	58.3%	37.5%	<0.001
		CT	9.9%	76.6%	13.5%	
		TT	35.8%	62.3%	1.9%	
	rs17708472	CC	18.1%	68.8%	13.1%	<0.001
		CT	6.1%	73.5%	20.4%	
		TT	0.0%	0.0%	100%	
CYP2C9	rs1799853	CC	14%	70.1%	15.9%	0.744
		CT	19.6%	63%	17.4%	
		TT	0.0%	100%	0.0%	
	rs4086116	CC	8.1%	73.2%	18.7%	0.012
		CT	24.1%	62.0%	13.9%	
		TT	30.0%	70.0%	0.0%	
	rs1057910	AA	8.8%	72.5%	18.7%	<0.001
		AC	41.5%	53.7%	4.9%	

* Chi-Square Test with *p*-value < 0.05 is considered significant.

Table 3. Frequencies of the haplotypes of *VKORC1* and *CYP2C9* genes among the 212 warfarin sensitive patients.

Gene	Haplotypes	Frequency * (%)	Odds Ratio (95% CI)	*p*-Value **
VKORC1	TGAG	0.512	0.00	——
	CCGG	0.324	0.32 (0.2–0.43)	<0.0001
	CCGA	0.129	0.38 (0.23–0.54)	<0.0001
	CGGG	0.028	0.34 (0.03–0.66)	0.034
	TCGG	0.007	0.21 (−0.38–0.8)	0.48
CYP2C9	CAC	0.767	0.00	——
	TAT	0.116	−0.05 (−0.21–0.11)	0.53
	TCC	0.094	−0.45 (−0.64–−0.27)	<0.0001
	TAC	0.021	0.01 (−0.34–0.37)	0.95
	TCT	0.002	−1.11 (−2.14–−0.08)	0.037

* Genetic haplotype frequency of 212 warfarin intake patients, ** *p*-value < 0.05 is considered significant.

3.3. *Effect of* CYP2C9 *and* VKORC1 *Polymorphisms on Warfarin Required Dose during Initiation Phase of Therapy*

Carriers of *CYP2C9* and *VKORC1* polymorphisms had a significantly increased required dose compared with wild-type subjects or carriers of only one polymorphism of *CYP2C9* or *VKORC1* (Table 4).

Table 4. Association of *VKORC1* and *CYP2C9* SNPs with variability on warfarin required doses and with INR treatment outcome.

SNP ID	Initiation Dose	*p*-Value *	Initiation INR	*p*-Value *
rs10871454	38.1 (23.02)	<0.001	2.46 (0.77)	0.006
rs8050894		<0.001		0.008
rs9934438		<0.001		0.009
rs17708472		<0.001		0.511
rs1799853		0.118		0.184
rs4086116		0.001		0.08
rs1057910		0.001		0.572

* Kurskal Wallis test with *p*-value < 0.05 is considered significant, Mean Standard deviation in square brackets.

3.4. *Effect of* CYP2C9 *and* VKORC1 *Polymorphisms on Warfarin Responsiveness during Initiation of Therapy*

There were no significant differences in patient responder groups regarding the *VKORC1* and *CYP2C9* SNPs except for the *VKORC1* rs17708472 ($p = 0.042$) and the *CYP2C9* rs4086116 ($p = 0.005$) SNPs (Table 5). However, significant associations were found between genetic haplotypes of CCGG *VKORC1* and TAT *CYP2C9* and warfarin sensitivity, with $p = 0.02$ and $p = 0.018$, respectively (Table 6).

3.5. *Effect of* CYP2C9 *and* VKORC1 *Polymorphisms on INR Treatment Outcome*

There were no significant differences observed between the *CYP2C9* SNP genotypes and INR values measured at start of treatment for 212 cardiovascular patients treated with warfarin. In contrast, significant differences were observed between INR values measured at the initiation phase of therapy and certain *VKORC1* SNPs, namely rs10871454 ($p = 0.006$), rs8050894 ($p = 0.007$), and rs9934438 ($p = 0.009$), as shown in Table 4.

Table 5. Association of *VKORC1* and *CYP2C9* SNPs with response to warfarin during the initiation phase of therapy of 212 cardiovascular patients.

Gene	SNP ID	Genotype	Poor Responder	Good Responder	Extensive Responder	p-Value *
VKORC1	rs10871454	CC	55.3%	36.2%	8.5%	0.171
		CT	40.9%	45.5%	13.6%	
		TT	30.9%	54.5%	14.5%	
	rs8050894	CC	53.5%	39.5%	7%	0.235
		CG	41.8%	43.6%	14.5%	
		GG	32.2%	54.2%	13.6%	
	rs9934438	CC	54.2%	37.5%	8.3%	0.226
		CT	40.5%	45%	14.4%	
		TT	32.1%	54.7%	13.2%	
	rs17708472	CC	38.1%	50.6%	11.3%	0.042
		CT	55.1%	28.6%	16.3%	
		TT	0.0%	66.7%	33.3%	
CYP2C9	rs1799853	CC	45.1%	44.5%	10.4%	0.076
		CT	28.3%	52.5%	19.6%	
		TT	50.0%	0.0%	50.0%	
	rs4086116	CC	45.5%	43.9%	10.6%	0.005
		CT	39.2%	49.4%	11.4%	
		TT	10.0%	40.0%	50.0%	
	rs1057910	AA	42.1%	45.0%	12.9%	0.910
		AC	39%	48.8%	12.2%	

* Chi-Square Test with p-value < 0.05 is considered significant.

Table 6. Frequencies of the haplotypes of *VKORC1* and *CYP2C9* genes among the 212 warfarin responsiveness patients.

Gene	Haplotypes	Frequency * (%)	Odds Ratio (95% CI)	p-Value **
VKORC1	TGAG	0.512	0.00	——
	CCGG	0.326	−0.18 (−0.33–−0.03)	0.02
	CCGA	0.129	−0.08 (−0.28–0.12)	0.46
	CGGG	0.026	−0.05 (−0.47–0.36)	0.8
	TCGG	0.007	0.55 (−0.22–1.32)	0.16
CYP2C9	CAC	0.767	0.00	——
	TAT	0.115	0.25 (0.04–0.45)	0.018
	TCC	0.094	0.06 (−0.17–0.3)	0.59
	TAC	0.021	0.44 (−0.01–0.89)	0.059
	TCT	0.003	0.4 (−0.9–1.71)	0.55

* Genetic haplotype frequency of 212 warfarin intake patients, ** p-value < 0.05 is considered significant.

3.6. Correlation Between Warfarin Dose and Clinical Data

Finally, there was no significant correlation between warfarin dose and body mass index, age, gender, co-morbidities, or the treatment indication ($p = 0.505$).

4. Discussion

Earlier studies on warfarin pharmacogenetics provide evidence that common *VKORC1* and *CYP2C9* polymorphisms with clinical and environmental factors are responsible for over half of the variability in warfarin required dose [23,24]. Genotyping patients who are carriers of *VKORC1* and

CYP2C9 variant alleles has been proven to reduce the risk of over-anticoagulation compared to the traditional initial dose approach [25,26].

In this study, our goal was to identify genetic factors associated with sensitivity and responsiveness to warfarin treatment during the initiation phase of treatment in Jordanian-Arab patients with cardiovascular disease. The results of the current pharmacogenetic study strongly suggest that there is a significant association of the *VKORC1* rs8050894, rs10871454, rs9934438, and rs17708472 SNPs and the *CYP2C9* rs4086116 and rs1057910 SNPs and their haplotypes with the required warfarin dosage and warfarin sensitivity. This study also reported that there is a genetic association between *VKORC1* rs17708472 SNP and CCGG genetic haplotype block and *CYP2C9* rs4086116 SNP and TAT genetic haplotype block with warfarin responsiveness during the initiation phase of therapy.

The allelic frequencies of *CYP2C9* and *VKORC1* SNPs in our population were similar to those found in other ethnic groups, as in the case of *CYP2C9**2*, with 10% in our population, 6% in American and European populations, and 1% in Africans [27]. However, allelic frequencies of *VKORC1* SNPs were found to differ drastically from other populations. For example, rs10871454 was 52% in our population compared to 41% in Americans, 39% in Europeans, and 6% in African populations [27]. With regard to the association of *CYP2C9* polymorphisms with warfarin sensitivity, our results are consistent with the study by Takahashi et al. (2001) which shows that *CYP2C9* *2 and *3 polymorphisms reduce warfarin clearance [28] as *CYP2C9* is the major metabolizing enzyme of warfarin, therefore, reduction of activity results in lower required doses needed to achieve the therapeutic INR. We found a strong association of *CYP2C9*3* (rs1057910 A>C) and *CYP2C9* (rs4086116 C>T) genotypes with warfarin sensitivity during the initiation stage of treatment with $p < 0.001$ and $p = 0.012$, respectively (Table 2). This study reported that individuals with one variant allele were associated with an increased risk of warfarin sensitivity. For example, 41.5% of the patients who carried the rs1057910 A>C variant allele were sensitive to warfarin, compared to 8.8% of the wild-type patients were sensitive. Moreover, carrying a *CYP2C9* TCC genetic haplotype block was significantly associated with warfarin sensitivity with $p < 0.0001$ (Table 3).

In disagreement with other studies, the *CYP2C9**2 variant did not show a significant association with warfarin sensitivity ($p = 0.744$). This can possibly be explained by the genotypic frequency having an impact on the association; in our population only two patients were homozygous for the variant allele (TT), 32 were heterozygous patients (CT), and 105 patients were homozygous for the wild-type allele (CC) (Table 2). Moreover, it has been proposed that patients who carry one *CYP2C9** 2 allele results in a dose reduction compared with the wild-type dose [14,29,30]. Although the allelic frequency of *CYP2C9**2 (rs1799853) in our samples was in agreement with the American and European populations [27], this study did not find significant differences between this SNP and variability in required doses in the initiation phase of therapy ($p = 0.366$) as shown in Table 4 and Figure 2.

Clinical pharmacogenetic studies suggested that patients who carry the *CYP2C9*3* (rs1057910) C allele leads to a dose reduction of 28–41% [12,29,30] in the Caucasian American population and from 12–38% of the Asian population compared to the wild-type [31–34]. In alignment with the aforementioned studies, we revealed that there is a 34.3% reduction in warfarin dose. Patients carrying one variant allele (C) required 41.75 mg/week, in comparison with the wild-type allele which required 27.43 mg/week ($p < 0.001$), as shown in Table 4 and Figure 2. Therefore, in our study the *CYP2C9*3* allele has a greater effect on variation in warfarin dose during the initiation phase of therapy compared with *CYP2C9**2. In the case of individuals carrying rs4086116 C>T variant allele, this resulted in 23.9% and 37.9% reduction on warfarin dose compared to wild-type with $p = 0.016$, as shown in Table 4 and Figure 2.

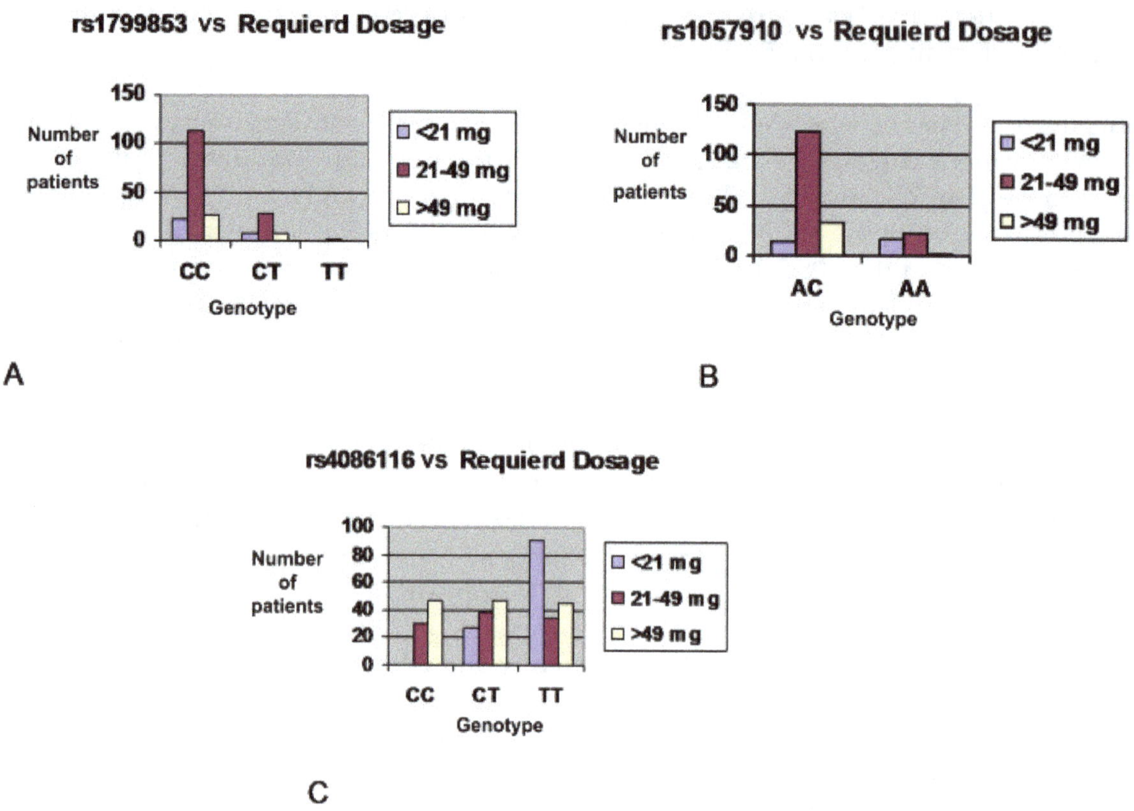

Figure 2. The distribution of warfarin dose by CYP2C9 genotypes during the initiation phase of therapy for 212 Jordanian cardiovascular patients: X axis represents different CYP2C9 genotypes, Y axis represents the proportion of patients across each genotype, Blue column represents a sensitive group who required the lowest warfarin dose (<21 mg/week), Purple column represents the intermediate group who required moderate warfarin dose ((21–49) mg/week), Yellow column represents a resistant group who required the highest warfarin dose (>49 mg/week). (**A**) Distribution of warfarin dose by rs1799853 variant. (**B**) Distribution of warfarin dose by rs1057910 variant. (**C**) Distribution of warfarin dose by rs4086116 variant.

For the four studied *VKORC1* SNPs, we observed a strong association of *VKORC1* SNPs with warfarin sensitivity ($p < 0.001$). For example, patients with the T allele for rs10871454 C>T showed a high risk of warfarin sensitivity with 25.5% (CT) and 48.3% (TT) reduction of the required dose, respectively. In this case, the drug target enzyme could be expressed in smaller amounts and, therefore, low doses of the drug can obtain a therapeutic INR in an initial phase of therapy (Table 2). Furthermore, *VKORC1* genetic haplotype analysis showed a significant association between three *VKORC1* genetic haplotype blocks and sensitivity to warfarin with $p < 0.0001$ (Table 3). Moreover, Schelleman et al. (2007) and Wadelius et al. (2005) reported that a correlation exists between *VKORC1* SNP 1173 C> T (rs9934438), and the variation in warfarin dose patients carrying the variant allele of this SNP is related to a reduction in the required dose compared to the wild-type [5,35]. In alignment with these results, we found that patients who carry one variant allele required an average dose of 39.47mg/week and two variant allele carriers needed an average of 26.82 mg/week, while patients carrying the wild type CC needed an average dose of 53.02 mg/week with $p < 0.001$ as shown in Figure 3. Limdi et al. (2007) and Shrif et al. (2011) showed that *VKORC1* rs8050894 (1542G>C) were associated with lower warfarin doses in European Americans and Sudanese patients, respectively [36,37]. Accordingly, our results found a significant association between lower required warfarin dose and this SNP at an initial phase of therapy with $p < 0.001$ as shown in Figure 3.

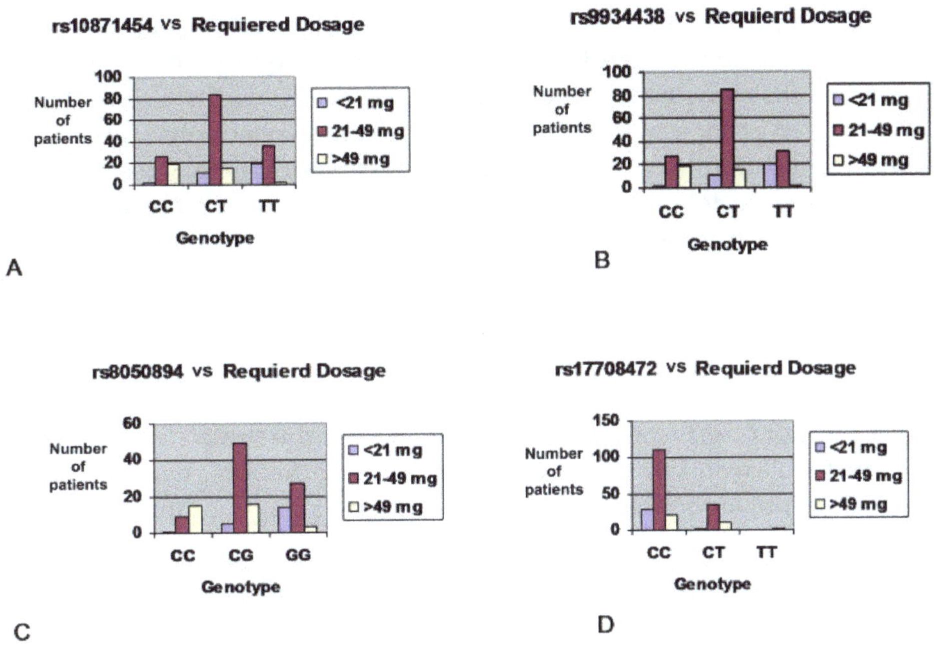

Figure 3. The distribution of warfarin dose by *VKORC1* genotypes during the initiation phase of therapy for 212 Jordanian cardiovascular patients: X axis represents different *VKORC1* genotypes, Y axis represents the proportion of patients across each genotype, Blue column represents a sensitive group who required the lowest warfarin dose (<21 mg/week), Purple column represents the intermediate group who required moderate warfarin dose ((21–49) mg/week), Yellow column represents a resistant group who required the highest warfarin dose (>49 mg/week). (**A**) Distribution of warfarin dose by rs10871454 variant. (**B**) Distribution of warfarin dose by rs9934438 variant. (**C**) Distribution of warfarin dose by rs8050894 variant. (**D**) Distribution of warfarin dose by rs17708472 variant.

For the last *VKORC1* SNP *VKORC1**4 C<T (rs17708472), our study is similar to the study by Haug et al. (2008), which reported that this SNP was associated with higher dose requirements [38]. Our results showed that this variant was associated with significant differences in initial warfarin required dose; patients who were homozygous for the variant allele (TT) genotype required an average dose of 57.8 mg/week, heterozygous (CT) patients required an average dose of 41.63 mg/week, while wild-type (CC) patients required an average dose of 33.65 with $p < 0.001$ (Table 4).

With regard to the correlation of *CYP2C9* and *VKORC1* SNPs and warfarin responsiveness, we compared SNP genotypes with the warfarin responder groups (poor, good, and extensive responders). Significant differences were found between *VKORC1* rs17708472 (C>T) genotypes and the three different responder groups (Table 5); 33.3% of the patients carrying the variant allele (TT) were within the extensive responder group (meaning this variant allele was associated with increased risk of over-anticoagulation), compared to 11.3% of the wild-type (CC) patients who were extensive responders ($p = 0.042$). Accordingly, Kringen et al. (2011) have also shown that patients who carry this SNP are associated with an increased risk of the existence of therapeutic INR (over-anticoagulation) [39]. Otherwise, *VKORC1* rs10871454, rs8050894, and rs9934438 alleles show no significant differences between SNP genotypes within the three responder groups in our population, with $p = 0.171$, 0.235, and 0.226, respectively (Table 5). In contrast, *VKORC1* CCGG genetic haplotype block showed a significant association with warfarin responsiveness with $p = 0.02$ (Table 6).

Moreover, significant differences were observed between *VKORC1* rs10871454, rs8050894, and rs9934438 SNPs and INR value during the initiation phase of therapy ($p = 0.006$, 0.007, and 0.009, respectively), while rs17708472 SNP showed no significant differences ($p = 0.493$). Therefore, in our population the *VKORC1* SNP genotypes are associated with the generation of a high or low INR during the initiation phase of therapy (Table 4).

Taube et al. (2000) reported that an individual carrying an allelic variant of *CYP2C9* was not associated with an increased incidence of severe over-coagulation during long-term treatment [40]. Correspondingly, our results show no significant differences between the *CYP2C9*2* and *3 genotypes within the three responder groups with $p = 0.076$ and 0.910, respectively (Table 5). Conversely, our study reported significant differences between the proportion of *CYP2C9* rs4086116 (C>T) genotype and the three different responder groups; 50% of TT carriers were within the extensive responder group compared with 10.6% of wild type CC carriers ($p = 0.005$), which means that TT carriers are associated with increased risk of over-anticoagulation (Table 5). Moreover, significant association was observed between *CYP2C9* TAT genetic haplotype block and warfarin responsiveness with $p = 0.018$ (Table 6).

In addition, we did not observe significant differences in the three studied SNPs (*CYP2C9*2, *3,* and *CYP2C9* (C> T) rs4086116) and the INR value during the initiation phase of therapy. Therefore, in our population *CYP2C9* is not associated with the generation of a high or low INR as shown in Table 4.

Confirmation of our results and ongoing research including additional factors will be accomplished in a larger patient cohort, including genetic factors such as *OATP* transporters (mediates the uptake of warfarin into hepatocytes), *CYP3A4*, *CYP1A1*, and *CYP1A2* enzymes (metabolizing of R-warfarin), or *GGCX* encoded *gamma-glutamyl carboxylase* (the reduced vitamin K–form to activate coagulation factors) [5,41]. Application for individualized warfarin treatment will be both beneficial and efficient for cardiovascular patients in the future. Finally, the majority of the population included in this study is elderly, with only 15% of the subjects under 40 years of age. Therefore, additional study is needed in children and young adults.

Author Contributions: L.N.A.-E. designed the study. L.N.A.-E., A.Y.A. and R.H.K. were responsible for clinical data and blood samples collection. L.N.A.-E. and A.Y.A. analyzed and interpreted the data. L.N.A.-E. and A.Y.A. prepared the manuscript. All authors helped in reviewing the manuscript.

Acknowledgments: We are grateful to Pharmacist Nadia Al-Omary, and engineer of Nutrition Miss Hanna from anticoagulation clinic for cooperation and providing excellent samples for this study and for coordinating the Anticoagulant Service, and Miss Diana, laboratory technician, for the blood collection and INR measurements.

References

1. Kim, Y.; Smith, A.; Wu, A. C3435T polymorphism of *MDR1* gene with warfarin resistance. *Clin. Chim. Acta* **2013**, *425*, 34–36. [CrossRef] [PubMed]
2. Motulsky, A.G.; Qi, M. Pharmacogenetics, pharmacogenomics and ecogenetics. *J. Zhejiang Univ. Sci. B.* **2006**, *7*, 169–170. [CrossRef] [PubMed]
3. Eriksson, N.; Wadelius, M. Prediction of warfarin dose: Why, when and how? *Pharmacogenomics* **2012**, *13*, 429–440. [CrossRef] [PubMed]
4. Sconce, E.A.; Khan, T.I.; Wynne, H.A.; Avery, P.; Monkhouse, L.; King, B.P.; Wood, P.; Kesteven, P.; Daly, A.K.; Kamali, F. The impact of *CYP2C9* and *VKORC1* genetic polymorphism and patient characteristics upon warfarin dose requirements: Proposal for a new dosing regimen. *Blood* **2005**, *106*, 2329–2333. [CrossRef] [PubMed]
5. Wadelius, M.; Chen, L.Y.; Downes, K.; Ghori, J.; Hunt, S.; Eriksson, N.; Wallerman, O.; Melhus, H.; Wadelius, C.; Bentley, D. Common *VKORC1* and *GGCX* polymorphisms associated with warfarin dose. *Pharmacogen. J.* **2005**, *5*, 262–270. [CrossRef] [PubMed]

6. Eichelbaum, M.; Ingelman-Sundberg, M.; Evans, W. Pharmacogenomics and individualized drug therapy. *Annu. Rev. Med.* **2006**, *57*, 119–137. [CrossRef] [PubMed]
7. D'Andrea, G.; D'Ambrosio, R.L.; Di Perna, P.; Chetta, M.; Santacroce, R.; Brancaccio, V.; Grandone, E.; Margaglione, M. A polymorphism in the *VKORC1* gene is associated with an interindividual variability in the dose-anticoagulant effect of warfarin. *Blood* **2005**, *105*, 645–649. [CrossRef] [PubMed]
8. Muszkat, M.; Blotnik, S.; Elami, A.; Krasilnikov, I.; Caraco, Y. Warfarin metabolism and anticoagulant effect: A prospective, observational study of the impact of *CYP2C9* genetic polymorphism in the presence of drug-disease and drug-drug interactions. *Clin. Ther.* **2007**, *29*, 427–437. [CrossRef]
9. Rendic, S. Summary of information on human CYP enzymes: Human P450 metabolism data. *Drug Metab. Rev.* **2002**, *34*, 83–448. [CrossRef] [PubMed]
10. Dean, L. *Warfarin Therapy and VKORC1 and CYP Genotype*; National Center for Biotechnology Information: Bethesda, MD, USA, 2012.
11. Zhou, S.; Zhou, Z.; Yang, L.; Cai, J. Substrates, inducers, inhibitors and structure-activity relationships of human cytochrome P450 2C9 and implications in drug development. *Curr. Med. Chem.* **2009**, *16*, 3480–3675. [CrossRef] [PubMed]
12. Kirchheiner, J.; Brockmoller, J. Clinical consequences of cytochrome P450 2C9 polymorphisms. *Clin. Pharmacol. Ther.* **2005**, *77*, 1–16. [CrossRef] [PubMed]
13. Zhou, Y.; Ingelman-Sundberg, M.; Lauschke, V.M. Worldwide distribution of cytochrome P450 alleles: A meta-analysis of population-scale sequencing projects. *Clin. Pharmacol. Ther.* **2017**, *102*, 688–700. [CrossRef] [PubMed]
14. Linder, M.W.; Homme, M.B.; Reynolds, K.K.; Gage, B.F.; Eby, C.; Silvestrov, N.; Valdes, R. Interactive modeling for ongoing utility of pharmacogenetic diagnostic testing: Application for warfarin therapy. *Clin. Chem.* **2009**, *55*, 1861–1868. [CrossRef] [PubMed]
15. Tie, J.K.; Stafford, D.W. Structural and functional insights into enzymes of the vitamin K cycle. *J. Thromb. Haemost.* **2016**, *14*, 236–247. [CrossRef] [PubMed]
16. Loebstein, R.; Dvoskin, I.; Halkin, H.; Vecsler, M.; Lubetsky, A.; Rechavi, G.; Amariglio, N.; Cohen, Y.; Ken-Dror, G.; Almog, S.; et al. A coding VKORC1 Asp36Tyr polymorphism predisposes to warfarin resistance. *Blood* **2007**, *109*, 2477–2480. [CrossRef] [PubMed]
17. Schalekamp, T.; De Boer, A. Pharmacogenetics of oral anticoagulant therapy. *Curr. Pharm. Des.* **2010**, *16*, 187–203. [CrossRef] [PubMed]
18. Wadelius, M.; Chen, L.Y.; Lindh, J.D.; Eriksson, N.; Ghori, M.J.; Bumpstead, S.; Holm, L.; McGinnis, R.; Rane, A.; Deloukas, P. The largest prospective warfarin-treated cohort supports genetic forecasting. *Blood* **2009**, *113*, 784–792. [CrossRef] [PubMed]
19. Lenzini, P.; Wadelius, M.; Kimmel, S.; Anderson, J.L.; Jorgensen, A.L.; Pirmohamed, M.; Caldwell, M.D.; Limdi, N.; Burmester, J.K.; Dowd, M.B.; et al. Integration of genetic, clinical, and INR data to refine warfarin dosing. *Clin. Pharmacol. Ther.* **2010**, *87*, 572–578. [CrossRef] [PubMed]
20. Gage, B.; Lesko, L. Pharmacogenetics of warfarin: Regulatory, scientific, and clinical issues. *J. Thromb. Thrombolysis* **2007**, *25*, 45–51. [CrossRef] [PubMed]
21. Kuruvilla, M.; Gurk-Turner, C. A review of warfarin dosing and monitoring. *Proc. Bayl. Univ. Med. Cent.* **2001**, *14*, 305–306. [CrossRef] [PubMed]
22. Hylek, E.; D'Antonio, J.; Evans-Molina, C.; Shea, C.; Henault, L.; Regan, S. Translating the results of randomized trials into clinical practice: The challenge of warfarin candidacy among hospitalized elderly patients with atrial fibrillation. *Stroke* **2006**, *37*, 1075–1080. [CrossRef] [PubMed]
23. Wiedermann, C.J.; Stockner, I. Warfarin-induced bleeding complications—Clinical presentation and therapeutic options. *Thromb. Res.* **2008**, *122*, S13–S18. [CrossRef]
24. Borgiani, P.; Ciccacci, C.; Forte, V.; Romano, S.; Federici, G.; Novelli, G. Allelic variants in the *CYP2C9* and *VKORC1* loci and interindividual variability in the anticoagulant dose effect of warfarin in Italians. *Pharmacogenomics* **2007**, *8*, 1545–1550. [CrossRef] [PubMed]
25. Hamberg, A.; Dahl, M.L.; Barban, M.; Scordo, M.G.; Wadelius, M.; Pengo, V.; Padrini, R.; Jonsson, E.N. A PK-PD model for predicting the impact of age, *CYP2C9*, and *VKORC1* genotype on individualization of warfarin therapy. *Clin. Pharmacol. Ther.* **2007**, *81*, 529–538. [CrossRef] [PubMed]

26. Teichert, M.; Van Schaik, R.H.N.; Hofman, A.; Uitterlinden, A.G.; de Smet, P.A.G.M.; Stricker, B.; Visser, L.E. Genotypes associated with reduced activity of *VKORC1* and *CYP2C9* and their modification of acenocoumarol anticoagulation during the initial treatment period. *Clin. Pharmacol. Ther.* **2009**, *85*, 379–386. [CrossRef] [PubMed]

27. 1000 Genomes Project Consortium. An integrated map of genetic variation from 1092 human genomes. *Nature* **2012**, *491*, 56–65. [CrossRef] [PubMed]

28. Takahashi, H.; Echizen, H. Pharmacogenetics of warfarin elimination and its clinical implications. *Clin. Pharmacokinet.* **2001**, *40*, 587–603. [CrossRef] [PubMed]

29. Kealey, C.; Chen, Z.; Christie, J.; Thorn, C.F.; Whitehead, A.S.; Price, M.; Samaha, F.F.; Kimmel, S.E. Warfarin and cytochrome P450 2C9 genotype: Possible ethnic variation in warfarin sensitivity. *Pharmacogenomics* **2008**, *8*, 217–225. [CrossRef] [PubMed]

30. Limdi, N.; McGwin, G.; Goldstein, J.; Beasley, T.; Arnett, D.; Adler, B.; Baird, M.; Acton, R. Influence of *CYP2C9* and *VKORC1 1173C/T* genotype on the risk of hemorrhagic complications in African-American and European-American patients on warfarin. *Clin. Pharmacol. Ther.* **2007**, *83*, 312–321. [CrossRef] [PubMed]

31. Ohno, M.; Yamamoto, A.; Ono, A.; Miura, G.; Funamoto, M.; Takemoto, Y.; Otsu, K.; Kouno, Y.; Tanabe, T.; Masunaga, Y.; et al. Influence of clinical and genetic factors on warfarin dose requirements among Japanese patients. *Eur. J. Clin. Pharmacol.* **2009**, *65*, 1097–1103. [CrossRef] [PubMed]

32. Huang, S.W.; Chen, H.S.; Wang, X.Q.; Huang, L.; Xu, D.L.; Hu, X.J.; Huang, Z.H.; He, Y.; Chen, K.M.; Xiang, D.K.; et al. Validation of *VKORC1* and *CYP2C9* genotypes on interindividual warfarin maintenance dose: A prospective study in Chinese patients. *Pharmacogenet. Genomics* **2009**, *19*, 226–234. [CrossRef] [PubMed]

33. Gan, G.; Phipps, M.; Ku, C.; Teh, A.; Sangkar, V. Genetic polymorphism of the CYP2C9 subfamily of 3 different races in warfarin maintenance dose. *Int. J. Hematol.* **2004**, *80*, 295–296. [CrossRef] [PubMed]

34. Tanira, M.; Al-Mukhaini, M.; Al-Hinai, A.; Al Balushi, K.; Ahmed, I. Frequency of CYP2C9 genotypes among Omani patients receiving warfarin and its correlation with warfarin dose. *Community Genet.* **2007**, *10*, 32–37. [CrossRef] [PubMed]

35. Schelleman, H.; Chen, Z.; Kealey, C.; Whitehead, A.S.; Christie, J.; Price, M.; Brensinger, C.M.; Newcomb, C.W.; Thorn, C.F.; Samaha, F.F.; et al. Warfarin response and vitamin K epoxide reductase complex 1 in African Americans and Caucasians. *Clin. Pharmacol. Ther.* **2007**, *81*, 742–747. [CrossRef] [PubMed]

36. Limdi, N.A.; Arnett, D.K.; Goldstein, J.A.; Beasley, T.M.; McGwin, G.; Adler, B.K.; Acton, R.T. Influence of *CYP2C9* and *VKORC1* on warfarin dose, anticoagulation attainment and maintenance among European Americans and African Americans. *Pharmacogenomics* **2008**, *9*, 511–526. [CrossRef] [PubMed]

37. Shrif, N.; Won, H.H.; Lee, S.T.; Park, J.H.; Kim, K.K.; Kim, M.J.; Kim, S.; Lee, S.Y.; Ki, C.S.; Osman, I.M.; et al. Evaluation of the effects of *VKORC1* polymorphisms and haplotypes, *CYP2C9* genotypes, and clinical factors on warfarin response in Sudanese patients. *Eur. J. Clin. Pharmacol.* **2011**, *67*, 1119–1130. [CrossRef] [PubMed]

38. Haug, K.B.; Sharikabad, M.N.; Kringen, M.K.; Narum, S.; Sjaatil, S.T.; Johansen, P.W.; Kierulf, P.; Seljeflot, I.; Arnesen, H.; Brørs, O. Warfarin dose and INR related to genotypes of CYP2C9 and VKORC1 in patients with myocardial infarction. *Thromb. J.* **2008**, *6*, 7. [CrossRef] [PubMed]

39. Kringen, M.K.; Haug, K.B.F.; Grimholt, R.M.; Stormo, C.; Narum, S.; Opdal, M.S.; Fosen, J.T.; Piehler, A.P.; Johansen, P.W.; Seljeflot, I.; et al. Genetic variation of VKORC1 and CYP4F2 genes related to warfarin maintenance dose in patients with myocardial infarction. *J. Biomed. Biotechnol.* **2011**, *2011*, 739–751. [CrossRef] [PubMed]

40. Taube, J.; Halsall, D.; Baglin, T. Influence of cytochrome P-450 CYP2C9 polymorphisms on warfarin sensitivity and risk of over-anticoagulation in patients on long-term treatment. *Blood* **2000**, *96*, 1816–1819. [PubMed]

41. Frymoyer, A. Effect of single-dose rifampin on the pharmacokinetics of warfarin in healthy volunteers. *Clin. Pharmacol. Ther.* **2010**, *88*, 540–547. [CrossRef] [PubMed]

9

Pharmacist-Initiated Pre-Emptive Pharmacogenetic Panel Testing with Clinical Decision Support in Primary Care: Record of PGx Results and Real-World Impact

Cathelijne H. van der Wouden [1,2], Paul C. D. Bank [1,2], Kübra Özokcu [3], Jesse J. Swen [1,2] and Henk-Jan Guchelaar [1,2,*]

1 Department of Clinical Pharmacy and Toxicology, Leiden University Medical Center, 2333 ZA Leiden, The Netherlands; j.j.swen@lumc.nl (J.J.S.)
2 Leiden Network for Personalised Therapeutics, 2333 ZA Leiden, The Netherlands
3 Division of Pharmacoepidemiology and Clinical Pharmacology, Utrecht Institute for Pharmaceutical Sciences (UIPS), Utrecht University, 3584 CG Utrecht, The Netherlands; K.Ozokcu@students.uu.nl
* Correspondence: H.J.Guchelaar@lumc.nl

Abstract: Logistics and (cost-)effectiveness of pharmacogenetic (PGx)-testing may be optimized when delivered through a pre-emptive panel-based approach, within a clinical decision support system (CDSS). Here, clinical recommendations are automatically deployed by the CDSS when a drug-gene interaction (DGI) is encountered. However, this requires record of PGx-panel results in the electronic medical record (EMR). Several studies indicate promising clinical utility of panel-based PGx-testing in polypharmacy and psychiatry, but is undetermined in primary care. Therefore, we aim to quantify both the feasibility and the real-world impact of this approach in primary care. Within a prospective pilot study, community pharmacists were provided the opportunity to request a panel of eight pharmacogenes to guide drug dispensing within a CDSS for 200 primary care patients. In this side-study, this cohort was cross-sectionally followed-up after a mean of 2.5-years. PGx-panel results were successfully recorded in 96% and 68% of pharmacist and general practitioner (GP) EMRs, respectively. This enabled 97% of patients to (re)use PGx-panel results for at least one, and 33% for up to four newly initiated prescriptions with possible DGIs. A total of 24.2% of these prescriptions had actionable DGIs, requiring pharmacotherapy adjustment. Healthcare utilization seemed not to vary among those who did and did not encounter a DGI. Pre-emptive panel-based PGx-testing is feasible and real-world impact is substantial in primary care.

Keywords: pre-emptive; pharmacogenetics; panel

---

1. Introduction

An individual's response to a drug can be predicted by their pharmacogenetic (PGx) profile [1,2]. Incorporation of an individual's PGx profile into drug prescribing promises a safer, more effective and thereby more cost-effective drug treatment [3,4]. Several randomized controlled trials (RCTs) demonstrate the clinical utility of pre-emptive single gene tests to guide dosing [5–7], and drug selection [8], for individual drug-gene interactions. These studies are perceived as a proof-of-concept supporting the clinical utility of pre-emptive PGx testing, and may therefore also be applied to other drug-gene interactions, for which evidence of the same rigour may lack [9,10]. The Dutch Pharmacogenetics Working Group (DPWG) was established in 2005 to devise clinical guidelines for individual drug-gene interactions based on a systematic review of literature [11,12]. These guidelines provide clinicians with recommendations on how to manage drug-gene interactions. To date, the DPWG has developed guidelines for 97 drug-gene interactions, of which 54 are actionable drug-gene interactions, many of which are encountered principally in primary care. In parallel, the Clinical Pharmacogenetics Implementation Consortium (CPIC) has also devised guidelines for more than 40 drugs [13]. The DPWG and CPIC guidelines have ongoing efforts to harmonize the two [14]. In the Netherlands, the DPWG guidelines are incorporated into a nationwide clinical decision support system, called the "G-standaard", providing pharmacists and general practitioners (GPs) with relevant clinical recommendations at the point of care when an actionable drug-gene interaction is encountered.

Significant debate persists regarding the optimal approach for implementing PGx testing in clinical care; where some support using a pre-therapeutic single gene approach and others a pre-emptive panel-based approach [15]. The pre-therapeutic single gene approach has several drawbacks. In this one-at-a-time strategy, an individual gene is tested in response to a first prescription of an interacting target drug. If, however, patients receive prescriptions for multiple interacting target drugs over time, they may require testing for multiple single genes. Here, pharmacotherapy may be delayed in awaiting the PGx results. Furthermore, the costs of single gene testing may be allocated a multitude of times, while the marginal cost of testing and interpreting additional pharmacogenes simultaneously is near-zero [16,17]. These logistical and cost-effectiveness issues may be overcome and optimized when delivering PGx in a panel-based approach [18]. Here, a panel of variants within multiple genes, which are associated with drug response, are tested and saved for later use in preparation of future prescriptions [15]. In this way, the panel-results can be reused over time, as multiple drugs which interact with multiple variants are prescribed [19]. When an interacting target drug is prescribed, the corresponding PGx guideline can be deployed by the clinical decision support system at the point of care, thereby providing clinicians with the necessary information to guide prescribing by PGx, without any delay. Alternatively, a combination of the two strategies may be the optimal approach for delivering PGx. Here, a panel test is ordered reactively in response to an incident prescription and is saved in the electronic medical record (EMR) for pre-emptive use in future prescriptions. However, in order for the clinical decision support system to be enabled, it is crucial that the PGx results are recorded and preserved in the EMR. If this fails, a potential drug-gene interaction may go unnoticed. As a result, the added value of testing multiple genes is lost. A recent study showed that PGx results for *CYP2D6* were sparsely recorded; only 3.1% and 5.9% of reported PGx results were recorded in EMRs by general practitioners (GPs) and pharmacists, respectively, within a mean follow-up of 862 days [20]. This indicates that correct record of PGx results in the EMR may be a remaining barrier preventing the realization of panel-based testing. However, this is yet undetermined when reporting the results for multiple genes simultaneously. Therefore, we sought to investigate whether pharmacists and GPs are able to record PGx panel testing results within their EMR, in order to enable life-long use of PGx results through a clinical decision support system.

Another barrier preventing implementation of panel-based PGx testing is the lack of evidence demonstrating its clinical utility. Although there is a firm evidence base supporting the clinical utility of pre-emptive single gene PGx testing, evidence of similar quality supporting a panel-based approach is lacking [21]. Even so, several smaller studies report promising results indicating that pre-emptive panel-based PGx guided prescribing is indeed (cost-)effective in preventing adverse drug reactions among polypharmacy and psychiatry patients. However, this is yet to be determined within primary care [22–27]. Alternatively, the clinical impact of population-wide panel-based testing has previously been modelled by using Medicare prescription data; indicating half of patients above 65 will use at least one of the drugs for which PGx guidelines are available during a four year period, and one fourth to one third, will use two or more of these drugs [28]. Another study showed that more than 60% of the population would benefit from PGx guided prescribing within a 5-year period [19]. However, the clinical impact is yet undetermined in a real-world setting. This may differ from modelled estimations since the patients selected by pharmacists to receive panel testing may differ from those included in prescription datasets. Therefore, we aim to quantify the potential real-world impact of implementation of PGx panel in a clinical decision support system within a side-study of the Implementation of Pharmacogenetics into Primary care Project (IP3 study). In this side-study, the primary outcome is the frequency at which patients receive newly initiated prescriptions, with possible drug-gene interactions, for which PGx results are available in the EMR. To explore which target groups may benefit most from panel testing, we aim to investigate which patient sub-groups may more frequently initiate newly prescribed drugs within follow-up. Secondary outcomes include their downstream impact on healthcare utilization. Firstly, we hypothesize that patients who encounter an actionable drug-gene interaction and adhered to the DPWG guidelines will have a similar healthcare utilization compared to those who did not encounter an actionable drug-gene interaction. Secondly, we hypothesize that patients who encounter an actionable drug-gene interaction, but did not adhere to the DPWG guidelines, have a higher healthcare utilization compared to those who did not encounter an actionable drug-gene interaction.

2. Materials and Methods

2.1. Study Design, Participants

We performed a cross-sectional follow-up of The Implementation of Pharmacogenetics into Primary care Project (IP3 study) cohort, as a side-study. The IP3 study is a prospective multicenter observational pilot study with the objective to test the feasibility of pharmacist-initiated pharmacogenetics testing within a clinical decision support system in primary care. The study design, rationale and main study findings have previously been described elsewhere [29]. In brief, community pharmacies in the vicinity of Leiden, The Netherlands, were invited to participate in the study. Pharmacists who agreed on participation were provided with the opportunity to request free PGx tests for a panel of 40 variants in eight pharmacogenes (see Supplementary Table S1), to guide drug dispensing based on the DPWG guidelines, for a maximum of 200 patients. The genes selected to be tested were based on genes for which DPWG guidelines are available and which are either included in the Affymetrix Drug Metabolizing and Transporters (DMET) array (*CYP2C9*, *CYP2C19*, *CYP2D6*, *CYP3A5*, *SLCO1B1*, *TPMT* and *VKORC1*) or determined in clinical care (*DPYD*). This panel can be used in combination with the DPWG guidelines to guide drug prescribing for 41 drugs. Here, a combination of reactive and pre-emptive panel testing is implemented. A PGx panel is ordered reactively in response to an incident prescription and is saved in the EMR for pre-emptive use is future prescriptions. Adult patients receiving a first prescription (defined as no prescription for the first drug within the preceding 12 months) for at least 28 days for one of 10 drugs (amitriptyline, atomoxetine, atorvastatin, (es)citalopram, clomipramine, doxepin, nortriptyline, simvastatin or venlafaxine) in routine care were eligible. Additional in- and exclusion criteria are reported elsewhere [29]. After identification of the patients through automated queries, the participating pharmacists manually checked whether patients fulfilled the in- and exclusion criteria. Finally, patients not recruited within 14 days after dispensing the first prescription were excluded. When patients were eligible, pharmacists were able to select these patients for ordering a PGx panel. The panel test result could be used reactively for the drug of enrolment and pre-emptively for future prescriptions of 41 drugs with potential drug-gene interactions.

2.2. Healthcare Setting

In the Dutch healthcare system, patients are typically listed with one GP and one pharmacy. The GP plays a gatekeeping role in the provision of healthcare. The GP is consulted for all initial healthcare problems and may refer to specialized care when appropriate. Typically, GPs maintain EMRs for their patients and contain prescription history, lab results, correspondence with specialized physicians and reports regarding ER (emergency room) visits and hospitalizations. In parallel, pharmacists maintain a separate EMR containing dispensing history, relevant contra-indications and drug allergies and are used for medication surveillance at drug dispensing.

In routine care, PGx testing is predominantly performed within hospital pharmacy or clinical chemistry laboratories. Hospitals additionally maintain a separate EMR for registered patients. Generated PGx results are typically recorded in the hospital's EMR and are communicated with requesting pharmacists of physicians in primary care by paper or electronic reports.

2.3. Ethics Approval

All subjects gave their written informed consent for enrolment before they participated in the study. The study was conducted in accordance with the Declaration of Helsinki, and the protocol was approved by the Ethics Committee of Leiden University Medical Center (LUMC) (P14.081). Patients provided informed consent for data collection regarding their medication and related outcomes from both pharmacy and GP EMRs within 3 years of enrolment.

2.4. DNA Collection, Isolation, Extraction and Genotyping

After providing signed informed consent, pharmacists collected a 2mL saliva sample from participating patients using the Oragene DNA OG-250 (DNA Genotek Inc). The samples were transported to the PGx laboratory in Leiden University Medical Center by research staff or mail. DNA was extracted in accordance to Oragene DNA OG-250 isolation procedure, where a solution volume of 100μL, instead of 200 μL, was used. The DNA concentration was quantified in each sample with NanoDropPhotometer (Thermo Fisher Scientific), and DNA quality was assessed with the use of the 260 nm/280 nm absorbance ratio. Genotypes of *CYP2C9*, *CYP2C19*, *CYP2D6*, *CYP3A5*, *DPYD*, *SLCO1B1*, *TPMT* and *VKORC1* were determined using the Drug Metabolizing and Transporters (DMET) Plus Array (Affymetrix, Santa Clara, CA). *CYP2D6* copy number variants were detected with qPCR (Thermo Fisher Scientific, Massachusetts, USA). The DMET array was supplemented with the *DPYD* 1236G>A and 2846A>T variants which were routinely tested in clinic at the LUMC. Validation of the assays is described elsewhere [29].

2.5. Translation of Genotype to Phenotype and Return of Results

Genotypes for the eight pharmacogenes were translated into predicted phenotypes using the DPWG guidelines. A paper report holding the genotypes, predicted phenotypes and the DPWG therapeutic recommendation for the drug of enrollment was devised and sent to the patients' general practitioner (GP) and pharmacist by mail and/or fax (see Supplementary Figure S1 for an example report). The report held the request to record the entire PGx profile in the EMR to enable the clinical decision support system when drug-gene interaction is encountered during drug prescribing or dispensing (see Figure 1). Predicted phenotypes must be recorded in the EMR in a contra-indication format to enable deployment of the relevant guideline through the clinical decision support system. Even if patients are predicted to be extensive metabolizers (EM), we recommend that they still be recorded as contra-indications to record the performance of this test. However, pharmacy EMRs can hold a maximum of 10 contra-indications. It is important to note that the pilot study is initiated through the pharmacists and therefore the GPs who receive the paper report may have had no prior knowledge about the existence of the IP3 pilot study.

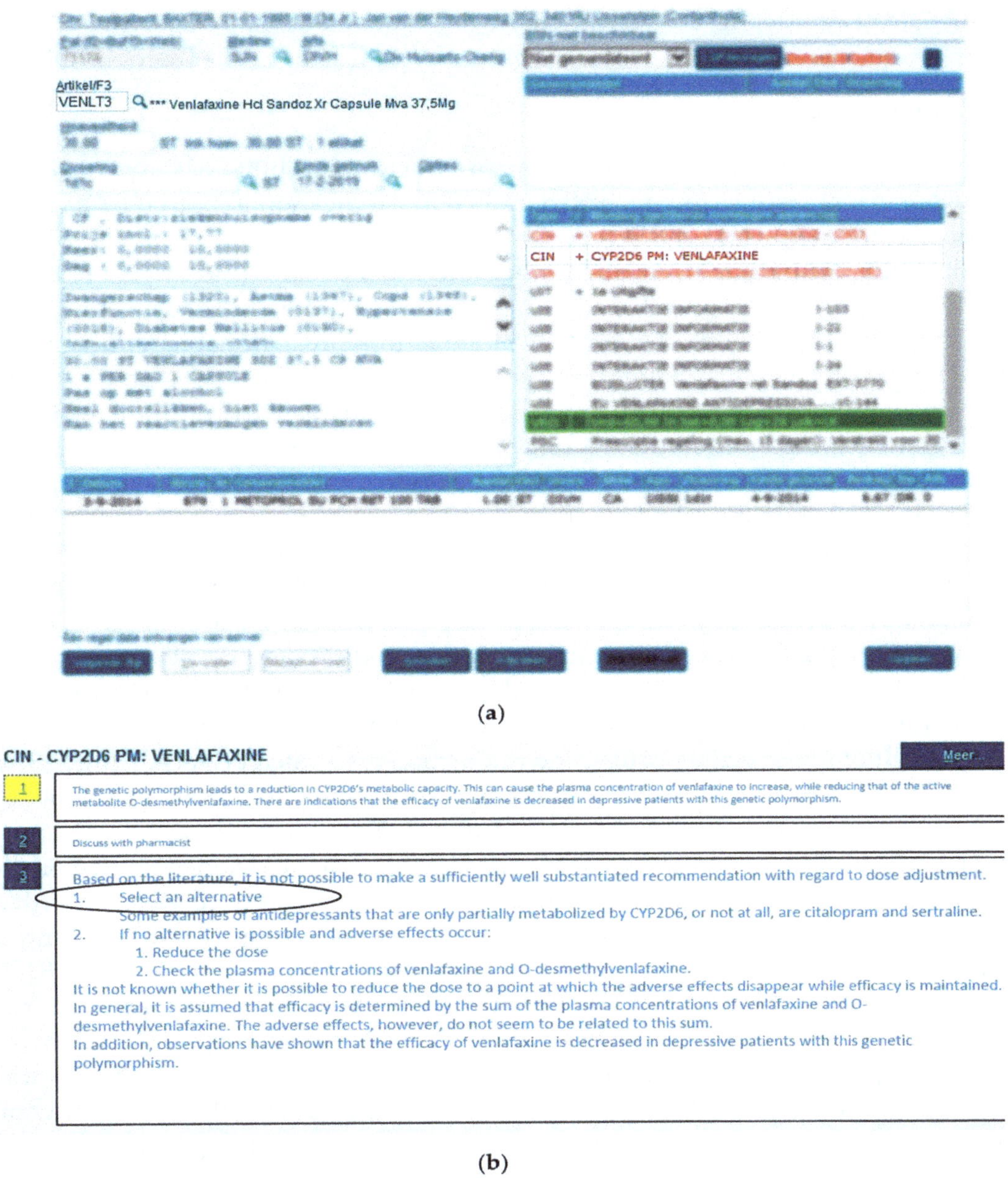
Artikel/F3
VENLT3
Venlafaxine Hcl Sandoz Xr Capsule Mva 37,5Mg
CIN + CYP2D6 PM: VENLAFAXINE
(a)
CIN - CYP2D6 PM: VENLAFAXINE
Meer...
1
The genetic polymorphism leads to a reduction in CYP2D6's metabolic capacity. This can cause the plasma concentration of venlafaxine to increase, while reducing that of the active metabolite O-desmethylvenlafaxine. There are indications that the efficacy of venlafaxine is decreased in depressive patients with this genetic polymorphism.
2
Discuss with pharmacist
3
Based on the literature, it is not possible to make a sufficiently well substantiated recommendation with regard to dose adjustment.
1. Select an alternative
Some examples of antidepressants that are only partially metabolized by CYP2D6, or not at all, are citalopram and sertraline.
2. If no alternative is possible and adverse effects occur:
1. Reduce the dose
2. Check the plasma concentrations of venlafaxine and O-desmethylvenlafaxine.
It is not known whether it is possible to reduce the dose to a point at which the adverse effects disappear while efficacy is maintained.
In general, it is assumed that efficacy is determined by the sum of the plasma concentrations of venlafaxine and O-desmethylvenlafaxine. The adverse effects, however, do not seem to be related to this sum.
In addition, observations have shown that the efficacy of venlafaxine is decreased in depressive patients with this genetic polymorphism.
(b)

Figure 1. Clinical decision support during drug dispensing. A patient who is *CYP2D6* PM (as noted in the electronic medical record (EMR) as contra-indication, as indicated by "CIN" (contra-indication) receives a prescription for venlafaxine (**a**) which triggers a pop-up with the relevant Dutch Pharmacogenetics Working Group (DPWG) recommendation directing selection of alternative drug (**b**).

2.6. Healthcare Provider Incorporation of PGx Results in Drug Prescribing and Dispensing

When an actionable drug-gene interaction is encountered, the DPWG guideline directs adjustment of drug, dose or vigilance of pharmacotherapy to avoid potential adverse drug reactions or lack of efficacy. However, pharmacists are free to choose whether to adhere to the DPWG guidelines. In The Netherlands, and within the IP3 study, pharmacists must discuss pharmacotherapy alteration, resulting from medication surveillance, with the prescribing physicians before the prescription can be altered.

2.7. Groups for Analysis

Patients have been stratified into three groups for comparison (see Table 1): 1) those who did not encounter an actionable drug-gene interaction for the drug of enrolment, 2) those who encountered an actionable drug-gene interaction for the drug of enrolment and whose health care providers chose to adhere to the DPWG guideline, and 3) those who encountered an actionable drug-gene interaction for the drug of enrolment and whose health care providers chose not to adhere to the DPWG guideline.

2.8. Outcomes and Analyses

In this side-study, the primary outcome for quantifying the feasibility of the panel-based approach is whether the PGx panel results were recorded as a contra-indication in both the GP and pharmacist EMRs at the time of follow-up.

In this side-study, the primary outcome for quantifying the real-world impact of the panel-based approach is the number of newly initiated drugs for which potential drug-gene interactions are encountered, since enrolment, and whether these interactions are actionable. A potential drug-gene interaction is encountered when a patient, regardless of their phenotype (e.g., *CYP2D6* PM, IM or EM), receives a new prescription for a drug for which an actionable DPWG guideline is available and the interacting gene was included in the IP3 panel (e.g., metoprolol-*CYP2D6* guideline). A potential drug-gene interaction becomes an actionable when the patient's predicted phenotype directs adjustment of pharmacotherapy, based on the relevant DPWG guideline (e.g., patient is *CYP2D6* PM and initiates metoprolol). See Supplementary Table S2 for a list of drugs for which actionable DPWG guidelines are available and IP3 panel results can be used to identify potential and actionable drug-gene interactions. To explore which target group may benefit most from panel testing, we investigate whether baseline demographic variables (gender, age, BMI, number of comorbidities and number of comedications) are associated with an increasing number of prescribed drugs with potential drug-gene interactions within follow-up by using univariate negative binomial regression. The secondary outcome is healthcare utilization as a result of pre-specified drug-gene interaction associated adverse drug reactions within 12 weeks of enrolment. This is a composite endpoint of GP consults (in person, by phone or by e-mail), emergency department (ED) visits, and hospitalizations. These drug-gene interactions associated adverse drug reactions were defined before data collection was initiated and are based on the literature underlying the DPWG guidelines. For example, if a patient enrolled on simvastatin with a *SLCO1B1* TC genotype consults their GP regarding muscle pain symptoms within 12 weeks of initiation, this is considered a drug-gene interaction associated adverse drug reactions since *SLCO1B1* TC and CC carriers are at higher risk for statin-induced myopathy [30]. See Supplementary Table S3 for an overview of pre-specified drug-gene interaction associated adverse drug reactions and underlying literature. We compare the frequency of the composite endpoint among patients who encounter an actionable drug-gene interaction and adhered to the DPWG guidelines (group 2) to those who did not encounter an actionable drug-gene interactions associated adverse drug reactions(group 1), using binomial logistic regression in a non-inferiority analysis. We have set a non-inferiority at a margin of 1.2. Secondly, we compare the frequency of the composite endpoint among patients who encounter an actionable drug-gene interaction, but did not adhere to the DPWG guidelines (group 3), to those who did not encounter an actionable drug-gene interaction (group 1), using binomial logistic regression.

3. Results

3.1. IP3 Cohort and Follow-Up

Overall 200 patients were enrolled in the IP3 study between November 2014 and July 2016. Patient characteristics are presented in Table 1. The database containing the genotypes and predicted phenotypes is available at https://databases.lovd.nl/shared/individuals (patient IDs 184080-184279). 62 (31.0%) patients encountered an actionable drug-gene interaction for the drug of enrolment, as previously reported by Bank et al. [29]. Of these, health care providers chose to adhere to the DPWG guideline in 49 (79.0%) cases. Data collection was performed retrospectively between April 2018 and September 2018 in both pharmacy and GP EMRs; from pharmacy EMRs between May 4th 2018 and May 29th 2018; and from GP EMRs between April 3rd 2018 and September 28th 2018. Data could be retrospectively collected cross-sectionally from 200 (100%) and 177 (88.5%) pharmacy and GP EMRs, respectively (see Figure 2). The mean follow-up from pharmacy EMRs was 933 days (range 649–1279), approximately 2.5 years. The mean follow-up from GP EMRs was 917 days (range 622–1238).

Table 1. Summary of patient characteristics in Implementation of Pharmacogenetics into Primary care Project (IP3) cohort stratified by groups for analysis

	Overall IP3 Study Cohort (n = 200)	Groups for Analysis		
			Actionable Drug-Gene Interaction for the Drug of Enrolment (n = 62, 31.0%)	
		1) No Drug-Gene Interaction for the Drug of Enrolment (n = 138, 69.0%)	2) Health Care Provider Adhered to DPWG Guideline (n = 49, 24.5%) *	3) Health Care Providers did not Adhere to DPWG Guideline (n = 9, 4.5%) *
Gender				
Female, n (%)	103 (51.5)	74 (53.6)	25 (51.0)	3 (33.3)
Male, n (%)	97 (48.5)	64 (46.4)	24 (49.0)	6 (66.8)
Age in years, Mean (SD)	61.6 (11.2)	62.3 (11.0)	60.9 (11.5)	56.8 (13.3)
BMI (kg/m^2), Mean (SD)	28.3 (14.9)	28.9 (17.7)	27.1 (4.5)	27.4 (2.4)
Self-reported ethnicity father, n (%)				
Caucasian	187 (93.5)	128 (92.8)	47 (95.9)	9 (100.0)
Other	13 (6.5)	10 (7.2)	2 (4.1)	0 (0.0)
Self-reported ethnicity mother, n (%)				
Caucasian	188 (94.0)	129 (93.5)	47 (95.9)	9 (100.0)
Other	12 (6.0)	9 (6.5)	2 (4.1)	0 (0.0)
Drug of enrolment, n (%)				
Amitriptyline	15 (7.5)	9 (6.5)	5 (10.2)	0 (0.0)
Atorvastatin	115 (57.5)	80 (58.0)	28 (57.1)	5 (55.6)
Citalopram	7 (3.5)	5 (3.6)	1 (2.0)	0 (0.0)
Escitalopram	3 (1.5)	2 (1.4)	1 (2.0)	0 (0.0)
Nortriptyline	17 (8.5)	10 (7.2)	5 (10.2)	2 (22.2)
Simvastatin	29 (14.5)	26 (18.8)	2 (4.1)	1 (11.1)
Venlafaxine	14 (7.0)	6 (4.3)	7 (14.3)	1 (11.1)
Number of comorbidities at baseline, Mean (SD) **	4.6 (2.5)	4.4 (2.4)	4.9 (2.6)	4.4 (2.3)
Number of comedications at baseline, Mean (SD) **	4.0 (3.3)	3.93 (3.4)	4.0 (2.9)	4.4 (3.0)

IP3: Implementation of Pharmacogenetics into Primary care Project; SD: standard deviation; BMI: body mass index; * Excluding others (n = 4): Recommendation given after drug was discontinued (n = 1); same dose (n = 1); dose increased and ECG unknown (n = 1); no drug-gene interaction and no action (n = 1). ** Based on n = 177 for whom data collection from GP records was completed.

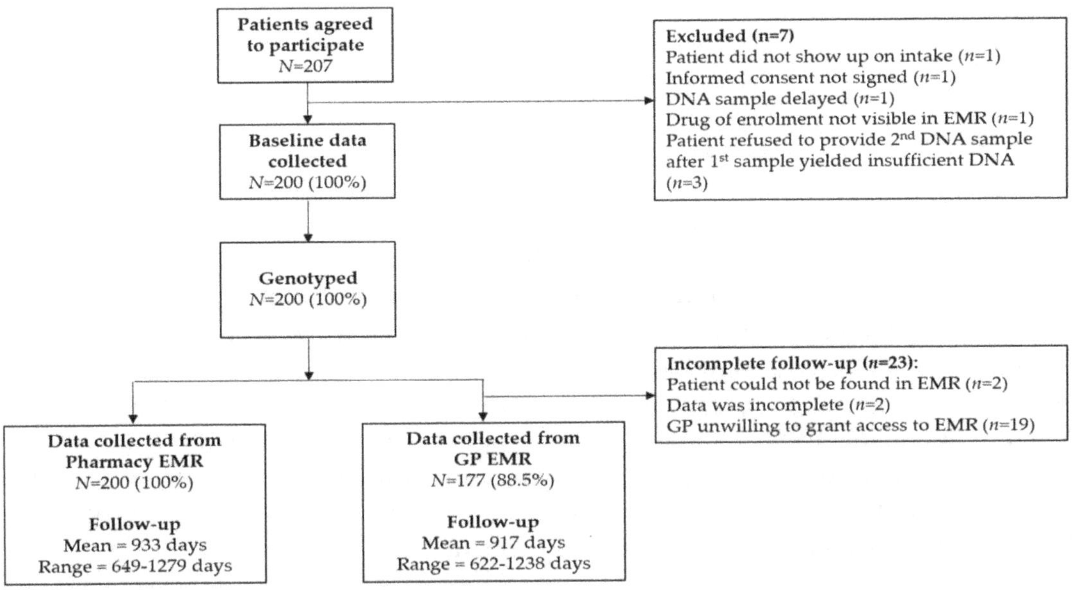

Figure 2. Flow chart or IP3 participant enrolment and follow-up.

3.2. Feasibility: Record of PGx Panel Results in the Pharmacy and GP EMRs

Record of PGx panel results by both pharmacists and GPs are shown in Figure 3. Pharmacists were able to record predicted phenotypes (including EMs) in 96.0% (n = 192) of pharmacy EMRs. In all cases they were recorded as contra-indications (100%, n = 192). Pharmacists failed to document the PGx results in 4.0% of cases (n = 8). The most common reason for failure of documentation (2.0%, n = 4) was merely due to PGx paper reports being lost in the pharmacy. The second most common reason was that the individual did not carry any aberrant variant, and was therefore predicted wildtype for all genes; this was the case for three patients (1.5%, n = 3). Pharmacists, therefore, felt it was not necessary to record EM phenotypes. Only one set of PGx results was failed to be documented in the EMR since the pharmacist did not know how to (0.5%). A discrepancy between the reported results and documented results was found in the records of two patients (1.0%). This was due to a manual error on account of the pharmacist.

General practitioners were able to record the PGx results in 67.8% (n = 120) of patient records. Of these, 34% (n = 59) were recorded as contra-indications and 35% (n = 61) in another format such as a PDF file.

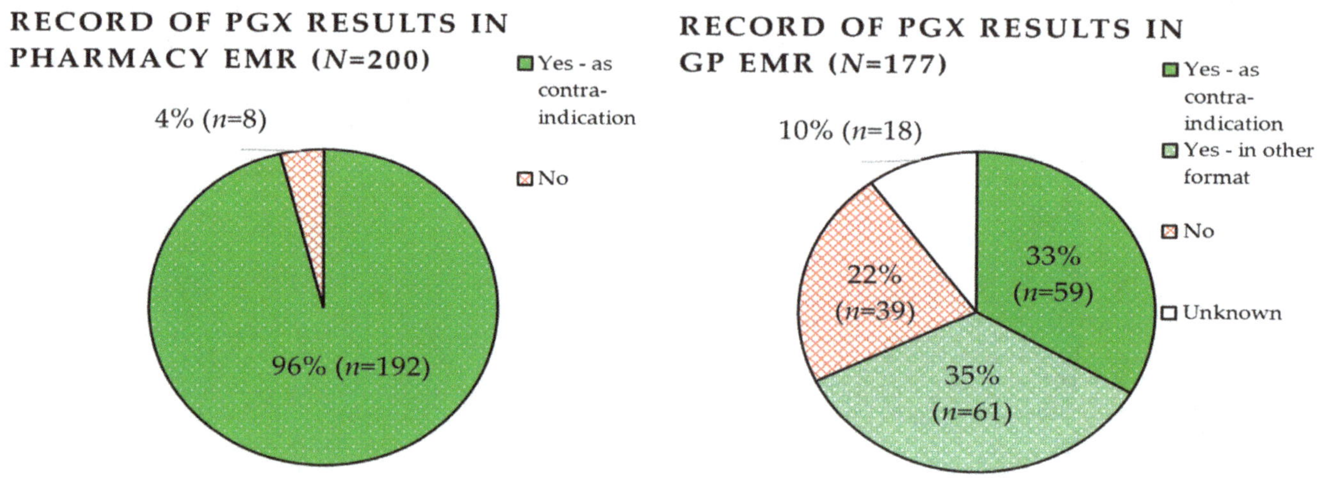

Figure 3. Record of pharmacogenetic panel results in the pharmacy and general practitioner (GP) electronic medical records (EMRs).

3.3. Real-World Impact: Frequency of Newly Prescribed Drugs for Which PGx Results Were Available in the EMR

Table 2 shows the frequency of newly initiated drugs for which there were potential drug-gene interactions and PGx results were available in the EMR. 97.0% (n = 194) of patients received at least one subsequent drug for which PGx results were in the EMR. Within the follow-up time, a mean of 2.71 drugs for which the PGx results were available were prescribed, of these 0.66 (24.2%) were actionable drug-gene interactions, requiring pharmacotherapy adjustment. The most commonly prescribed drugs for which PGx results were available were atorvastatin (14.4%), simvastatin (9.4%) and pantoprazole (9.4%). The most common drugs which were actionable drug-gene interactions, however, were atorvastatin (28.2%), metoprolol (13.0%) and amitriptyline (8.4%). To explore who may benefit most from PGx-panel testing, Table 3 presents baseline demographics stratified by an increasing number of newly initiated drugs for which there were potential drug-gene interaction. It seems that the number of newly initiated prescriptions increases with age, number of comorbidities and number of comedications, but this could not be statistically concluded.

Table 2. Frequency of newly initiated drugs for which there were potential drug-gene interactions in subsequent prescriptions after pharmacogenetics panel in 200 primary care patients with a mean follow-up of 933 days (=2.56 years).

	Number of Patients (%)	Three Most Commonly Prescribed with Potential Drug-Gene Interaction, N (%)	Actionable Drug-Gene Interaction (%)	Three Most Commonly Prescribed with Actionable Drug-Gene Interactions, N (%)
Subsequent drug 1	194 (97%)	1. atorvastatin, 69 (35.6%) 2. omeprazole, 26 (13.4%) 3. pantoprazole, 20 (10.3%)	47 (24.2%)	1. atorvastatin, 19 (40.4%) 2. amitriptyline, 11 (23.4%) 3. citalopram, 6 (12.8%)
Subsequent drug 2	166 (83%)	1. atorvastatin, 32 (19,3%) 2. metoprolol, 29 (17.5%) 3. simvastatin, 21 (12.7%)	46 (27.7%)	1. atorvastatin, 14 (30.4%) 2. metoprolol, 10 (21.7%) 3. codeine, 6 (13.0%)
Subsequent drug 3	115 (57.5%)	1. pantoprazole, 20 (17.4%) 2. omeprazole, 19 (16.5%) 3. simvastatin, 15 (13.0%)	23 (20.0%)	1. metoprolol, 7 (30.4%) 2. simvastatin, 4 (17.4%) 3. codeine/venlafaxine, 3 (13.0%)
Subsequent drug 4	66 (33%)	1. simvastatin, 15 (22.7%) 2. pantoprazole, 11 (16.7%) 3. atorvastatin, 9 (13.6%)	15 (22.7%)	1. atorvastatin, 4 (26.7%) 2. venlafaxine/simvastatin/ clopidogrel, 2 (13.3%) 3. citalopram/omeprazole/codeine/ flecainide/metoprolol, 1 (6.7%)
Overall	**541**	**1. atorvastatin, 78 (14.4%)** **2. simvastatin, 51 (9.4%)** **3. pantoprazole, 51 (9.4%)**	**131 (24.2%)**	**1. atorvastatin, 37 (28.2%)** **2. metoprolol, 17 (13.0%)** **3. amitriptyline, 11 (8.4%)**
Mean per patient (SD)	**2.71 (1.1)**	-	**0.66 (0.8)**	-

SD: standard deviation.

Table 3. IP3 cohort stratified by number of newly initiated drugs with a potential drug-gene interaction within follow-up.

	Overall IP3 Study Cohort (n = 200)	0 (n = 6, 3%)	1 (n = 27, 13.5%)	2 (n = 52, 26%)	3 (n = 50, 25%)	≥4 (n = 65, 32.5%)	p-Value *
Gender							
Female, n (%)	103 (51.5)	4 (66.7)	12 (44.4)	24 (46.2)	27 (54.0)	36 (55.4)	0.775
Male, n (%)	97 (48.5)	2 (33.3)	15 (55.6)	28 (53.8)	23 (46.0)	29 (44.6)	
Age in years, Mean (SD)	61.6 (11.2)	53.3 (16.3)	59.4 (10.6)	61.0 (11.5)	63.0 (10.5)	62.8 (11.1)	0.442
BMI (kg/m^2), Mean (SD)	28.3 (14.9)	25.6 (2.6)	29.1 (5.8)	27.4 (4.5)	27.6 (4.8)	29.6 (25.2)	0.854
Number of comorbidities at baseline, Mean (SD) **	4.6 (2.5)	3.4 (1.1)	4.0 (2.2)	4.0 (2.5)	4.6 (2.3)	5.4 (2.6)	0.232
Number of comedications at baseline, Mean (SD) **	4.0 (3.3)	3.0 (2.1)	3.4 (3.4)	3.3 (3.4)	3.8 (2.7)	5.1 (3.4)	0.279

SD: standard deviation; BMI: body mass index; * Univariate negative binomial regression; ** Based on n = 177 for whom data collection from GP records was completed.

3.4. Real-World Impact: Downstream Effects of Actionable Drug-Gene Interactions on Healthcare Utilization

Table 4 shows that patients who encountered an actionable drug-gene interaction and whose health care providers adhered to the DPWG guidelines had a similar healthcare utilization as a result of a drug-gene interactions associated adverse drug reaction (40.0%) to those who did not carry an actionable drug-gene interaction (30.0%). This in line with our initial hypothesis. The 95%-CIs of the incidence of composite endpoint drug-gene interactions associated adverse drug reaction of groups 1 and 2 overlap. We therefore observe that there is no difference between the two groups. However, we cannot demonstrate non-inferiority since the upper limit of the 95%-CI of the OR of group 1 is not lower than the non-inferiority margin of 1.2.

We observed a much lower healthcare utilization as a result of a drug-gene interactions associated adverse drug reactions among patients carrying an actionable drug-gene interaction but whose health care providers did not adhere to the DPWG guidelines (0.0%) to those who did not carry an actionable drug-gene interaction (30.0%). This is in contrast to our initial hypothesis.

Table 4. Healthcare utilization as a result of drug-gene interaction associated adverse drug reactions within 12 weeks of enrolment.

	Overall IP3 Study Cohort $n = 200$	1) No Drug-Gene Interaction for the Drug of Enrolment $n = 138$ (69.0%)	Actionable Drug-Gene Interaction for the Drug of Enrolment: 2) Health Care Provider Adhered to DPWG Guideline $n = 49$ (24.5%)	Actionable Drug-Gene Interaction for the Drug of Enrolment: 3) Health Care Provider did not Adhere to DPWG Guideline $n = 9$ (4.5%)
GP EMR follow-up completed (%)	177 (88.5%)	120 (87.0%)	45 (91.8%)	8 (88.9%)
Number of patients experiencing drug-gene interactions associated adverse drug reactions	56 (31.6%)	37 (30.8%)	19 (43.2%)	0 (0.0%)
Composite endpoint drug-gene interactions associated adverse drug reactions				
Number of patients, n (%)	**54 (30.5%)**	**36 (30.0%)**	**18 (40.0%)**	**0 (0.0%)**
95% CI		**66.0%–80.6%**	**47.1%–73.7%**	
GP consults as a result of drug-gene interactions associated adverse drug reactions				
Number of patients, n (%)	52 (29.4%)	35 (29.2%)	17 (37.8%)	0 (0.0%)
Number of GP consults, Mean (SD)	53, 2.19 (2.11)	35, 2.06 (1.99)	18, 2.44 (2.36)	0, 0 (0)
ER visit as a result of drug-gene interactions associated adverse drug reactions				
Number of patients, n (%)	3 (1.7%)	1 (0.8%)	2 (4.4%)	0 (0%)
Number of ER visits, Mean (SD)	3, 1 (1)	1, 1 (1)	2, 1 (1)	0, 0 (0)
Hospitalization as a result of drug-gene interactions associated adverse drug reactions				
Number of patients, n (%)	1 (0.6%)	1 (0.6%)	0 (0.0%)	0 (0.0%)
Number of hosp., Mean (SD)	1, 1 (1)	1, 1 (1)	0, 0 (0)	0, 0 (0)
Binomial Logistic Regression (group 1 and 2) OR [95%CI] *		**1.81 [0.89, 3.67]**		

GP: general practitioner; OR: odd ratio; CI: confidence interval; * Including gender, age, and BMI as covariates.

4. Discussion

We report what is, to our knowledge, the first assessment of the real-world impact of pharmacist-initiated pre-emptive panel-based testing in primary care. This side-study demonstrates that recording of PGx panel results in the EMR is feasible and enables health care providers to (re)use these results to inform pharmacotherapy of newly initiated prescriptions. 96% of PGx panel results were successfully recorded in the pharmacy EMR, enabling 97% of patients to (re)use these results for at least one, and 33% of patients for up to four newly initiated prescriptions, within a relatively short 2.5-year follow-up. Of all newly initiated prescriptions with a potential drug-gene interaction (n = 541), 24.2% (n = 131) were actionable drug-gene interactions, requiring pharmacotherapy adjustment. We expect the potential impact of pre-emptive panel-based testing to further increase with time as the likelihood of additional subsequent prescriptions increases.

With their dedication to medication surveillance, pharmacists are leading candidates to manage requesting of PGx testing, recording of PGx results and application of the PGx guidelines. This is confirmed by other pilot studies performed in pharmacy settings [31–35]. However, we found that both pharmacists and GPs are very able to record PGx results in their EMRs as contra-indications (96% and 33% of pharmacists and GPs, respectively); enabling deployment of relevant guidelines by the clinical decision support system when a drug-gene interaction is encountered both at prescribing and dispensing. An advantage of applying this double-verification is the minimization of the risk of missing a drug-gene interaction. As a result, it is not disastrous that GPs also recorded them in other formats, thereby not enabling the clinical decision support system at prescribing, in 35% of cases. In contrast, a recent study showed that genotyping results were sparsely communicated and recorded correctly; only 3.1% and 5.9% of reported genotyping results were recorded by GPs and pharmacists, respectively, within a similar follow-up time [20]. The discrepancy between these could be due to the pilot study setting or differences in PGx reporting methods. IP3 study researchers have visited the participating IP3 pharmacies multiple times within the follow-up period; possibly unintentionally reminding or motivating pharmacists to record PGx results, which they may otherwise have not performed. However, it is important to note that GPs were outside the scope of the pilot study setting, as they were not the enrolling health care providers, and therefore provide a less biased perspective on recording frequency. Still, it is much higher than that reported by Simoons et al. [20]. Surprisingly, 1.5% of PGx results were not recorded by pharmacists because they did not include actionable genotypes. However, it is still of importance to document these results to avoid unnecessary re-testing of the patient. Finally, the fact that discrepancies between reported results and the recorded result were only observed in 1% of pharmacy EMR cases, indicates that the current manual system of recording is error prone. Regardless of the low error rate, PGx results are static and therefore life-long. It is therefore imperative that errors in the recording of PGx results are avoided. Future initiatives should focus on the development of automated sharing of PGx results across EMRs. In the Netherlands, such an initiative has been the launched but requires patient consent before it can be utilized. The National Exchange Point ("Landelijk Schakel Punt" (LSP)) is a nationwide secured EMR infrastructure to which nearly health care providers access [36]. Only when a patient has provided written consent for the LSP, can a professional summary of the local pharmacy or GP EMR, including PGx results, be downloaded by another treating health care provider in the same region; unless the patient chose to shield this information. Alternatively, providing the PGx results directly to patients may resolve the issue in terms of communicating and recording PGx results; for example, utilizing the Medication Safety-Code card [37,38].

In the face of a time in which health care providers are confronted with an increasing number of variables to optimize clinical decision making, it is of utmost importance that this information is presented in a structured fashion; this is achieved by a clinical decision support system [39,40]. PGx testing results differ from other laboratory testing results because they remain applicable over a patient's lifetime. We have demonstrated that, even within a relatively short follow-up, the real-world impact of a panel-based approach combined with a clinical decision support system is immense; almost all (97%) of patients used PGx results for at least one, and 33% of patients for up to four prescriptions within a relatively short 2.5-year follow-up. Of these, 24.2% (n = 131) were actionable drug-gene interactions. Similar proportions of actionable drug-gene interactions in primary care were found by Bank et al. (unpublished) [41]. Here, investigators overlaid the frequencies of phenotypes as observed within the IP3 cohort with nationwide prescription data spanning one year and found that 3.6 million incident prescriptions encountered a potential drug-gene interactions and of these, 856,002 (23.6%) encountered an actionable drug-gene interaction [41]. We observed drugs for which results were useful; these were primarily statins and proton pump inhibitors. This finding is in accordance with Samwald et al. [28]. The observed frequencies of potential drug-gene interactions, however, are much higher than reported by others previously [19,28]. Samwald et al. indicated half of the patients above 65 will use at least one of the drugs for which PGx guidelines are available during a four year period, and one fourth to one third will use two or more of these drugs [28]. Schildcrout et al. reported that 60% of the population would benefit from PGx guided prescribing within a 5-year period [19]. The higher frequency we observed could be a result of different target populations and drugs. Our sample consisted of patients selected by pharmacist and who initiated one of ten drugs, and therefore at higher risk for initiating subsequent drugs. Several promising studies indicate the effectiveness and effect of PGx panel-based testing on healthcare utilization in psychiatry and polypharmacy [22–27]. For example, Brixner et al. studied the effect of panel-based PGx testing with 6 genes on the healthcare utilization within polypharmacy patients. Results showed that the

PGx screened cohort had a lower rate of ER visits (RR = 0.29, 95% confidence interval (CI) = 0.15–0.55, $p = 0.0002$) and a lower rate of hospitalizations (relative risk (RR) of 0.61, 95% CI = 0.39–0.95, $p = 0.027$). With this decrease in ER visits and hospitalizations, the authors concluded that PGx panel-based testing could potentially lead to cost-savings [23]. These cost savings may be potentially higher than that observed in primary care since polypharmacy patients have a higher a priori risk of hospitalization, as it increases with the number of comedications [42]. In this study we aimed to assess the downstream effects of an actionable drug-gene interaction on healthcare utilization. Although we did not observe a statistically significant difference between groups 1 (40%) and 2 (30%), we were not able to conclude non-inferiority, since this is a side-study by design and therefore was underpowered for a non-inferiority analysis. In contrast to our initial hypothesis we observed a much lower healthcare utilization among group 3 (0%) patients when compared to group 2 (30%). However, this cannot be concluded, since the adherence rate of HCPs was high, thereby resulting in a relatively low number of patients carrying an actionable DGI but whose HCPs did not adhere to the DPWG guidelines. Another limitation to this analysis is the retrospectively collected data from GP EMRs, which is prone to reporting bias. Nonetheless, gold-standard evidence demonstrating (cost-)effectiveness of this approach is required to convince stakeholders of population-wide implementation. An RCT aiming to generate such evidence is underway [21].

However, questions regarding who should be tested, and when it is most cost effective to perform pre-emptive panel testing, remain unanswered. In this side-study, we have chosen to perform pre-emptive panel testing among those who received a first prescription for one of ten drugs. Here, there is an initial delay of PGx testing results for the first prescription, but PGx results can be used uninterrupted, if recorded in the EMR, when future drug-gene interactions are encountered. On the one hand, it may be more cost-effective to perform population-wide testing at birth, to ensure maximization of instances in which a PGx result is available when a drug-gene interaction is encountered. In contrast to our approach, not one prescription will be delayed as a result of PGx testing. On the other hand, some may never encounter drug-gene interactions, thereby unintentionally wasting resources on PGx testing. To shed light on this issue, some have predicted which patients may benefit from PGx testing in the near future algorithmically and using prescription data [43,44]. Others have modelled the cost-effectiveness of testing a 40-year old for life-long prevention of adverse drug reactions using a Markov model [45]. Overall, a consensus has not been reached regarding whom and when to test [16]. Within this side-study we observe the number of newly initiated prescriptions, and thus potential benefit of panel testing, increases with age, number of comorbidities and number of comedications, although this was not statistically significant. However, since 97% of this cohort made re-use of their panel results, we may conclude that the in- and exclusion criteria of this study may be successful criteria in selecting patients who will further benefit from panel testing. The most cost-effective target groups applicable for panel testing must be further investigated.

In addition to unanswered timing and application of testing, the variants selected to be included in a PGx panel also require additional curation. Recently, the DPWG has provided a suggested panel (van der Wouden et al., unpublished) [46]. Here, variants included in the panel reflect the entire set of existing DPWG guidelines and are continuously updated as the field of PGx expands. It will be of utmost importance to record the version number of the tested panel, so that it can be retrieved which variants were tested within a specific gene. Moreover, the most cost-effective technique used to determine the PGx profile is also undetermined. As the cost of next-generation sequencing decreases, we envision a future in which we may be able to extract relevant PGx variant alleles from sequencing data [47], possibly making genotype based testing redundant. If this is to come into fruition, the determining the cost-effectiveness of implementing PGx testing will become redundant, as the information on PGx variants become secondary findings, free of additional costs. In this case, only effectiveness will be of interest. Overall, the cost-effectiveness of a panel-approach is a dependant on many variables including the target population, timing, tested variants and testing technique.

5. Conclusions

Both pharmacists and GPs are very able to record PGx results into their respective EMRs, thereby maximizing the potential benefits of PGx results when deployed by the clinical decision support system in future prescriptions. Within this cohort, almost all patients were able to benefit from the availability of the PGx-panel results in their EMR, indicating that the real-world impact of a panel approach is immense. The downstream impact on healthcare utilization was unable to be concluded due to the small sample size. Ongoing research will quantify the effects of pre-emptive panel-based testing on patient outcomes [21]. Future research should focus on assessing the most cost-effective approach regarding timing, target population, variants and techniques for PGx testing. Regardless, we argue that in terms of logistics, delivery through a clinical decision support system is most feasible.

Author Contributions: Conceptualization, C.H.v.d.W., P.C.D.B., K.O., J.J.S. and H.J.G..; methodology, C.H.v.d.W., P.C.D.B., K.O., J.J.S. and H.J.G..; formal analysis, C.H.v.d.W., P.C.D.B., K.O., J.J.S. and H.J.G.; writing—original draft preparation, C.H.v.d.W.; writing—review and editing, C.H.v.d.W., P.C.D.B., K.O., J.J.S. and H.J.G.; visualization, C.H.v.d.W., P.C.D.B., K.O., J.J.S. and H.J.G.; supervision, J.J.S. and H.J.G.; project administration, C.H.v.d.W., P.C.D.B., K.O., J.J.S. and H.J.G.; funding acquisition, P.C.D.B., J.J.S., H.J.G.

Acknowledgments: We would like to thank Stefan Böhringer for providing statistical advice. We would like to thank Rowena Schaap, Daniëlle Klootwijk, and Renée Baak-Pablo for their assistance in sample handling and analysis. We would also like to thank Noortje Stijntjes for her assistance in the collection of the follow-up data from pharmacy records. Finally, we would also like to thank Stephan Joosten for providing Figure 1.

References

1. Relling, M.V.; Evans, W.E. Pharmacogenomics in the clinic. *Nature* **2015**, *526*, 343–350. [CrossRef] [PubMed]
2. Weinshilboum, R.; Wang, L. Pharmacogenomics: Bench to bedside. *Nat. Rev. Drug Discov.* **2004**, *3*, 739–748. [CrossRef]
3. Wu, A.H. Pharmacogenomic testing and response to warfarin. *Lancet* **2015**, *385*. [CrossRef]
4. Pirmohamed, M. Personalized pharmacogenomics: Predicting efficacy and adverse drug reactions. *Annu. Rev. Genom. Hum. Genet.* **2014**, *15*, 349–370. [CrossRef]
5. Pirmohamed, M.; Burnside, G.; Eriksson, N.; Jorgensen, A.L.; Toh, C.H.; Nicholson, T.; Kesteven, P.; Christersson, C.; Wahlstrom, B.; Stafberg, C.; et al. A randomized trial of genotype-guided dosing of warfarin. *N. Engl. J. Med.* **2013**, *369*, 2294–2303. [CrossRef] [PubMed]
6. Verhoef, T.I.; Ragia, G.; de Boer, A.; Barallon, R.; Kolovou, G.; Kolovou, V.; Konstantinides, S.; Le Cessie, S.; Maltezos, E.; van der Meer, F.J.; et al. A randomized trial of genotype-guided dosing of acenocoumarol and phenprocoumon. *N. Engl. J. Med.* **2013**, *369*, 2304–2312. [CrossRef] [PubMed]
7. Coenen, M.J.; de Jong, D.J.; van Marrewijk, C.J.; Derijks, L.J.; Vermeulen, S.H.; Wong, D.R.; Klungel, O.H.; Verbeek, A.L.; Hooymans, P.M.; Peters, W.H.; et al. Identification of patients with variants in TPMT and dose reduction reduces hematologic events during thiopurine treatment of inflammatory bowel disease. *Gastroenterology* **2015**, *149*, 907–917. [CrossRef]
8. Mallal, S.; Phillips, E.; Carosi, G.; Molina, J.M.; Workman, C.; Tomazic, J.; Jagel-Guedes, E.; Rugina, S.; Kozyrev, O.; Cid, J.F.; et al. HLA-B*5701 screening for hypersensitivity to abacavir. *N. Engl. J. Med.* **2008**, *358*. [CrossRef]
9. Altman, R.B. Pharmacogenomics: "Noninferiority" is sufficient for initial implementation. *Clin. Pharmacol. Ther.* **2011**, *89*, 348–350. [CrossRef] [PubMed]

10. Pirmohamed, M.; Hughes, D.A. Pharmacogenetic tests: The need for a level playing field. *Nat. Rev. Drug Discov.* **2013**, *12*, 3–4. [CrossRef]
11. Swen, J.J.; Nijenhuis, M.; de Boer, A.; Grandia, L.; Maitland-van der Zee, A.H.; Mulder, H.; Rongen, G.A.; van Schaik, R.H.; Schalekamp, T.; Touw, D.J.; et al. Pharmacogenetics: From bench to byte—An update of guidelines. *Clin. Pharmacol. Ther.* **2011**, *89*, 662–673. [CrossRef]
12. Swen, J.J.; Wilting, I.; de Goede, A.L.; Grandia, L.; Mulder, H.; Touw, D.J.; de Boer, A.; Conemans, J.M.; Egberts, T.C.; Klungel, O.H.; et al. Pharmacogenetics: From bench to byte. *Clin. Pharmacol. Ther.* **2008**, *83*, 781–787. [CrossRef] [PubMed]
13. Relling, M.V.; Klein, T.E. CPIC: Clinical pharmacogenetics implementation consortium of the pharmacogenomics research network. *Clin. Pharmacol. Ther.* **2011**, *89*. [CrossRef] [PubMed]
14. Bank, P.; Caudle, K.E.; Swen, J.J.; Gammal, R.S.; Whirl-Carrillo, M.; Klein, T.E.; Relling, M.V.; Guchelaar, H.J. Comparison of the guidelines of the clinical pharmacogenetics implementation consortium and the dutch pharmacogenetics working group. *Clin. Pharmacol. Ther.* **2018**, *103*, 599–618. [CrossRef] [PubMed]
15. Weitzel, K.W.; Cavallari, L.H.; Lesko, L.J. Preemptive panel-based pharmacogenetic testing: The time is now. *Pharm. Res.* **2017**, *34*, 1551–1555. [CrossRef]
16. Roden, D.M.; Van Driest, S.L.; Mosley, J.D.; Wells, Q.S.; Robinson, J.R.; Denny, J.C.; Peterson, J.F. Benefit of preemptive pharmacogenetic information on clinical outcome. *Clin. Pharmacol. Ther.* **2018**, *103*, 787–794. [CrossRef]
17. Verbelen, M.; Weale, M.E.; Lewis, C.M. Cost-effectiveness of pharmacogenetic-guided treatment: Are we there yet? *Pharmacogenom. J.* **2017**. [CrossRef] [PubMed]
18. Swen, J.J.; Nijenhuis, M.; van Rhenen, M.; de Boer-Veger, N.J.; Buunk, A.-M.M.; Houwink, E.J.F.J.F.; Mulder, H.; Rongen, G.A.; van Schaik, R.H.N.H.N.; van der Weide, J.; et al. Pharmacogenetic information in clinical guidelines: The European perspective. *Clin. Pharmacol. Ther.* **2018**, *103*, 795–801. [CrossRef] [PubMed]
19. Schildcrout, J.S.; Denny, J.C.; Bowton, E.; Gregg, W.; Pulley, J.M.; Basford, M.A.; Cowan, J.D.; Xu, H.; Ramirez, A.H.; Crawford, D.C.; et al. Optimizing drug outcomes through pharmacogenetics: A case for preemptive genotyping. *Clin. Pharmacol. Ther.* **2012**, *92*, 235–242. [CrossRef] [PubMed]
20. Simoons, M.; Mulder, H.; Schoevers, R.A.; Ruhe, H.G.; van Roon, E.N. Availability of CYP2D6 genotyping results in general practitioner and community pharmacy medical records. *Pharmacogenomics* **2017**, *18*, 843–851. [CrossRef]
21. Van der Wouden, C.H.; Cambon-Thomsen, A.; Cecchin, E.; Cheung, K.C.; Dávila-Fajardo, C.L.; Deneer, V.H.; Dolžan, V.; Ingelman-Sundberg, M.; Jönsson, S.; Karlsson, M.O.; et al. Implementing pharmacogenomics in Europe: Design and implementation strategy of the ubiquitous pharmacogenomics consortium. *Clin. Pharmacol. Ther.* **2017**, *101*, 341–358. [CrossRef]
22. Elliott, L.S.; Henderson, J.C.; Neradilek, M.B.; Moyer, N.A.; Ashcraft, K.C.; Thirumaran, R.K. Clinical impact of pharmacogenetic profiling with a clinical decision support tool in polypharmacy home health patients: A prospective pilot randomized controlled trial. *PLoS ONE* **2017**, *12*, e0170905. [CrossRef] [PubMed]
23. Brixner, D.; Biltaji, E.; Bress, A.; Unni, S.; Ye, X.; Mamiya, T.; Ashcraft, K.; Biskupiak, J. The effect of pharmacogenetic profiling with a clinical decision support tool on healthcare resource utilization and estimated costs in the elderly exposed to polypharmacy. *J. Med. Econ.* **2015**, *19*, 213–228. [CrossRef]
24. Finkelstein, J.; Friedman, C.; Hripcsak, G.; Cabrera, M. Potential utility of precision medicine for older adults with polypharmacy: A case series study. *Pharmacogenom. Pers. Med.* **2016**, *9*, 31–45. [CrossRef]
25. Saldivar, J.-S.; Taylor, D.; Sugarman, E.; Cullors, A.; Garces, J.; Oades, K.; Centeno, J. Initial assessment of the benefits of implementing pharmacogenetics into the medical management of patients in a long-term care facility. *Pharmacogenom. Pers. Med.* **2016**, *9*, 1–6. [CrossRef]
26. Pérez, V.; Salavert, A.; Espadaler, J.; Tuson, M.; Saiz-Ruiz, J.; Sáez-Navarro, C.; Bobes, J.; Baca-García, E.; Vieta, E.; Olivares, J.M.M.; et al. Efficacy of prospective pharmacogenetic testing in the treatment of major depressive disorder: Results of a randomized, double-blind clinical trial. *BMC Psychiatry* **2017**, *17*, 250. [CrossRef] [PubMed]
27. Espadaler, J.; Tuson, M.; Lopez-Ibor, J.M.; Lopez-Ibor, F.; Lopez-Ibor, M.I. Pharmacogenetic testing for the guidance of psychiatric treatment: A multicenter retrospective analysis. *CNS Spectr.* **2017**, *22*, 315–324. [CrossRef] [PubMed]

28. Samwald, M.; Xu, H.; Blagec, K.; Empey, P.E.; Malone, D.C.; Ahmed, S.M.; Ryan, P.; Hofer, S.; Boyce, R.D. Incidence of exposure of patients in the United States to multiple drugs for which pharmacogenomic guidelines are available. *PLoS ONE* **2016**, *11*, e0164972. [CrossRef]
29. Bank, P.C.; Swen, J.J.; Schaap, R.D.; Klootwijk, D.B.; Baak-Pablo, R.F.; Guchelaar, H.J. A pilot study of the implementation of pharmacogenomic pharmacist initiated pre-emptive testing in primary care. *Eur. J. Hum. Genet.* **2019**. Accepted.
30. Link, E.; Parish, S.; Armitage, J.; Bowman, L.; Heath, S.; Matsuda, F.; Gut, I.; Lathrop, M.; Collins, R. SLCO1B1 variants and statin-induced myopathy—A genomewide study. *N. Engl. J. Med.* **2008**, *359*, 789–799. [CrossRef] [PubMed]
31. Dawes, M.; Aloise, M.N.; Ang, S.J.; Cullis, P.; Dawes, D.; Fraser, R.; Liknaitzky, G.; Paterson, A.; Stanley, P.; Suarez-Gonzalez, A.; et al. Introducing pharmacogenetic testing with clinical decision support into primary care: A feasibility study. *CMAJ Open* **2016**, *4*. [CrossRef] [PubMed]
32. Swen, J.J.; van der Straaten, T.; Wessels, J.A.; Bouvy, M.L.; Vlassak, E.E.; Assendelft, W.J.J.; Guchelaar, H.J.J. Feasibility of pharmacy-initiated pharmacogenetic screening for CYP2D6 and CYP2C19. *Eur. J. Clin. Pharmacol.* **2012**, *68*, 363–370. [CrossRef] [PubMed]
33. Ferreri, S.P.; Greco, A.J.; Michaels, N.M.; O'Connor, S.K.; Chater, R.W.; Viera, A.J.; Faruki, H.; McLeod, H.L.; Roederer, M.W. Implementation of a pharmacogenomics service in a community pharmacy. *J. Am. Pharm. Assoc.* **2014**, *54*, 172–180. [CrossRef] [PubMed]
34. Haga, S.B.; LaPointe, N.M.; Cho, A.; Reed, S.D.; Mills, R.; Moaddeb, J.; Ginsburg, G.S. Pilot study of pharmacist-assisted delivery of pharmacogenetic testing in a primary care setting. *Pharmacogenomics* **2014**, *15*, 1677–1686. [CrossRef]
35. Murray, M.E.; Barner, J.C.; Pope, N.D.; Comfort, M.D. Impact and feasibility of implementing a systematic approach for medication therapy management in the community pharmacy setting: A pilot study. *J. Pharm. Pract.* **2018**. [CrossRef]
36. Track your own healthcare with 'Volgjezorg'. Available online: https://www.volgjezorg.nl/en (accessed on 18 January 2019).
37. Samwald, M.; Minarro-Giménez, J.A.A.; Blagec, K.; Adlassnig, K.-P.P. Towards a global IT system for personalized medicine: The Medicine Safety Code initiative. *Stud. Health Technol. Inform.* **2014**, *205*, 261–265.
38. Blagec, K.; Koopmann, R.; Crommentuijn-van Rhenen, M.; Holsappel, I.; van der Wouden, C.H.; Konta, L.; Xu, H.; Steinberger, D.; Just, E.; Swen, J.J.; et al. Implementing pharmacogenomics decision support across seven European countries: The Ubiquitous Pharmacogenomics (U-PGx) project. *J. Am. Med. Inform. Assoc.* **2018**. [CrossRef]
39. Overby, C.L.; Erwin, A.L.; Abul-Husn, N.S.; Ellis, S.B.; Scott, S.A.; Obeng, A.O.; Kannry, J.L.; Hripcsak, G.; Bottinger, E.P.; Gottesman, O. Physician attitudes toward adopting genome-guided prescribing through clinical decision support. *J. Pers. Med.* **2014**, *4*. [CrossRef]
40. Bell, G.C.; Crews, K.R.; Wilkinson, M.R.; Haidar, C.E.; Hicks, J.K.; Baker, D.K.; Kornegay, N.M.; Yang, W.; Cross, S.J.; Howard, S.C.; et al. Development and use of active clinical decision support for preemptive pharmacogenomics. *J. Am. Med. Inform. Assoc.* **2014**. [CrossRef]
41. Bank, P.; Swen, J.; Guchelaar, H.J. Nation-wide impact of implementing a pre-emptive pharmacogenetics panel approach to guide drug prescribing in primary care in The Netherlands (in submission). **2019**.
42. Leendertse, A.J.; Van Den Bemt, P.M.; Poolman, J.B.; Stoker, L.J.; Egberts, A.C.; Postma, M.J. Preventable hospital admissions related to medication (HARM): Cost analysis of the HARM study. *Value Health* **2011**, *14*, 34–40. [CrossRef]
43. Pulley, J.M.; Denny, J.C.; Peterson, J.F.; Bernard, G.R.; Jones, C.L.; Ramirez, A.H.; Delaney, J.T.; Bowton, E.; Brothers, K.; Johnson, K. Operational implementation of prospective genotyping for personalized medicine: The design of the Vanderbilt PREDICT project. *Clin. Pharmacol. Ther.* **2012**, *92*, 87–95. [CrossRef]
44. Grice, G.R.; Seaton, T.L.; Woodland, A.M.; McLeod, H.L. Defining the opportunity for pharmacogenetic intervention in primary care. *Pharmacogenomics* **2006**, *7*, 61–65. [CrossRef]
45. Alagoz, O.; Durham, D.; Kasirajan, K. Cost-effectiveness of one-time genetic testing to minimize lifetime adverse drug reactions. *Pharmacogenom. J.* **2015**, *16*, 129–136. [CrossRef]

46. Van der Wouden, C.H.; Van Rhenen, M.H.; Jama, W.; Ingelman-Sundberg, M.; Lauschke, V.M.; Konta, L.; Schwab, M.; Swen, J.; Guchelaar, H.J. Development of the PGx-passport: A panel of actionable germline genetic variants for pre-emptive pharmacogenetic testing (manuscript in preparation). 2019.
47. Yang, W.; Wu, G.; Broeckel, U.; Smith, C.A.; Turner, V.; Haidar, C.E.; Wang, S.; Carter, R.; Karol, S.E.; Neale, G.; et al. Comparison of genome sequencing and clinical genotyping for pharmacogenes. *Clin. Pharmacol. Ther.* **2016**, *100*. [CrossRef]

10

Outcome Definition Influences the Relationship between Genetic Polymorphisms of *ERCC1*, *ERCC2*, *SLC22A2* and Cisplatin Nephrotoxicity in Adult Testicular Cancer Patients

Zulfan Zazuli [1,2,3], Leila S. Otten [3], Britt I. Drögemöller [4,5], Mara Medeiros [6,7], Jose G. Monzon [8], Galen E. B. Wright [4,9], Christian K. Kollmannsberger [10], Philippe L. Bedard [11], Zhuo Chen [12], Karen A. Gelmon [10], Nicole McGoldrick [13], Abhijat Kitchlu [14], Susanne J. H. Vijverberg [1], Rosalinde Masereeuw [3], Colin J. D. Ross [4,5], Geoffrey Liu [12], Bruce C. Carleton [13,15,†] and Anke H. Maitland-van der Zee [1,†,*]

1 Department of Respiratory Medicine, Amsterdam University Medical Centers, University of Amsterdam, 1105 AZ Amsterdam, The Netherlands; z.zazuli@amc.uva.nl (Z.Z.); s.j.vijverberg@amsterdamumc.nl (S.J.H.V.)
2 Department of Pharmacology-Clinical Pharmacy, School of Pharmacy, Bandung Institute of Technology, Bandung 40132, Indonesia
3 Division of Pharmacology, Utrecht Institute for Pharmaceutical Sciences, Utrecht University, 3512 JE Utrecht, The Netherlands; l.s.otten@students.uu.nl (L.S.O.); R.Masereeuw@uu.nl (R.M.)
4 British Columbia Children's Hospital Research Institute, Vancouver, BC V5Z 4H4, Canada; bdrogemoller@cmmt.ubc.ca (B.I.D.); gwright@cmmt.ubc.ca (G.E.B.W.); colin.ross@ubc.ca (C.J.D.R.)
5 Faculty of Pharmaceutical Sciences, The University of British Columbia, Vancouver, BC V6T 1Z4, Canada
6 Nephrology Research Unit, Hospital Infantil de México Federico Gómez, Mexico City 06720, Mexico; medeiro.mara@gmail.com
7 Departamento de Farmacología, Facultad de Medicina, Universidad Nacional Autónoma de México, Mexico City 04510, Mexico
8 Department of Medical Oncology, Tom Baker Cancer Centre, Calgary, AB T2N 4N2, Canada; jgmonzon@ucalgary.ca
9 Department of Medical Genetics, University of British Columbia, Vancouver, BC V6T 1Z4, Canada
10 BC Cancer Agency and University of British Columbia, Vancouver, BC V6T 1Z4, Canada; ckollmannsberger@bccancer.bc.ca (C.K.K.); kgelmon@bccancer.bc.ca (K.A.G.)
11 Princess Margaret Cancer Centre and University of Toronto, Toronto, ON M5S, Canada; philippe.bedard@uhn.ca
12 Medical Oncology and Hematology, Department of Medicine, Princess Margaret Cancer Centre-University Health Network and University of Toronto, Toronto, ON M5S, Canada; Zhuo.Chen@uhnresearch.ca (Z.C.); Geoffrey.Liu@uhn.ca (G.L.)
13 Pharmaceutical Outcomes Programme, BC Children's Hospital, Vancouver, BC V6H 3N1, Canada; nicolemcgoldrick@hotmail.com (N.M.); bcarleton@popi.ubc.ca (B.C.C.)
14 Division of Nephrology, Department of Medicine, University Health Network and University of Toronto, Toronto, ON M5S, Canada; Abhijat.Kitchlu@uhn.ca
15 Division of Translational Therapeutics, Department of Pediatrics, Faculty of Medicine, University of British Columbia, Vancouver, BC V6T 1Z4, Canada
* Correspondence: a.h.maitland@amsterdamumc.nl
† These authors contributed equally to this work.

Abstract: Although previous research identified candidate genetic polymorphisms associated with cisplatin nephrotoxicity, varying outcome definitions potentially contributed to the variability in the effect size and direction of this relationship. We selected genetic variants that have been significantly associated with cisplatin-induced nephrotoxicity in more than one published study (*SLC22A2* rs316019; *ERCC1* rs11615 and rs3212986; *ERCC2* rs1799793 and rs13181) and performed a replication analysis to confirm associations between these genetic polymorphisms and cisplatin nephrotoxicity using various outcome definitions. We included 282 germ cell testicular cancer patients treated with cisplatin from 2009–2014, aged >17 years recruited by the Canadian Pharmacogenomics Network for Drug Safety. Nephrotoxicity was defined using four grading tools: (1) Common Terminology Criteria for Adverse Events (CTCAE) v4.03 for acute kidney injury (AKI) or CTCAE-AKI; (2) adjusted cisplatin-induced AKI; (3) elevation of serum creatinine; and (4) reduction in the estimated glomerular filtration rate (eGFR). Significant associations were only found when using the CTCAE v4.03 definition: genotype CA of the *ERCC1* rs3212986 was associated with decreased risk of cisplatin nephrotoxicity ($OR_{adj} = 0.24$; 95% CI: 0.08–0.70; $p = 0.009$) compared to genotype CC. In contrast, addition of allele A at *SLC22A2* rs316019 was associated with increased risk ($OR_{adj} = 4.41$; 95% CI: 1.96–9.88; $p < 0.001$) while genotype AC was associated with a higher risk of cisplatin nephrotoxicity ($OR_{adj} = 5.06$; 95% CI: 1.69–15.16; $p = 0.004$) compared to genotype CC. Our study showed that different case definitions led to variability in the genetic risk ascertainment of cisplatin nephrotoxicity. Therefore, consensus on a set of clinically relevant outcome definitions that all such studies should follow is needed.

Keywords: pharmacogenetics; cisplatin; nephrotoxicity; kidney injury; genetic polymorphisms

---

1. Introduction

Cisplatin remains one of the most widely prescribed antineoplastic therapies due to its effectiveness as a component of first-line regimens against various types of cancers, including carcinomas, germ cell tumours, lymphomas and sarcomas [1,2]. In Europe, the 1- and 5-years survival rate in testicular cancer patients was 98% and 97%, respectively [3]. However, the dose-limiting toxicities of cisplatin, such as nausea and vomiting, hematotoxicity, ototoxicity and nephrotoxicity, hinder its potential antineoplastic effect. Nephrotoxicity is the most prevalent of these adverse effects caused by cisplatin, resulting in a two-fold risk of acute kidney injury and an increase in serum creatinine levels [4,5]. Approximately one third of all patients treated with cisplatin develop renal dysfunction after a single dosage of cisplatin (50–100 mg/m^2) [6]. In addition, concerns about long-term renal side effects are rising especially in cancers that occur in young patients and have a high chance of being successfully treated such as testicular cancer [7]. A previous study suggested that circulating platinum is still detectable in the plasma of testicular cancer survivors even 20 years after the last administration of cisplatin [8].

Cisplatin is mainly excreted through the kidneys. Therefore, renal tubular injury is a common clinical manifestation of cisplatin accumulation in renal tubular cells. Cisplatin levels in tubular epithelial cells may increase up to five times higher levels than blood levels [9]. After uptake via organic cation transporter 2 (OCT2) and high-affinity copper transporter 1 (CTR1) in the renal tubules, multiple mechanisms lead to cytotoxicity: complex intracellular pathways lead to DNA damage and cell death and an inflammatory response speeds up renal damage even more [10]. Cisplatin may induce vascular injury as well, which accelerates tubular cell death. These multifactorial processes lead to tubular necrosis and eventually loss of kidney function [10]. This loss of function manifests itself in multiple ways: acute kidney injury (as measured by decreased glomerular filtration rate (GFR)), decreased magnesium and potassium levels and increased serum creatinine (SCr) are paramount but cisplatin may also cause hypocalcaemia, renal salt wasting and even chronic kidney disease [10]. Various patient-related (e.g., age, gender, chronic comorbid illness, pre-existing kidney disease) and treatment-related factors (cisplatin dose per cycle, cumulative dosage, hydration) have been associated with cisplatin nephrotoxicity [11]. In addition, previous studies also suggest that variations in genes involved in cisplatin pharmacodynamics and pharmacokinetics contribute to cisplatin nephrotoxicity [12–18].

Genetic variations have been reported to play a role both as protective and as risk factors for cisplatin nephrotoxicity. In a recent systematic review we reported that variants in *ERCC1*, *ERCC2* and *SLC22A2* genes were associated with cisplatin nephrotoxicity and replicated in at least one other study [19]. *ERCC1* and *ERCC2* polymorphisms have been associated with alterations of DNA repair process in cells [20–22] including possibly the nephron following cisplatin exposure [19]. In addition, *ERCC1* polymorphisms may alter cell sensitivity to cisplatin [23]. Polymorphisms in *SLC22A2*, a gene which product is the organic cation transporter OCT2 responsible for cellular cisplatin uptake in renal proximal tubule cells [24,25], affects the severity of tubular injury process due to cisplatin accumulation. However, variability in effect size and direction of association have been reported. Consequently, this complicates the understanding of the true impact of genetic variants. Differences in clinical characteristics for example, age, type of cancer, cisplatin dose and ethnicity might be related to variability of results. We expect that differences in how cisplatin nephrotoxicity is defined contribute to the variability in results as no widely accepted single cisplatin nephrotoxicity definition exists.

Our aim is to validate the use of already associated genetic variants to predict cisplatin nephrotoxicity and to determine if different cisplatin nephrotoxicity definitions contributed to the variability in effect size and direction of already published associations between these genetic polymorphisms and cisplatin nephrotoxicity. This approach was important to highlight the need of consensus on a set of clinically relevant cisplatin nephrotoxicity definitions that future studies is able to follow.

2. Materials and Methods

This study is reported according to Strengthening the Reporting of Genetic Association Studies (STREGA) guidelines [26].

2.1. Study Design and Participants

The retrospective study included males (≥17 years old) diagnosed with germ cell testicular cancer treated with cisplatin between January 1979 and February 2013. These patients were part of a previously conducted study on cisplatin-induced adverse events and were recruited through the Canadian Pharmacogenomics Network for Drug Safety (CPNDS) in multiple Canadian centres in Ontario and British Columbia from 2009–2013 [27].

Patients were included if they had normal kidney function, were treatment-naïve and had received 100 mg/m^2 cisplatin per cycle. Patients suffering from other diseases than testicular cancer, non-genotyped patients, patients with pre-existing electrolyte disorders or patients that had received abdominal radiation were excluded from this study. All subjects gave their informed consent for inclusion prior their participation in the study. The study was conducted in accordance with the Declaration of Helsinki and the protocol was approved by the UBC C&W Research Ethics Board (ethics certificate no. H04-70358).

2.2. Clinical Data Collection

Information concerning co-medication, chemotherapy protocols, duration of the treatment, cumulative dosage of platinum, serum magnesium levels (Mg), serum potassium levels (K), serum sodium levels (Na), serum phosphate levels (PO4) and serum creatinine (SCr) levels was obtained from the medical records. The glomerular filtration rate (GFR) was not available in all patient records. Therefore, estimated glomerular filtration rate (eGFR) was calculated using the CKD-EPI equation [28] as per the KDIGO recommendation [29].

Only cisplatin-induced nephrotoxicity related variables were included as covariates in our analysis (i.e., disease-related variables were excluded). Height and body weight were not included as covariates, as the dosage was already adjusted for this (mg/m^2). Alcohol consumption, family history of cancer, prior surgery and albumin levels were not available in the medical records and were therefore not be included in the genetic association analyses. All patients in our cohort were cisplatin-naïve at the time of testicular cancer diagnosis.

Age was calculated at the start date of cisplatin treatment. Ethnicity was analysed through ancestry proportions and principal components (PCs) using EIGENSOFT v.5.0 (Harvard and Massachusetts Institute of Technology, Cambridge, MA, USA) and ADMIXTURE. Cardiovascular disease and diabetes data were not available in the database and were for that reason determined based on co-medications [30–34]. Potentially nephrotoxic co-medications were identified from the start until the end date of cisplatin treatment and grouped according to their mechanism of action [35]. The amount of hydration depended on standardized chemotherapy regimen and was derived from Canadian protocols for testicular cancer [36,37]. Cumulative dose was assessed and where carboplatin had been substituted for cisplatin, a conversion factor of 1:4 for cisplatin: carboplatin was used [1,38]. For the baseline SCr and electrolyte measurement, the measurement closest to the start date within 30 days prior to start was taken.

2.3. *Outcome Definition*

To assess the relationship between cisplatin-induced nephrotoxicity and genetic variants, multiple outcomes were studied. Multiple outcomes were used to determine if different cisplatin nephrotoxicity definitions contributed to the variability in effect size and direction of already published associations between these genetic polymorphisms and cisplatin nephrotoxicity. A new tailored definition for cisplatin-induced nephrotoxicity was formulated based on expert opinions to optimize clinical relevance (see below "Adjusted Acute Kidney Injury" Outcome Definition). Since the results for this definition were not comparable with previously published studies, CTCAE-AKI grading and the differences in SCr and eGFR before and after cisplatin-treatment (ΔSCr and ΔeGFR) were assessed as well.

2.3.1. "Adjusted Acute Kidney Injury" (Adjusted-AKI) Outcome Definition

The definition of cisplatin-induced nephrotoxicity combines SCr-based staging and electrolyte disturbances (i.e., National Cancer Institute Common Terminology Criteria for Adverse Events (NCI-CTCAE) v.4.03 definitions for electrolyte disturbances) [39] (Table 1). Measurements from start date up to 90 days after the end of cisplatin treatment were collected. The measurement closest to the start date with a cut-off of 30 days was taken as the baseline value when calculating the increase in SCr.

Hyperhydration during administration may cause a hypervolemic state which may provoke hyponatremia [40]. To increase sensitivity and decrease false-positive or overestimated results, hyponatremia must have persisted for longer than two consecutive months. For further statistical analyses, these categories were divided into case, control and ambiguous groups (Table 2). Two separate investigators designated the patients in one of three categories and discrepancies were resolved through discussion between a clinical pharmacologist and nephrologist.

Table 1. Adjusted Acute Kidney Injury (Adjusted-AKI) grading.

Grade	Definition	Characteristic(s)
0	An increase in serum creatinine, up to 1.5 times baseline value AND Electrolyte disorders grade 0 CTCAE: • Hypomagnesemia: ≥LLN–1.2 mg/dL; <LLN–0.5 mmol/L, OR • Hypokalaemia: ≥LLN–3.0 mmol/L, OR • Hypophosphatemia: ≥LLN–2.5 mg/dL; <LLN–0.8 mmol/L, OR • Hyponatremia: ≥LLN–130 mmol/L (>2 months)	Asymptomatic
1	Between 1.5–1.9 times baseline SCr OR ≥0.3 mg/dL (≥26.5 μmol/L) increase in SCr OR Electrolyte disorders grade 1 CTCAE: • Hypomagnesemia: <LLN–1.2 mg/dL; <LLN–0.5 mmol/L, OR • Hypokalaemia: <LLN–3.0 mmol/L, OR • Hypophosphatemia: <LLN–2.5 mg/dL; <LLN–0.8 mmol/L, OR • Hyponatremia: <LLN–130 mmol/L (>2 months)	Possible Symptomatic
2	An increase in serum creatinine between 2.0–2.9 times baseline SCr ORElectrolyte disorders grade 2 CTCAE: • Hypomagnesemia: <1.2–0.9 mg/dL; <0.5–0.4 mmol/L, OR • Hypokalaemia: <LLN–3.0 mmol/L, OR • Hypophosphatemia: <2.5–2.0 mg/dL; <0.8–0.6 mmol/L, OR • Hyponatremia: <LLN–130–120 mmol/L (>2 months)	Clinically relevant, required intervention
3	An increase in serum creatinine at least 3.0 times baseline OR Increase in serum creatinine to ≥4.0 mg/dL (≥353.6 μmol/L) OR Initiation of renal replacement therapy, OR OR Electrolyte disorders ≥grade 3 CTCAE: • Hypomagnesemia: <0.9 mg/dL; <0.4 mmol/L, OR • Hypokalaemia: <3.0 mmol/L; hospitalization indicated, OR • Hypophosphatemia: <2.0 mg/dL; <0.6 mmol/L, OR • Hyponatremia: <LLN–120 mmol/L (>2 months)	Required close monitoring

Table 2. Case-control designation according to Adjusted-AKI outcome definition.

Case	Control	Ambiguous
Acute nephrotoxicity ≥ grade 1 OR Received electrolyte supplementation	Acute nephrotoxicity < grade 1 AND No supplementation	No lab values available during the time frame (3 months before initiation and 3 months after the last administration of cisplatin) OR Incomplete data e.g., initiation and end date of cisplatin therapy OR Pre-existing renal disease (electrolyte disturbances, not SCr or eGFR)

SCr: serum creatinine; eGFR: estimated glomerular filtration rate.

2.3.2. CTCAE-AKI Outcome Definition

The SCr-based CTCAE v.4.03 definition of "Acute Kidney Injury" was also used to define cisplatin-induced nephrotoxicity [39]. Patients were divided into cases (≥grade 1) and controls (<grade 1) (Table 3). The lowest SCr measurement up to 30 days before start of cisplatin treatment was taken as baseline. The follow up value used was the highest SCr value within 90 days after the end of cisplatin treatment.

Table 3. Case-control designation according to Common Terminology Criteria for Adverse Events (CTCAE)-AKI Outcome Definition.

Case	Control	Ambiguous
Acute kidney injury ≥ grade 1	Acute kidney injury < grade 1	No lab values available during the time frame (3 months before initiation and 3 months after the last administration of cisplatin) OR Incomplete data e.g., initiation and end date of cisplatin therapy

2.3.3. "ΔSCr and ΔeGFR" Outcome Definition

To calculate the differences between baseline and follow up SCr and eGFR (ΔSCr and ΔeGFR), the same procedure of creatinine serum measurements was applied as with the CTCAE outcome definition.

2.4. Genotype Data

2.4.1. Candidate Genes

The list of candidate genes and related variants was selected from a systematic review [19]. Candidate genes were included if they were found to be significantly associated with nephrotoxicity (any outcome definition) in a published study and the relationship had been replicated at least once. The following five single nucleotide polymorphisms (SNPs) meeting these criteria were included in this study: *ERCC1* rs11615 (chr19:45420395; A>G; a synonymous variant) and rs3212986 (chr19:45409478; C>A/C>G/C>T; non-coding transcript variant), *ERCC2* rs13181 (chr19:45351661; T>A/T>G; stop gained) and rs1799793 (chr19:45364001; C>A/C>T; a missense variant)) and *SLC22A2* rs316019 (chr6:160249250; A>C; a missense variant).

2.4.2. Genotyping

DNA was collected from saliva using Oragene collection kits (DNK Genotek Inc., Ottawa, ON, Canada) and was extracted according to the manufacturer's protocol. Genomic DNA samples for all patients were genotyped for 7907 variants located within absorption, distribution, metabolism, excretion (ADME) gene regions using the Illumina Infinium Panel (Illumina, San Diego, CA, USA), according to the manufacturer's instructions at the Canadian Pharmacogenomics Network for Drug Safety at the University of British Columbia. The genotyping details and the ADME custom panel used have been described in previously [27].

2.4.3. Quality Control of Genotype Data

Variants are filtered on SNP call rate (>95%), sample call rate (samples missing ≥2 SNPs excluded), Hardy-Weinberg equilibrium (HWE, p-value > 0.05, in controls) and minor allele frequency (MAF, >0.05, in patients with a European proportion ancestry ≥80%). HWE was calculated using Fisher's exact test.

2.5. Statistical Analyses

The genetic association between SNPs and the categorical clinical outcomes reflecting nephrotoxicity (i.e., adjusted-AKI and CTCAE-AKI) were examined using logistic regression assuming an additive model. MAFs for the whole cohort in both designations were calculated for each SNP. An allele frequency lower than 0.5 indicated the minor allele and was also classified as the risk allele. Power analyses were performed assuming a 0.05 significance level, assuming 5% MAF and with an OR > 3 as effect size with the goal of achieving a power of at least 80%. To assess differences between cases and controls (adjusted AKI and CTCAE-AKI designation) for continuous clinical variables, a Mann-Whitney U test was used. The differences between categorical clinical variables and cases and controls (adjusted AKI and CTCAE-AKI designation) were evaluated using a Chi-squared tests. A logistic regression model analysis that included potential confounders (counting subject ancestry) was used to calculate adjusted odds ratios (OR) and the 95% confidence intervals (95% CI) separately for outcomes defined using an adjusted-AKI and CTCAE-AKI designation. Cochran-Armitage trend test was conducted to test the assumption of an additive genetic model. Multiple linear regression was performed to assess the association between genetic variants and the continuous variables ΔeGFR and ΔSCr, adjusting for potential confounders. Key assumptions for multiple linear regression analysis—for example, multivariate normality, no multicollinearity and homoscedasticity—were fulfilled. Clinical variables which caused changes of the crude regression coefficient by 10% or more is considered a confounder and is added to the model. Multiple testing was accounted for using Bonferroni adjustments ($p = 0.05/5 = 0.01$). Statistical analyses were performed using SPSS v.25 (IBM Corporation, Armonk, NY, USA).

3. Results

3.1. Study Population

The study included 282 testicular-cancer patients from five adult oncology centres in British Columbia and Ontario through active surveillance of the Canadian Pharmacogenomics Network for Drug Safety (CPNDS) [41]. Ambiguous patients (Tables 2 and 3) or patients with missing SCr or eGFR data were excluded from further analyses. From the primary cohort, 72 patients were excluded because they were not genotyped (N = 61), had received abdominal radiation (N = 4) or because they were not diagnosed with testicular cancer (N = 7). From the secondary cohort (N = 210), 47 patients were excluded for the adjusted-AKI analyses due to pre-existing renal disease, incomplete data regarding the start- and/or end date of cisplatin therapy or absence of laboratory values. For the CTCAE-AKI outcome and ΔSCr analyses, 51 patients were excluded due to lack of SCr data. For the ΔeGFR analyses, 52 patients were excluded due to lack of eGFR data.

For genetic association analyses 167, 159, 158 and 159, patients were eligible for the adjusted AKI designation, the CTCAE-AKI designation and ΔeGFR and ΔSCr analyses, respectively (Figure 1). These patient cohorts were similar with respect to baseline characteristics. The mean age (± standard deviation) of the testicular-cancer patients was 31.8 ± 10.2 (Table 4). European has the highest ancestry proportion in our dataset (0.72 ± 0.26) followed by South Asian, East Asian, American and African. The detailed of ancestry analysis has been published elsewhere [27]. Patients had a low number of comorbidities: 1.0% (N = 2) suffered from diabetes and 3.3% (N = 7) from a cardiovascular disease. Only 2.9% (N = 6) of the patients received carboplatin within 90 days after cisplatin treatment ended (these dosages were included in the calculation of total platinum exposure). A majority of patients received the regimen of cisplatin with bleomycin and etoposide (BEP; 65%, N = 136). Because data on phosphate levels were missing for 207 patients, this electrolyte was excluded from further analyses.

3.2. Genotyping Results

The lowest SNP call rate was 97.5% for *SLC22A2* rs316019 (Table S2). HWE was fulfilled in the control group of all evaluated SNPs for adjusted-AKI outcome ($p > 0.05$) but not in the control group of *ERCC1* rs1799793 for the CTCAE-AKI outcome ($p = 0.013$) (Tables S1 and S2).

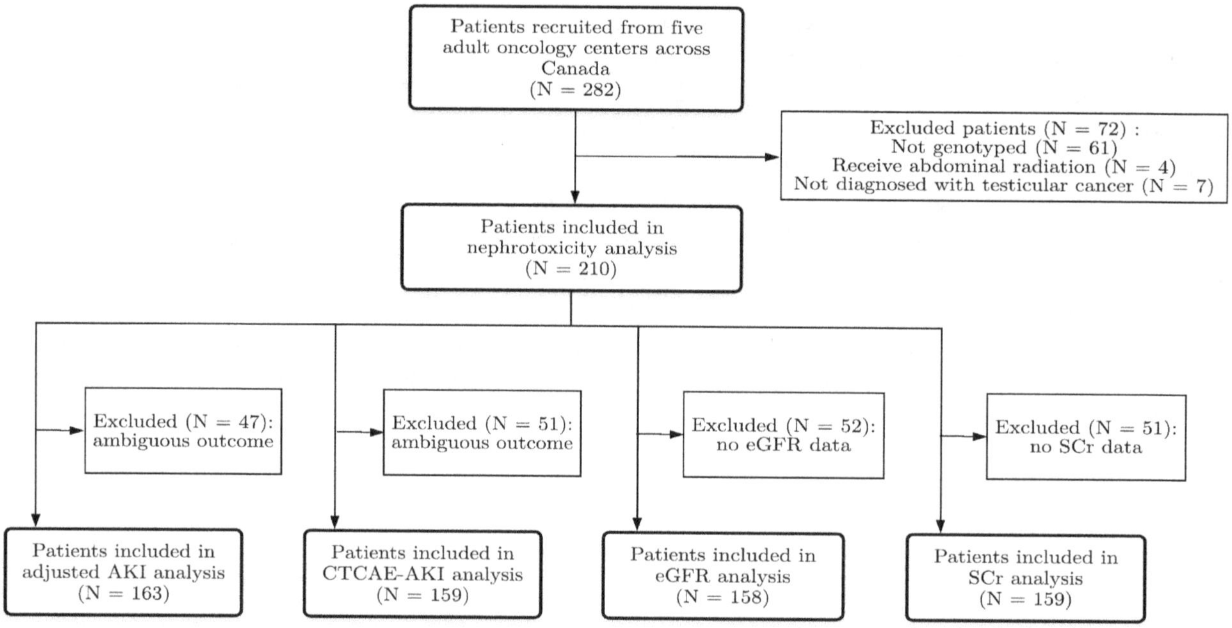

Figure 1. Flowchart of patient inclusion in statistical analyses.

Table 4. Clinical characteristics testicular cancer patients included in nephrotoxicity analyses (N = 210).

Characteristics		
Age at start treatment, mean ± SD, years		31.8 ± 10.2
Ancestry, mean ± SD, proportion	European	0.72 ± 0.26
	East-Asian	0.09 ± 0.23
	American	0.05 ± 0.10
	African	0.03 ± 0.03
	South-Asian	0.11 ± 0.15
Cardiovascular disease, no. (%)		7 (3.3)
Diabetes, no. (%)		2 (1.0)
Potentially nephrotoxic co-medications, mean ± SD, total number per patient		2 ± 2
Potentially nephrotoxic co-medications, no. (%)	ACEIs [a]	3 (1.4)
	Aminoglycosides	4 (1.9)
	ARBs [b]	1 (0.5)
	Benzodiazepines	30 (14)
	NSAIDs [c]	6 (2.9)
	Betalactams	26 (12)
	PPIs [d]	25 (12)
	Quinolones	29 (14)
	Statins	2 (1.0)
	Acetaminophen	29 (14)
	Other	104 (50)
Baseline [SCr], mean ± SD, umol/L		84 ± 16
Baseline [K^+], mean ± SD, mmol/L		4.1 ± 0.4
Baseline [Mg^{2+}], mean ± SD, mmol/L		0.85 ± 0.10
Baseline [Na^+], mean ± SD, mmol/L		138 ± 2.49
Baseline [$PO4^-$], mean ± SD, mmol/L		1.09 ± 0.23
Cumulative platinum dose, mean ± SD, mg/m^2		380 ± 123
Duration cisplatin treatment, mean ± SD	Weeks	8.7 ± 3.3
	Cycles	3.8 ± 1.1
Chemotherapy protocol, no. (%), BEP		136 (65)
Chemotherapy hydration, mean ± SD, L/cycle		10.7 ± 0.5

[a] ACEIs: Angiotensin-converting enzyme inhibitors, [b] ARBs: Angiotensin-II-Receptor Blockers, [c] NSAIDs: non-steroidal anti-inflammatory drugs, [d] PPIs: proton-pump inhibitors, BEP: bleomycin, etoposide, and cisplatin.

3.3. Adjusted AKI Analysis

For this outcome, 75 cases and 88 controls were identified (Table S3). Cases had significantly lower baseline magnesium compared to controls (0.83 vs. 0.88 mmol/L, $p = 0.008$). Quinolone usage was significantly higher in cases versus controls (24% vs. 5.7%, $p = 0.001$). Cases received significantly more platinum (400 vs. 300 mg/m^2, $p = 0.001$) and were treated longer with platinum (4 vs. 3 cycles, $p = 0.001$) compared to controls.

Genetic association analyses on the adjusted AKI designation were corrected for quinolone usage, cumulative dose, baseline magnesium and ancestry using principal components (PC's) to account for population structure. None of the genetic variants were found to be significantly associated with the risk of nephrotoxicity using this definition (Tables 5 and 6). In addition, Cochran-Armitage trend test also showed no significant trend to confirm the additive effect of minor allele (Table 6).

Table 5. Strength of genotypic association between genetic polymorphisms and cisplatin nephrotoxicity in adjusted-AKI outcome (N = 163).

Gene–SNP	OR	95% CI	*p*-Value	OR$_{adj}$	95% CI$_{adj}$	*p*-Value$_{adj}$
			ERCC1 rs11615			
GG	1 #			1 #		
GA	1.30	0.63–2.67	0.48	1.45	0.64–3.27	0.38
AA	1.24	0.51–3.02	0.63	1.47	0.50–4.28	0.48
			ERCC1 rs3212986			
CC	1 #			1 #		
CA	0.71	0.37–1.36	0.31	0.63	0.30–1.34	0.23
AA	1.00	0.30–3.37	1.00	1.44	0.32–6.43	0.63
			ERCC2 rs13181			
AA	1 #			1 #		
CA	0.84	0.42–1.66	0.61	0.59	0.26–1.33	0.20
CC	1.60	0.65–3.93	0.31	1.43	0.50–4.07	0.51
			ERCC2 rs1799793			
AA	1 #			1 #		
CA	1.00	0.49–2.03	1.00	0.92	0.40–2.15	0.85
CC	0.50	0.21–1.17	0.11	0.55	0.21–1.43	0.22
			SLC22A2 rs316019			
CC	1 #			1 #		
AC	1.15	0.51–2.57	0.71	1.10	0.43–2.79	0.85
AA	2.46	0.22–27.78	0.47	1.70	0.11–25.57	0.70

$_{adj}$ Adjusted for: cumulative dose, quinolone usage, all ancestries (from four PCs) and baseline magnesium.
Reference category.

Table 6. Odds ratio of minor allele addition in adjusted-AKI outcome (N = 163) and Cohcran-Armitage trend test result for additive model assumption.

Gene–SNP	OR	95% CI	*p*-Value	OR$_{adj}$	95% CI$_{adj}$	*p*-Value$_{adj}$	Cohcran-Armitage Trend Test *p*-Value
ERCC1 rs11615 GG vs. GA vs. AA	1.13	0.73–1.75	0.586	1.23	0.73–2.05	0.436	0.586
ERCC1 rs3212986 AA vs. CA vs. CC	0.86	0.54–1.40	0.551	0.89	0.51–1.54	0.669	0.537
ERCC2 rs13181 CC vs. CA vs. AA	1.19	0.75–1.88	0.461	1.04	0.61–1.78	0.875	0.497
ERCC2 rs1799793 CC vs. CA vs. AA	0.70	0.45–1.09	0.114	0.73	0.44–1.19	0.206	0.280
SLC22A2 rs316019 AA vs. CA vs. CC	1.28	0.64–2.59	0.488	1.17	0.53–2.60	0.702	0.502

$_{adj}$ Adjusted for: cumulative dose, quinolone usage, all ancestries (as PC's) and baseline magnesium.

3.4. CTCAE-AKI Analysis

For this outcome, 36 cases and 123 controls were identified (Table S4). Cases were significantly older compared to controls (35 vs. 29 years old, $p = 0.002$) and differed from controls in ancestry: cases had a lower proportion who were of East-Asian ancestry (0 vs. 0.023, $p = 0.041$) and higher proportion who were of European ancestry (0.853 vs. 0.811, $p = 0.017$). Cases used proton-pump inhibitors (PPIs) significantly more often compared to controls (25% vs. 8%, $p = 0.015$). Cases received significantly more platinum (400 vs. 300 mg/m^2, $p = 0.005$) and were treated longer with platinum (4 vs. 3 cycles, $p = 0.007$) compared to controls. Furthermore, therapy regimens varied between cases and controls: cases were less often treated with a bleomycin-etoposide-platinum (BEP) protocol (53% vs. 72%, $p = 0.041$) and cases received chemotherapy hydration less often (10.75 (IQR = 10.50–10.75) vs. 10.75 (IQR = 0) L/cycle, $p = 0.004$).

The results of genotypic logistic regression are provided in Table 7. When corrected for age, ancestry from four PCs, chemotherapy protocol, cumulative dosage, hydration and PPI usage, patients carrying *ERCC1* rs3212986 heterozygous genotypes were found to have fewer nephrotoxicity events when compared with patients carrying the homozygous wildtype ($OR_{adj} = 0.24$, CI = 0.08–0.70, $p = 0.009$). Patients carrying *SLC22A2* rs316019 heterozygous genotypes were found to have a greater number of nephrotoxicity events than patients who carrying the wildtype (normal) genotype before and after adjusting for the same covariates ($OR_{adj} = 5.06$, CI = 1.69–15.16, $p = 0.004$). Besides this, the *SLC22A2* rs316109 homozygous variant carriers had more nephrotoxicity events than patients carrying the wildtype genotype, however after Bonferroni correction this was no longer statistically significant ($OR_{adj} = 38.12$, CI = 1.89–767.51, $p = 0.017$).

Table 7. Strength of genotypic association between genetic polymorphisms and cisplatin nephrotoxicity in CTCAE-AKI designation (N = 159).

Gene–SNP	OR	95% CI	*p*-Value	OR_{adj}	95% CI_{adj}	*p*-$Value_{adj}$
			ERCC1 rs11615			
GG	1 #			1 #		
GA	1.30	0.57–2.99	0.55	1.23	0.45–3.39	0.68
AA	0.48	0.14–1.65	0.24	0.53	0.12–2.37	0.41
			ERCC1 rs3212986			
CC	1 #			1 #		
CA	0.45	0.20–1.02	0.06	0.24	0.08–0.70	0.009 *
AA	0.48	0.10–2.36	0.37	0.43	0.07–2.47	0.34
			ERCC2 rs13181			
AA	1 #			1 #		
CA	1.16	0.49–2.73	0.74	0.59	0.20–1.76	0.37
CC	3.16	1.17–8.58	0.02	1.72	0.53–5.65	0.35
			ERCC2 rs1799793			
AA	1 #			1 #		
CA	1.52	0.65–3.54	0.33	2.39	0.84–6.77	0.10
CC	0.57	0.18–1.79	0.33	0.66	0.16–2.64	0.56
			SLC22A2 rs316019			
CC	1 #			1 #		
AC	3.24	1.36–7.74	0.008 *	5.06	1.69–15.16	0.004 *
AA	9.18	0.80–105.80	0.08	38.12	1.89–767.51	0.02

adj Adjusted for: age, all ancestries (as PC's), chemotherapy protocol, cumulative dosage, hydration and PPI usage, # Reference category, * significant ($p < 0.01$).

Additive effect of risk allele was found significant only on *SLC22A2* rs316109. The OR was even higher after adjustment ($OR_{adj} = 4.41$, CI = 1.96–9.88, $p < 0.001$). In contrast, addition of minor allele on *ERCC1* rs3212986 produce protective effect although the result was not significant ($OR_{adj} = 0.52$,

CI = 0.26–1.07, p = 0.076). The additive effect of minor allele was confirmed by Cochran-Armitage trend test but only for *SLC22A2* rs316019 and *ERCC2* rs13181 (Table 8).

Table 8. Odds ratio of minor allele addition in CTCAE-AKI designation (N = 159) and Cohcran-Armitage trend test result for additive model assumption.

Gene–SNP	OR	95% CI	p-Value	OR_{adj}	95% CI_{adj}	p-$Value_{adj}$	Cohcran-Armitage Trend Test p-Value
ERCC1 rs11615 GG vs. GA vs. AA	0.78	0.46–1.33	0.364	0.92	0.50–1.68	0.777	0.368
ERCC1 rs3212986 AA vs. CA vs. CC	0.57	0.30–1.06	0.077	0.52	0.26–1.07	0.076	0.067
ERCC2 rs13181 CC vs. CA vs. AA	1.84	1.07–3.15	0.027	1.39	0.75–2.58	0.293	0.039 *
ERCC2 rs1799793 CC vs. CA vs. AA	0.81	0.48–1.38	0.447	0.85	0.47–1.53	0.578	0.473
SLC22A2 rs316019 AA vs. CA vs. CC	3.29	1.60–6.81	0.001 **	4.41	1.96–9.88	<0.001 **	0.001 **

$_{adj}$ Adjusted for: age, all ancestries (as PC's), chemotherapy protocol, cumulative dosage, hydration and PPI usage, * significant ($p < 0.05$); proof of trend, ** significant ($p < 0.01$).

3.5. ΔSCr and ΔeGFR Analysis

Multiple linear regression was used to predict ΔSCr and ΔeGFR based on genotype for each SNP before and after adjustment for confounding variables. The analysis did not reveal any statistically significant results (Table 9). However, there was a very slight trend for the *ERCC1* rs3212986 variant to be protective and the *SLC22A2* rs316019 homozygous variant to be a risk factor, based on box-plots (Figures S1 and S2).

Table 9. Multiple linear regression analysis results between genetic polymorphisms and ΔSCr and ΔeGFR.

Gene–SNP	ΔSCr [a]				ΔeGFR [b]			
	R^2	p-Value	R^2_{adj}	p-Value $_{adj}$	R^2	p-Value	R^2_{adj}	p-Value $_{adj}$
ERCC1 rs11615 GG vs. GA vs. AA	0.01	0.218	0.055	0.17	0.006	0.347	0.042	0.20
ERCC1 rs3212986 AA vs. CA vs. CC	0.008	0.268	0.058	0.16	0.013	0.167	0.052	0.12
ERCC2 rs13181 CC vs. CA vs. AA	0.001	0.652	0.046	0.28	0	0.796	0.035	0.29
ERCC2 rs1799793 CC vs. CA vs. AA	0.001	0.77	0.046	0.27	0.001	0.668	0.036	0.29
SLC22A2 rs316019 AA vs. CA vs. CC	0.002	0.599	0.047	0.27	0.006	0.343	0.039	0.25

[a] adjusted for cardiovascular disease, duration (weeks), aminoglycoside users and baseline magnesium, [b] adjusted for duration (weeks), baseline potassium and beta-lactams use.

4. Discussion

4.1. Main Findings

Previous studies assessing the associations between *ERCC1* rs3212986 and *SLC22A2* rs316019 genotypes and cisplatin-induced nephrotoxicity have reported conflicting results. In this study, associations between genetic variants and multiple definitions of cisplatin-induced nephrotoxicity were analysed in the same dataset and demonstrated that different definitions of cisplatin nephrotoxicity contributed to variability of results. We could not reproduce the same genetic associations that were previously reported, when using the adjusted-AKI or continuous outcomes [13,16,18,42]. In contrast, when using the CTCAE-AKI outcome in the same patient sample, the *ERCC1* rs3212986 heterozygous genotype was reno-protective whilst the *SLC22A2* rs316019 homozygous genotype was a risk factor for cisplatin-induced nephrotoxicity. We also found that additive effect of risk allele was found significant only on *SLC22A2* rs316109.

Several published studies could not detect any significant associations between the CTCAE-AKI outcome definition of cisplatin-induced nephrotoxicity and *ERCC1* rs3212986 [14,43–45]; the reasons for this lack of association include lack of study power, population stratification or phenotypic heterogeneity. However, studies carried out by Tzvetkov et al. and Khrunin et al. did reveal associations between *ERCC1* rs3212986 genotypes and cisplatin-induced nephrotoxicity. Tzvetkov et al. found that homozygous variants were not associated with a decrease of eGFR, while the C allele carriers (major allele) had mean decrease of 11.5 ± 1.8% of eGFR ($p = 0.004$) [13]. By applying the same genetic model, we also found that the C allele carriers of this SNP have higher mean eGFR reduction than the homozygous variant subjects although the result was not statistically significant (18.9 ± 22.6 vs. 13.5 ± 23.0 mL/min/1.73 m^2; $p = 0.412$). This finding suggested protective effect of the variant genotype of rs3212986. Furthermore, we found that variant genotypes were protective against cisplatin nephrotoxicity when applying the CTCAE-AKI definition of nephrotoxicity: heterozygous carriers of the *ERCC1* rs3212986 had an OR_{adj} of 0.24 (95% CI: 0.08–0.70) while the homozygous variant had an OR_{adj} of 0.43 (95% CI: 0.07–2.47; $p = 0.341$). Addition of minor allele on this SNP produce protective effect although the result was not significant (ORadj = 0.52, CI = 0.26–1.07, $p = 0.076$). In contrast to these findings, Khrunin et al. reported a higher prevalence of cisplatin-induced nephrotoxicity among heterozygous genotypes compared with homozygous wildtype (OR = 3.29, 95% CI = 1.40–7.73, $p = 0.009$) [12].

The relationship between *SLC22A2* rs316019 genotypes and cisplatin-induced nephrotoxicity has been assessed in multiple studies. Filipski et al. reported a significant increase in SCr compared to baseline in homozygous wildtype patients after the first cycle ($p = 0.0009$) but found no significant increase in heterozygous patients ($p = 0.12$) [18]. Iwata et al. reported a significant higher increase in SCr in homozygous wildtype patients compared to heterozygous patients (0.34 ± 0.33 vs. 0.14 ± 0.12 mg/dL, $p = 0.04$, respectively) [16]. In addition, Zhang et al. observed a higher increase of cystatin C in homozygous wildtype patients compared to heterozygous and homozygous variant patients (0.043 ± 0.107 vs. −0.013 ± 0.120 mmol/L, $p = 0.009$, respectively) [46]. These results indicate that the homozygous wildtype genotype may be a risk factor for developing cisplatin-induced nephrotoxicity. In contrast, our results suggest that both homozygous and heterozygous variant carriers have an increased risk of cisplatin-induced nephrotoxicity when using the CTCAE-AKI definition. This finding also supported by significant additive effect of risk allele on *SLC22A2* rs316109 when applying additive genetic model. However, our study identified a possible greater risk of nephrotoxicity as defined by ΔSCr in patients carrying the homozygous variant (Figure S1); these data are consistent with Zhang et al. and Hinai et al., who reported a higher increase of SCr in heterozygous and homozygous variant than in homozygous wildtype subjects, although the result is not statistically significant (0.83 ± 7.39 vs. 2.09 ± 6.30 mmol/L, $p = 0.35$ and 0.30 ± 0.30 vs. 0.40 ± 0.53 mg/dL, $p = 0.25$, respectively) [46].

Other factors could also contribute to the discrepancy in results between our study and previous studies. Our results suggest that cisplatin-induced nephrotoxicity is confounded by ethnic origin. The CTCAE-AKI outcome was related to East-Asian and European ancestry. Our results suggest that East-Asian ancestry may be a protective factor and European ancestry may be a risk factor for cisplatin-induced nephrotoxicity. This may also explain the differences of results between our study and the studies of Iwata et al. and Hinai et al. that included subjects of East Asian ancestry. Discrepancies regarding the ΔSCr—and hence, ΔeGFR—among those studies could also be explained by the age of the population. Hinai et al. and Iwata et al. both studied an older population: 68.0 ± 9.7 and 65.8 ± 7.7 years old (mean ± SD) [16,42]. As highlighted before, older age could attribute to a higher increase in SCr [47]. This may explain the elevated SCr levels in the wildtype homozygous group of *SLC22A2* rs316019 found by Iwata et al. and Hinai et al. compared to our study. Furthermore, our population received a high dose cisplatin (100 mg/m^2 per cycle) compared to dosages used in other indications and compared to the other studies [16,42]: patients analysed by Hinai et al. received 80 mg/m^2 per cycle and Iwata et al. treated their patients with 60–80 mg/m^2 cisplatin per cycle. The higher cisplatin-dose in our study could have attributed to a possible higher incidence of cisplatin-induced nephrotoxicity.

This study further shows that different outcome definitions produce different results. The main difference in the outcomes definitions is the inclusion of electrolyte disturbances in the adjusted AKI outcome definition (Table 10). Our results suggest that the genetic associations were found when the SCr based definition was used but not when using an electrolyte-based definition that forms the adjusted AKI outcome definition. Acute kidney injury caused by cisplatin mainly manifests itself as renal tubular injury and is therefore characterized earlier by electrolyte abnormalities (phosphate, magnesium, potassium and sodium) [48]. However, incorporating serum abnormalities with creatinine serum levels in one single definition of cisplatin nephrotoxicity should be further validated.

Table 10. Multiple outcome definitions of cisplatin-induced nephrotoxicity used in this study.

	Adjusted-AKI	CTCAE-AKI	ΔeGFR	ΔSCr
Basis of Determination	SCr + Mg/K/PO_4/Na	SCr	CKD-EPI equation (SCr+age+sex+ethnicity)	SCr
Data Characteristics	Categorical	Categorical	Continuous	Continuous
Advantage	Tailored on cisplatin-induced nephrotoxicity	• Mostly used in clinics and studies in cancer subjects • Easily calculated	• Easily calculated • CKD-EPI is the equation recommended by KDIGO	• Routinely measured in patients
Disadvantage	• Not comparable with other studies • Not validated yet	• Is ≥ grade 1 cut-off clinically relevant? • SCr often increase late resulting in failing to detect early stage nephrotoxicity	• Could not correct for cystatin-C due to unavailable data in routine practice • Disregarding the clinical value of baseline eGFR	• Highly influenced by various individual factors (e.g., age, gender, body weight, diet etc.) • SCr often increase late resulting in failing to detect early stage nephrotoxicity • Disregarding the clinical value of baseline SCr

4.2. Gene Expression and Regulation

ERCC1 rs3212986, located at the 3′ UTR (non-coding region) was not associated with changes in protein and mRNA expression [49,50]. However, the tissue expression quantitative trait loci (eQTL) analysis from the Genotype-Tissue Expression (GTEx) Project reported a significant association between rs3212986 and gene expression in various tissues [51]. Unfortunately, no association has been found between rs3212986 and ERCC1 expression in kidney cortex tissue. *SLC22A2* rs316019, a nonsynonymous missense mutation (p.270Ala>Ser), is the only common coding polymorphism of *SLCC2A2* with an allele frequency ranging from 9–16% and is reported to cause changes in transporter function [52]. No significant eQTLs were found for rs316019 in the eQTL tissues database [51]. Specific functional validation of *ERCC1* rs3212986 and *SLC22A2* rs316019 in kidney tubular tissue is needed to elucidate their role in cisplatin nephrotoxicity and how they affect protein expression involved in cisplatin nephrotoxicity pathway (e.g., OCT2).

4.3. Strength and Limitations of the Study

Compared to the previously published studies, our study was conducted in an appropriate population of relatively young adult male patients, who had a low number of comorbidities. By studying a dataset of testicular cancer patients, we minimized the influence of gender, older age, comorbidities and long-term use of medications that could have affected the renin-angiotensin systems (e.g., angiotensin converting enzyme inhibitors and angiotensin receptor blockers) and nephrotoxic compounds (e.g., non-steroidal anti-inflammatory drugs).

Our study had several limitations. The retrospective design led to several potential but unavoidable bias. Since laboratory measurements that were available were mostly measured in patients who were monitored more intensively, any missing data was non-random. Hence, the measurements that were available more likely to found individuals who were prone to cisplatin-induced nephrotoxicity. This resulted in selection bias and a possible overestimation of the amount of cases. The relatively small sample size was also a possible cause of failing to detect an association in this candidate gene study. A large prospective cohort study with a genome-wide approach is recommended to explore additional genetic variants that might be of importance. Furthermore, slightly different number of cohorts were used for each outcome. This may also have influenced the associations observed with each outcome.

5. Conclusions

In conclusion, the results of this study imply that the use of different outcome definitions lead to altered results. Consensus on a set of clinically relevant outcome definitions that future studies can follow are needed. The adjusted acute kidney injury definition that includes electrolyte imbalances seems more appropriate for cisplatin-induced nephrotoxicity. However, further validation of the definition and staging is necessary before it can be applied in further research or clinical settings. Furthermore, this study provides more evidence for associations between genetic variants and cisplatin-induced nephrotoxicity by using serum creatinine-based grading. These findings imply that genetic variations are involved in the inter-individual susceptibility to cisplatin-induced nephrotoxicity. Thus, in the future genotyping will make it possible to optimize therapy with cisplatin for the individual patients by improving cisplatin dosage selection–lower doses for patients prone to renal toxicity and higher doses for patient not susceptible to developing renal toxicity.

Author Contributions: Conceptualization, Z.Z., B.I.D., S.J.H.V., R.M., G.L., B.C.C. and A.H.M.-v.d.Z.; Data curation, G.E.B.W., N.M., C.J.D.R. and B.C.C.; Formal analysis, Z.Z., L.S.O., B.I.D. and B.C.C.; Funding acquisition, B.C.C. and Z.Z.; Investigation, Z.Z., L.S.O., B.I.D., M.M., J.G.M., G.E.B.W., C.K.K., P.L.B., Z.C., K.A.G., N.M., C.J.D.R., G.L., B.C.C. and A.H.M.-v.d.Z.; Methodology, Z.Z., B.I.D., M.M., A.K., S.J.H.V., C.J.D.R., B.C.C. and A.H.M.-v.d.Z.; Project administration, B.C.C. and A.H.M.-v.d.Z.; Resources, J.G.M., G.E.B.W., C.K.K., P.L.B., Z.C., K.A.G., C.J.D.R., G.L. and B.C.C.; Supervision, B.I.D., S.J.H.V., R.M., B.C.C. and A.H.M.-v.d.Z.; Visualization, Z.Z. and L.S.O.; Writing—original draft, Z.Z. and L.S.O.; Writing—review & editing, Z.Z., L.S.O., B.I.D., M.M., J.G.M., G.E.B.W., C.K.K., P.L.B., Z.C., K.A.G., N.M., A.K., S.J.H.V., R.M., C.J.D.R., G.L., B.C.C. and A.H.M.-v.d.Z.

Acknowledgments: We gratefully acknowledge the participation of all patients and families who took part in this study. We also acknowledge the contributions of the Canadian Pharmacogenomics Network for Drug Safety (CPNDS) Consortium.

References

1. Dasari, S.; Tchounwou, P.B. Cisplatin in cancer therapy: Molecular mechanisms of action. *Eur. J. Pharmacol.* **2014**, *740*, 364–378. [CrossRef]
2. Rancoule, C.; Guy, J.B.; Vallard, A.; Ben Mrad, M.; Rehailia, A.; Magne, N. 50th anniversary of cisplatin. *Bull. Cancer* **2017**, *104*, 167–176. [CrossRef]
3. Hoffmann, R.; Plug, I.; McKee, M.; Khoshaba, B.; Westerling, R.; Looman, C.; Rey, G.; Jougla, E.; Lang, K.; Parna, K.; et al. Innovations in health care and mortality trends from five cancers in seven European countries between 1970 and 2005. *Int. J. Public. Health* **2014**, *59*, 341–350. [CrossRef]
4. Sakaeda, T.; Kadoyama, K.; Okuno, Y. Adverse event profiles of platinum agents: Data mining of the public version of the FDA adverse event reporting system, AERS and reproducibility of clinical observations. *Int. J. Med. Sci.* **2011**, *8*, 487–491. [CrossRef]
5. Arany, I.; Safirstein, R.L. Cisplatin nephrotoxicity. *Semin. Nephrol.* **2003**, *23*, 460–464. [CrossRef]
6. Sahni, V.; Choudhury, D.; Ahmed, Z. Chemotherapy-associated renal dysfunction. *Nat. Rev. Nephrol.* **2009**, *5*, 450–462. [CrossRef]
7. Chovanec, M.; Abu Zaid, M.; Hanna, N.; El-Kouri, N.; Einhorn, L.H.; Albany, C. Long-term toxicity of cisplatin in germ-cell tumor survivors. *Ann. Oncol.* **2017**, *28*, 2670–2679. [CrossRef] [PubMed]

8. Gietema, J.A.; Meinardi, M.T.; Messerschmidt, J.; Gelevert, T.; Alt, F.; Uges, D.R.A.; Sleijfer, D.T. Circulating plasma platinum more than 10 years after cisplatin treatment for testicular cancer. *Lancet* **2000**, *355*, 1075–1076. [CrossRef]
9. Bajorin, D.F.; Bosl, G.J.; Alcock, N.W.; Niedzwiecki, D.; Gallina, E.; Shurgot, B. Pharmacokinetics of cis-diamminedichloroplatinum(II) after administration in hypertonic saline. *Cancer Res.* **1986**, *46*, 5969–5972. [PubMed]
10. Pabla, N.; Dong, Z. Cisplatin nephrotoxicity: Mechanisms and renoprotective strategies. *Kidney Int.* **2008**, *73*, 994–1007. [CrossRef]
11. Manohar, S.; Leung, N. Cisplatin nephrotoxicity: A review of the literature. *J. Nephrol.* **2018**, *31*, 15–25. [CrossRef]
12. Khrunin, A.V.; Moisseev, A.; Gorbunova, V.; Limborska, S. Genetic polymorphisms and the efficacy and toxicity of cisplatin-based chemotherapy in ovarian cancer patients. *Pharmacogenomics J.* **2010**, *10*, 54–61. [CrossRef]
13. Tzvetkov, M.V.; Behrens, G.; O'Brien, V.P.; Hohloch, K.; Brockmoller, J.; Benohr, P. Pharmacogenetic analyses of cisplatin-induced nephrotoxicity indicate a renoprotective effect of ERCC1 polymorphisms. *Pharmacogenomics* **2011**, *12*, 1417–1427. [CrossRef]
14. Windsor, R.E.; Strauss, S.J.; Kallis, C.; Wood, N.E.; Whelan, J.S. Germline genetic polymorphisms may influence chemotherapy response and disease outcome in osteosarcoma: A pilot study. *Cancer* **2012**, *118*, 1856–1867. [CrossRef] [PubMed]
15. Powrozek, T.; Mlak, R.; Krawczyk, P.; Homa, I.; Ciesielka, M.; Koziol, P.; Prendecka, M.; Milanowski, J.; Malecka-Massalska, T. The relationship between polymorphisms of genes regulating DNA repair or cell division and the toxicity of platinum and vinorelbine chemotherapy in advanced NSCLC patients. *Clin. Transl. Oncol.* **2016**, *18*, 125–131. [CrossRef]
16. Iwata, K.; Aizawa, K.; Kamitsu, S.; Jingami, S.; Fukunaga, E.; Yoshida, M.; Yoshimura, M.; Hamada, A.; Saito, H. Effects of genetic variants in SLC22A2 organic cation transporter 2 and SLC47A1 multidrug and toxin extrusion 1 transporter on cisplatin-induced adverse events. *Clin. Exp. Nephrol.* **2012**, *16*, 843–851. [CrossRef]
17. Zhang, L.; Gao, G.; Li, X.; Ren, S.; Li, A.; Xu, J.; Zhang, J.; Zhou, C. Association between single nucleotide polymorphisms (SNPs) and toxicity of advanced non-small-cell lung cancer patients treated with chemotherapy. *PLoS ONE* **2012**, *7*, e48350. [CrossRef]
18. Filipski, K.K.; Mathijssen, R.H.; Mikkelsen, T.S.; Schinkel, A.H.; Sparreboom, A. Contribution of organic cation transporter 2 (OCT2) to cisplatin-induced nephrotoxicity. *Clin. Pharmacol. Ther.* **2009**, *86*, 396–402. [CrossRef] [PubMed]
19. Zazuli, Z.; Vijverberg, S.; Slob, E.; Liu, G.; Carleton, B.; Veltman, J.; Baas, P.; Masereeuw, R.; Maitland-van der Zee, A.H. Genetic Variations and Cisplatin Nephrotoxicity: A Systematic Review. *Front. Pharmacol.* **2018**, *9*, 1111. [CrossRef]
20. Giachino, D.F.; Ghio, P.; Regazzoni, S.; Mandrile, G.; Novello, S.; Selvaggi, G.; Gregori, D.; DeMarchi, M.; Scagliotti, G.V. Prospective assessment of XPD Lys751Gln and XRCC1 Arg399Gln single nucleotide polymorphisms in lung cancer. *Clin. Cancer Res.* **2007**, *13*, 2876–2881. [CrossRef]
21. Friboulet, L.; Olaussen, K.A.; Pignon, J.P.; Shepherd, F.A.; Tsao, M.S.; Graziano, S.; Kratzke, R.; Douillard, J.Y.; Seymour, L.; Pirker, R.; et al. ERCC1 isoform expression and DNA repair in non-small-cell lung cancer. *N. Engl. J. Med.* **2013**, *368*, 1101–1110. [CrossRef]
22. Xiong, Y.; Huang, B.Y.; Yin, J.Y. Pharmacogenomics of platinum-based chemotherapy in non-small cell lung cancer: Focusing on DNA repair systems. *Med. Oncol.* **2017**, *34*, 48. [CrossRef] [PubMed]
23. Han, Y.; Liu, J.; Sun, M.; Zhang, Z.; Liu, C.; Sun, Y. A Significant Statistical Advancement on the Predictive Values of ERCC1 Polymorphisms for Clinical Outcomes of Platinum-Based Chemotherapy in Non-Small Cell Lung Cancer: An Updated Meta-Analysis. *Dis. Markers* **2016**, *2016*, 7643981. [CrossRef]
24. Miller, R.P.; Tadagavadi, R.K.; Ramesh, G.; Reeves, W.B. Mechanisms of Cisplatin nephrotoxicity. *Toxins* **2010**, *2*, 2490–2518. [CrossRef]
25. Wensing, K.U.; Ciarimboli, G. Saving ears and kidneys from cisplatin. *Anticancer Res.* **2013**, *33*, 4183–4188. [PubMed]

26. Little, J.; Higgins, J.P.; Ioannidis, J.P.; Moher, D.; Gagnon, F.; von Elm, E.; Khoury, M.J.; Cohen, B.; Davey-Smith, G.; Grimshaw, J.; et al. Strengthening the reporting of genetic association studies (STREGA): An extension of the STROBE Statement. *Hum. Genet.* **2009**, *125*, 131–151. [CrossRef] [PubMed]
27. Drogemoller, B.I.; Monzon, J.G.; Bhavsar, A.P.; Borrie, A.E.; Brooks, B.; Wright, G.E.B.; Liu, G.; Renouf, D.J.; Kollmannsberger, C.K.; Bedard, P.L.; et al. Association Between SLC16A5 Genetic Variation and Cisplatin-Induced Ototoxic Effects in Adult Patients With Testicular Cancer. *JAMA Oncol.* **2017**, *3*, 1558–1562. [CrossRef]
28. Levey, A.S.; Stevens, L.A.; Schmid, C.H.; Zhang, Y.L.; Castro, A.F., 3rd; Feldman, H.I.; Kusek, J.W.; Eggers, P.; Van Lente, F.; Greene, T.; et al. A new equation to estimate glomerular filtration rate. *Ann. Intern. Med.* **2009**, *150*, 604–612. [CrossRef] [PubMed]
29. Group, K.D.I.G.O.K.C.W. KDIGO 2012 Clinical Practice Guideline for the Evaluation and Management of Chronic Kidney Disease. *Kidney Int. Suppl.* **2013**, *3*, 1–150.
30. Winkelmayer, W.C.; Levin, R.; Setoguchi, S. Associations of kidney function with cardiovascular medication use after myocardial infarction. *Clin. J. Am. Soc. Nephrol.* **2008**, *3*, 1415–1422. [CrossRef]
31. Becquemont, L.; Bauduceau, B.; Benattar-Zibi, L.; Berrut, G.; Bertin, P.; Bucher, S.; Corruble, E.; Danchin, N.; al-Salameh, A.; Derumeaux, G.; et al. Association between Cardiovascular Drugs and Chronic Kidney Disease in Non-Institutionalized Elderly Patients. *Basic Clin. Pharmacol. Toxicol.* **2015**, *117*, 137–143. [CrossRef]
32. Aronow, W.S.; Frishman, W.H.; Cheng-Lai, A. Cardiovascular drug therapy in the elderly. *Cardiol. Rev.* **2007**, *15*, 195–215. [CrossRef]
33. Shlipak, M.G.; Smith, G.L.; Rathore, S.S.; Massie, B.M.; Krumholz, H.M. Renal function, digoxin therapy and heart failure outcomes: Evidence from the digoxin intervention group trial. *J. Am. Soc. Nephrol.* **2004**, *15*, 2195–2203. [CrossRef]
34. Diabetes Canada Clinical Practice Guidelines Expert, C.; Lipscombe, L.; Booth, G.; Butalia, S.; Dasgupta, K.; Eurich, D.T.; Goldenberg, R.; Khan, N.; MacCallum, L.; Shah, B.R.; et al. Pharmacologic Glycemic Management of Type 2 Diabetes in Adults. *Can. J. Diabetes* **2018**, *42*, S88–S103.
35. Awdishu, L.; Mehta, R.L. The 6R's of drug induced nephrotoxicity. *BMC Nephrol.* **2017**, *18*, 124. [CrossRef]
36. BCCA Genitourinary Chemotherapy Protocols. BC Cancer, Provincial Health Services Authority. Available online: http://www.bccancer.bc.ca/health-professionals/clinical-resources/chemotherapy-protocols/genitourinary#Testicular (accessed on 21 February 2018).
37. CCA Genitourinary Cancer Guidelines and Advice. Cancer Care Ontario. Available online: https://www.cancercareontario.ca/en/guidelines-advice/types-of-cancer/genitourinary?f%5B0%5D=field_type_of_cancer%3A656&f%5B1%5D=field_type_of_cancer%3A681 (accessed on 21 February 2018).
38. Rantanen, V.; Grenman, S.; Kulmala, J.; Grenman, R. Comparative evaluation of cisplatin and carboplatin sensitivity in endometrial adenocarcinoma cell lines. *Br. J. Cancer* **1994**, *69*, 482–486. [CrossRef]
39. Common Terminology Criteria for Adverse Events (CTCAE) Version 4.0. National Cancer Institute. Available online: https://evs.nci.nih.gov/ftp1/CTCAE/About.html (accessed on 15 February 2018).
40. Castillo, J.J.; Vincent, M.; Justice, E. Diagnosis and management of hyponatremia in cancer patients. *Oncologist* **2012**, *17*, 756–765. [CrossRef]
41. CPNDS. Welcome to The Canadian Pharmacogenomics Network for Drug Safety (CPNDS). Available online: http://cpnds.ubc.ca/ (accessed on 8 January 2019).
42. Hinai, Y.; Motoyama, S.; Niioka, T.; Miura, M. Absence of effect of SLC22A2 genotype on cisplatin-induced nephrotoxicity in oesophageal cancer patients receiving cisplatin and 5-fluorouracil: Report of results discordant with those of earlier studies. *J. Clin. Pharm. Ther.* **2013**, *38*, 498–503. [CrossRef]
43. KimCurran, V.; Zhou, C.; Schmid-Bindert, G.; Shengxiang, R.; Zhou, S.; Zhang, L.; Zhang, J. Lack of correlation between ERCC1 (C8092A) single nucleotide polymorphism and efficacy/toxicity of platinum based chemotherapy in Chinese patients with advanced non-small cell lung cancer. *Adv. Med. Sci.* **2011**, *56*, 30–38. [CrossRef]
44. Goekkurt, E.; Al-Batran, S.E.; Hartmann, J.T.; Mogck, U.; Schuch, G.; Kramer, M.; Jaeger, E.; Bokemeyer, C.; Ehninger, G.; Stoehlmacher, J. Pharmacogenetic analyses of a phase III trial in metastatic gastroesophageal adenocarcinoma with fluorouracil and leucovorin plus either oxaliplatin or cisplatin: A study of the arbeitsgemeinschaft internistische onkologie. *J. Clin. Oncol.* **2009**, *27*, 2863–2873. [CrossRef] [PubMed]

45. Erculj, N.; Kovac, V.; Hmeljak, J.; Dolzan, V. The influence of platinum pathway polymorphisms on the outcome in patients with malignant mesothelioma. *Ann. Oncol.* **2012**, *23*, 961–967. [CrossRef]
46. Zhang, J.; Zhou, W. Ameliorative effects of SLC22A2 gene polymorphism 808 G/T and cimetidine on cisplatin-induced nephrotoxicity in Chinese cancer patients. *Food Chem. Toxicol.* **2012**, *50*, 2289–2293. [CrossRef] [PubMed]
47. Tiao, J.Y.; Semmens, J.B.; Masarei, J.R.; Lawrence-Brown, M.M. The effect of age on serum creatinine levels in an aging population: relevance to vascular surgery. *Cardiovasc. Surg.* **2002**, *10*, 445–451. [CrossRef]
48. McMahon, K.R.; Rod Rassekh, S.; Schultz, K.R.; Pinsk, M.; Blydt-Hansen, T.; Mammen, C.; Tsuyuki, R.T.; Devarajan, P.; Cuvelier, G.D.; Mitchell, L.G.; et al. Design and Methods of the Pan-Canadian Applying Biomarkers to Minimize Long-Term Effects of Childhood/Adolescent Cancer Treatment (ABLE) Nephrotoxicity Study: A Prospective Observational Cohort Study. *Can. J. Kidney Health Dis.* **2017**, *4*, 2054358117690338. [CrossRef] [PubMed]
49. Woelfelschneider, A.; Popanda, O.; Lilla, C.; Linseisen, J.; Mayer, C.; Celebi, O.; Debus, J.; Bartsch, H.; Chang-Claude, J.; Schmezer, P. A distinct ERCC1 haplotype is associated with mRNA expression levels in prostate cancer patients. *Carcinogenesis* **2008**, *29*, 1758–1764. [CrossRef] [PubMed]
50. Zhuo, Z.J.; Liu, W.; Zhang, J.; Zhu, J.; Zhang, R.; Tang, J.; Yang, T.; Zou, Y.; He, J.; Xia, H. Functional Polymorphisms at ERCC1/XPF Genes Confer Neuroblastoma Risk in Chinese Children. *EBioMedicine* **2018**, *30*, 113–119. [CrossRef] [PubMed]
51. Consortium, G. *The Genotype-Tissue Expression (GTEx)*, GTEx Consortium, 2017.
52. Zolk, O. Disposition of metformin: variability due to polymorphisms of organic cation transporters. *Ann. Med.* **2012**, *44*, 119–129. [CrossRef] [PubMed]

11

Pharmacogenetics in the Treatment of Cardiovascular Diseases and its Current Progress Regarding Implementation in the Clinical Routine

Cristina Lucía Dávila-Fajardo [1,*], Xando Díaz-Villamarín [1], Alba Antúnez-Rodríguez [2], Ana Estefanía Fernández-Gómez [1], Paloma García-Navas [1], Luis Javier Martínez-González [2], José Augusto Dávila-Fajardo [3] and José Cabeza Barrera [1]

1 Department of Clinical Pharmacy, San Cecilio University Hospital, Institute for Biomedical Research, ibs.GRANADA, 18016 Granada, Spain; xandodv@gmail.com (X.D.-V.); estefania_fergo@hotmail.com (A.E.F.-G.); palomichi_96@hotmail.com (P.G.-N.); jose.cabeza.sspa@juntadeandalucia.es (J.C.B.)

2 Genomics Unit, Centro Pfizer-Universidad de Granada-Junta de Andalucía de Genómica e Investigación Oncológica (Genyo), 18016 Granada, Spain; albantunez@gmail.com (A.A.-R.); luisjavier.martinez@genyo.es (L.J.M.-G.)

3 English Department, Official Language School Leganes, 28915 Leganés, Madrid, Spain; josehood11@hotmail.com

* Correspondence: cristinal.davila.sspa@juntadeandalucia.es

Abstract: There is a special interest in the implementation of pharmacogenetics in clinical practice, although there are some barriers that are preventing this integration. A large part of these pharmacogenetic tests are focused on drugs used in oncology and psychiatry fields and for antiviral drugs. However, the scientific evidence is also high for other drugs used in other medical areas, for example, in cardiology. In this article, we discuss the evidence and guidelines currently available on pharmacogenetics for clopidogrel, warfarin, acenocoumarol, and simvastatin and its implementation in daily clinical practice.

Keywords: pharmacogenetics; clopidogrel; warfarin; acenocoumarol

---

1. Introduction

In recent years, there have been important advances to understand how genetic variations are associated with the efficacy and/or toxicity of medicines. Some of these studies have been randomized clinical trials (RCT) for a variety of drug–gene combinations that have shown that the performance of pharmacogenetic tests before prescribing a medication can improve patient health outcomes [1–5]. For this reason, nowadays, there is an important need to generalize the clinical implementation of genomic medicine and pharmacogenetics (PGx).

There are some barriers that are preventing the integration of PGx in daily clinical practice [6]. Among them, we can highlight the lack of correlation between the different PGx guidelines and those published by other professional organizations (oncology, cardiology, etc.) [7], the lack of a clinically relevant PGx test panel, the need for training of health personnel and patients, and the lack of information on cost-effectiveness studies [8,9]. All of those reasons prevent physicians from demanding a proactive approach to PGx.

The most important PGx-based drug dosing guidelines are published by the Clinical Pharmacogenetics Implementation Consortium (CPIC), the Royal Dutch Association for the Advancement of Pharmacy—Pharmacogenetics Working Group (DPWG), and the Canadian Pharmacogenomics Network for Drug Safety (CPNDS). In general, there is enough agreement between the guidelines in terms of pharmacotherapeutic recommendations, but there are some aspects in which there are discrepancies due to the methodology used to support the dose recommendations that should be taken into account [10]. A large part of these PGx tests are focused on drugs used in oncology, antiviral drugs [11], and psychiatry fields. However, the scientific evidence is also high for other drugs used in other medical areas, for example, in cardiology. In our opinion, clinical pharmacists are ideal candidates to translate the PGx to clinical practice since they are qualified to lead efforts to guide optimal drug selection and drug dosing based on those results. However, most of them are not fully aware of the advance in the knowledge of PGx and some advanced pharmacist functions in applying clinical pharmacogenetic may require specialized education, training, or experience.

In this article we discuss the most relevant evidence currently available on PGx of cardiovascular drugs, focusing on those drugs with available PGx information and genetic tests, and its implementation into daily clinical practice. In order to provide a thorough analysis, we chose well-defined criteria. We decided to use the Pharmacogenomics Knowledgebase (PharmGKB) [12], where strength of evidence is rated in levels ranging from 1–4, with level 1 meeting the highest criteria. Thus, for this review, we focused on clopidogrel, warfarin, acenocoumarol, and simvastatin, as all of them are considered as level 1 for at least one variant (Table 1).

Table 1. Drug-genes interactions reported in this article and the corresponding PGx guidelines and the level of evidence. CPIC: Clinical Pharmacogenetics Implementation Consortium, DPWG: Dutch Pharmacogenetics Working Group, CPNDS: Canadian Pharmacogenomics Network for Drug Safety.

Drugs	Genes	PGx Guidelines	Level of Evidence
Clopidogrel	*CYP2C19*	CPIC, DPWG	1A
Warfarin	*CYP2C9, VKORC1*	CPIC, CPNDS	1A
Acenocoumarol	*CYP2C9, VKORC1, CYP4F2*	DPWG	1B
Simvastatin	*SLCO1B1*	CPIC	1A

2. The Most Relevant Evidence in Pharmacogenetics of Drugs Used in Cardiology

2.1. Clopidogrel

Clopidogrel is a prodrug used as an antiplatelet in combination with acetylsalicylic acid in the treatment of acute coronary syndrome (ACS), including patients undergoing stent implantation after percutaneous coronary intervention (PCI) [13,14]. However, there is significant interpatient variability in the response of clopidogrel as a significant number of patients show high incidence of secondary cardiovascular events [15]. Several mechanisms were proposed for explaining the variable response to the drug, particularly when patients undergo PCI [16]. Subsequently, different genetic variants were associated with variability in response to the drug. The higher level of evidence is focused on the *CYP2C19* polymorphisms [17–21].

After absorption, 85% of the prodrug is inactivated by plasma esterases, and the remaining prodrug is activated in the liver by hepatic cytochrome isoenzymes. The conversion to its active metabolite depends partially on the CYP2C19 enzyme. Loss of function (LOF) *CYP2C19* alleles (*2 (rs424485), *3 (rs4986893), *4 (rs28399504), *5 (rs56337013), *6 (rs72552267), *7 (rs72558186), *8 (rs41291556), *9 (rs17884712), *10 (rs6413438), *22 (rs140278421), *24 (rs118203757), and *35 (rs12769205), mainly the *CYP2C19**2 variant due to the higher frequency, were associated with lower levels of active clopidogrel metabolite, reduced platelet inhibition, and higher rates of cardiovascular events [22]. The variant *CYP2C19**17 (rs12248560) is associated with a higher enzymatic activity, which means a lower on-treatment platelet reactivity [23–26] in response to clopidogrel when compared with homozygous wild-type carriers. However, *CYP2C19**2/*17 carriers exhibited an increased platelet reactivity in response to clopidogrel, as compared with *CYP2C19**1/*1 carriers [27], although data need to be consistently replicated.

For this reason, in 2010, The US Food and Drug Administration (FDA)-approved drug label for clopidogrel warned that tests are available to identify patients who were CYP2C19 poor metabolizers and suggested an alternative treatment in these patients, as they may have reduced effectiveness of the drug, therefore increasing the chance of secondary cardiovascular event rates in ACS and PCI patients, compared with patients with normal CYP2C19 function [28]. The European Medicines Agency (EMA) was positioned in a very similar way.

Nowadays, there have been some published clinical trials, meta-analyses, intervention studies, and many observational studies supporting the evidence of genotyping patients for clopidogrel use in ACS and PCI (Tables 2 and 3).

Table 2. Main characteristics from the large scale clopidogrel studies included in this review. MACE: major adverse cardiovascular events, CV: cardiovascular, LOF: loss of function alleles, ST: stent thrombosis, PCI: percutaneous coronary intervention.

Ref	Year	Ethnic	Population Studied	*n*	PCI-Stent (%)	Follow up	Endpoint	Polymorphisms	Outcomes (LOF vs. no LOF)
					High-risk patients (PCI-stent)				
Collet [29]	2009	Europeans	ACS	259	86	>4 years	MACE (CV death, ACS, urgent PCI)	*CYP2C19*2*	HR 5.38 (2.32-12.47) $p \leq 0.0001$
							ST definite	*CYP2C19*2*	HR 6.04 (1.75-20.80) $p = 0.004$
Mega [22]	2009	84% Europeans	ACS stent (TRITON)	1477	100	15 months	MACE (CV death, ACS, stroke)	*CYP2C19*2*	HR 1.53 (1.07-2.19) $p = 0.01$
							ST definite	*CYP2C19*2*	HR 3.09 (1.19-8.0) $p = 0.02$
Mega [17]	2010	84% Europeans	ACS stent (TRITON)	2905	100	15 months	MACE (CV death, ACS, stroke)	*CYP2C19*2* and *ABCB1*	*ABCB1* TT vs. CT/CC: HR 1.72 (1.22-2.44) $p = 0.002$ *CYP2C19*2* + *ABCB1* HR 1.97 (1.38-2.82) $p = 0.0002$
Simon [30]	2009	Europeans	ACS	2208	68.7	12 months	MACE (death any cause, ACS, stroke)	*CYP2C19* and *ABCB1*	*CYP2C19*: HR 1.98 (1.10-3.58) *ABCB1*: HR 1.72 (1.20-2.47)
Sorich [31]	2010	84% Europeans	ACS stent (TRITON)	13608	100	15 months	MACE (CV death, ACS, stroke)	*CYP2C19* LOF	OR 1.63 (1.45-1.81) $p < 0.0001$
Shuldiner [32]	2009	Europeans	PCI	227	100	12 months	MACE (CV death, ACS, stroke, PCI)	*CYP2C19*2*	HR 2.42 (1.18-4.99) $p = 0.02$
Wallentin [33]	2010	Europeans	ACS	10285	60	12 months	MACE (CV death, ACS, stroke)	*CYP2C19*	HR at 30 days: $p = 0.028$
								CYP2C19 and *ABCB1*	HR 1.2 (1.0-1.4) $p = 0.047$**
					Low-risk patients				
Pare [34]	2010	Europeans-latin american	ACS stable	5059	14.5	12 months	MACE (CV death, ACS, stroke)	*CYP2C19*2*	$p = 0.32$

Data are showed as: OR: odds ratio, HR: hazard ratio, (95%CI), *p*-value, ** Data obtained from the frequencies of the groups.

Table 3. Main characteristics from the non RCT and RCT about clopidogrel included in this review. MACE: major adverse cardiovascular events, CV: cardiovascular, LOF: loss of function alleles, ST: stent thrombosis, MI: myocardial infarction.

Ref	Year	Ethnic	Population Studied	n	PCI-Stent (%)	Follow up	Endpoint	Polymorphisms	Outcomes (Intervention Group vs. Control Group)
						Non RCT			
Sánchez-Ramos [35]	2016	Europeans	ACS-PCI-stent	719	100	1 year	MACE (CV death, ACS, stroke)	*CYP2C19**2, *3 and *ABCB1*	HR 0.63 (0.41-0.97) $p = 0.037$ HR 0.61 (0.39-0.94) $p = 0.02$**
							ST definite	*CYP2C19* *2, *3 and *ABCB1*	HR 1.27 (0.08-20.2) $p = 0.87$
							Urgent revascularization*	CYP2C19 *2, *3 and ABCB1	HR 0.63 (0.31-1.28) $p = 0.20$
						RCT			
Shen [36]	2016	Asians	CAD-PCI	628	100	1 month 6 months 12 months	MACE (composite of death from any cause, myocardial infarction, or target vessel revascularization)	*CYP2C19**2	1.3% vs. 5.6%, $p = 0.003$ 3.2% vs. 7.8%, $p = 0.012$ 4.2% vs. 9.4%, $p = 0.010$
Roberts (Rapid Gene) [37]	2012	Europeans	ACS or stable angina/ stent	187	100	7 days	high on-treatment platelet reactivity	*CYP2C19**2	0% vs. 30% $p = 0.0092$
Roberts (RAPID STEMI study) [38]	2016	Europeans	STEMI- stent	102	100	1 month	high on-treatment platelet reactivity	*CYP2C19**2, *17 and *ABCB1* TT	OR=0.15 $p = 0.03$
Xie [39]	2013	Asians	CAD-PCI	600	100	180 days	MACE (death from any cause, MI, stroke, ischemia)	*CYP2C19**2,*3	1.0% and 6.2%, $p < 0.01$
Notarangelo Pharmclo [40]	2018	Europeans	ACS	888	No data	12 months	MACE (CV death, nonfatal IM, nonfatal stroke)	*CYP2C19**2, *17 and *ABCB1*	HR 0.58 (0.43-0.78) $p < 0.001$
Bergmeijer (Popular genetics) [41]	ongoing	Europeans	STEMI-stent	2500	100	15 months	MACE (CV death, ACS, stroke)	*CYP2C19**2, *3	
Tailor-PCI (NCT01742117)	ongoing	Europeans	ACS or CAD/ stent	5000	100	12 months	MACE (non-fatal MI, non-fatal stroke, severe recurrent ischemia, CV death, and ST)	*CYP2C19**2,*17	

Data are showed as: OR: odds ratio, HR: hazard ratio, (95%CI), p-value, * Urgent revascularization non related with ST, ** adjusted in multivariate analysis.

2.1.1. Large-Scale Studies in High-Risk Patients

Several large-scale studies in high-risk patients (PCI–stent) have evaluated the clinical implications of genetic variations in patients with coronary artery disease (CAD). In an article published at the beginning of 2009, Collet et al. [29] examined 259 patients <45 years with a first ACS with clopidogrel for at least one month, with 73% undergoing PCI. *CYP2C19**2 carriers had a higher risk of death, ACS, and urgent revascularization ($p = 0.0005$, HR = 3.69) compared with non-carriers.

During this period, 2208 patients were enrolled in the French Registry of Acute ST-elevation and non-ST-elevation Myocardial Infarction (FAST-MI) [30], with 68.7% undergoing PCI. They evaluated whether some genes previously associated with altered pharmacokinetics of clopidogrel were also associated with cardiovascular events during the first year after ACS. Patients with two allelic variations *ABCB1* (TT) had a higher risk of cardiovascular events than those without allelic variation (CC) (Hazard ratio, HR = 1.72, 95%CI: 1.20–2.47). The risk of death, ACS, or stroke in patients with PCI was 3.58 times higher in patients who carry two copies *CYP2C19* LOF alleles compared to subjects without this allele.

In a Genome Wide Association Study (GWAS) performed in a large Amish population [32], it was seen that patients with increased age, greater BMI, higher triglycerides levels, and lower high-density lipoprotein cholesterol were associated with a poorer clopidogrel response; these variables explained less than 10% of the variation. In contrast, the heritability of ADP-stimulated platelet aggregation in response to clopidogrel was 73%, suggesting a substantial genetic component. They showed that in 277 ACS–PCI patients, the *CYP2C19**2 polymorphism was associated with poorer cardiovascular outcomes (HR = 2.42, 95%CI: 1.18–4.99, $p = 0.02$).

Genetic Post-Hoc Substudies of the TRITON 38 Trial

The efficacies of clopidogrel and prasugrel were compared in the TRITON 38 trial [42] where 13,608 ACS–PCI–stent patients were included. Prasugrel reduced the percentage of cardiovascular death, ACS, or stroke at 15 months post-ACS, although it increased cases of bleeding.

Two genetic post-hoc studies of the TRITON-TIMI trial have been published by Mega et al. [17,22]. In a first approach [22], they evaluated the association between genetic polymorphisms in *CYP450* and secondary cardiovascular events in the clopidogrel subgroup. Patients who carried LOF alleles showed higher risk of cardiovascular death, ACS, or stroke compared with non-carriers (HR 1.53, 95%IC: 1.07–2.19, $p = 0.01$) and a higher risk of stent thrombosis (HR = 3.09, 95%CI: 1.19–8.00, $p = 0.02$). Months later, in a second article [17], they assessed the effect of the *ABCB1* polymorphism by itself and alongside variants in *CYP2C19* on cardiovascular outcomes. Both variants (*CYP2C19**2 and *ABCB1*) were significant independent predictors of cardiovascular death, ACS, or stroke (*ABCB1* 3435 TT vs. CT/CC, HR 2.01, 95% CI: 1.30–3.11, $p = 0.0017$; *CYP2C19* LOF alleles carriers vs. non-carriers, HR 1.77, IC95%: 1.11–2.80, $p = 0.0155$). When the participants were divided into four groups on the basis of *ABCB1* 3435 C > T and *CYP2C19* status, those who did not carry at-risk genotypes in either gene had a significantly lower rate of cardiovascular death, ACS, or stroke at 15 months compared to those who were either carriers of *CYP2C19* LOF alleles, *ABCB1* 3435 TT homozygotes, or both ($p = 0.0002$).

During this period, another post-hoc study was published by Sorich et al. [31]. Individuals with a *CYP2C19* LOF genotype had a higher risk of cardiovascular death, ACS, or stroke than non-carriers in the clopidogrel group (RR 1.62, 95%CI: 1.27–2.06).

Genetics Post-Hoc Substudy of PLATO

In the PLATO trial [43], ticagrelor and clopidogrel were compared in patients with ACS, of whom only 64% had undergone PCI. In the genetic substudy including 10285 [33], PLATO demonstrated an increased rate of cardiovascular events in *CYP2C19* LOF carriers in the first 30 days of treatment with clopidogrel than in those with normal alleles, but they didn't find significant difference in outcomes over the full follow-up period. Although *ABCB1* polymorphism was also genotyped, the combination of both variants (*CYP2C19* and *ABCB1*) comparing LOF carriers versus non-carriers in the clopidogrel group was not compared.

2.1.2. Meta-Analyses of Large-Scale Studies

These studies and others were combined in several meta-analyses. In 2015, a systematic review of them was published by Osnabrugge et al. [44]. Most of the studies included in the meta-analysis showed statistical significance between polymorphisms and clinical endpoints, e.g., major adverse cardiovascular events (MACE) and stent thrombosis. However, the meta-analysis concluded that the association between *CYP2C19* LOF alleles and clinical efficacy of clopidogrel differed widely with regard to assessment, interpretation of high heterogeneity, and publication bias. Also, personalizing antiplatelet management based on genotyping is not supported by the currently available evidence [44].

2.1.3. Non-Randomized Clinical Trials

Others prospective, non-RCTs of *CYP2C19* genotype-guided clopidogrel therapy with clinical outcomes have been performed. In 2016, our group published a study with the aim of analyzing if the *CYP2C19/ABCB1* genotype-guided approach, in which the choice of antiplatelet therapy is based on the genetic test, could reduce the rates of cardiovascular events and bleeding compared to a non-tailored approach in 719 patients (more than 86% with ACS) who had undergone PCI with stent [35,45]. The primary endpoint (composite of cardiovascular death, ACS, or stroke during 12 months after intervention) occurred in 10.1% in the genotyping group and in 14.1% in the control group (HR 0.63, 95% CI (0.41–0.97), $p = 0.037$). The results showed that there was no difference in major and minor bleeding between the two groups (4.1% vs. 4.7%, HR = 0.80, 95%CI (0.39–1.63), $p = 0.55$) [35].

2.1.4. Clinical Trials

In 2016, Shen et al. published a study where 628 CAD patients undergoing PCI were divided into a control group (n = 319) and an intervention group ($n = 309$), which were tested for *CYP2C19* [36]. In the intervention group, extensive metabolizer patients received 75 mg daily of clopidogrel, intermediate metabolizer patients received 150 mg daily of clopidogrel, and poor metabolizer patients received ticagrelor 90 mg twice daily. The control group received clopidogrel 75 mg daily. The rates of MACE in the intervention group were lower than those in the control group at 1, 6, and 12 months ($P = 0.010$). There were no differences in the rates of bleeding between both groups ($P > 0.05$).

In 2012, a clinical trial testing this strategy was published (RAPID GENE Study, NCT01184300) using a novel point-of-care genetic test to identify carriers of the *CYP2C19**2 allele, which aimed to assess a pharmacogenetic approach to dual antiplatelet treatment after PCI [37]. The *CYP2C19**2-pharmacogenetic strategy after PCI was effective in reducing high on-treatment platelet reactivity at day 7 in *CYP2C19**2 carriers. Recently, the same group confirmed that the identification of these genetic variants in patients with STEMI receiving PCI is feasible at the bedside and demonstrated that treatment of *CYP2C19**2, *17, and *ABCB1* TT carriers with prasugrel resulted in a significant reduction in high platelet reactivity after 1 month compared to an augmented dosing of clopidogrel [38].

In 2013, 600 patients with CAD undergoing PCI randomly received a personalized antiplatelet therapy or conventional antiplatelet treatment and followed for the 180-day period after randomization. In the intervention group, the antiplatelet therapy was chosen according to CYP2C19 phenotype. In the control group, the patients received conventional antiplatelet treatment. The incidence of the primary end point (MACE) was 9.03% for patients assigned to conventional treatment and 2.66% for patients assigned to personalized therapy ($p < 0.01$), without differences in bleeding events between the 2 groups [39].

The PHARMCLO RCT is another clopidogrel pharmacogenetic study published in 2018 [40]. It is a prospective, multicenter RCT achieved in Italy between 2013 and 2015. 888 patients hospitalized for ACS were randomly assigned to standard of care or the PGx intervention arm, which included the genotyping of *ABCB1*, *CYP2C19**2, and *CYP2C19**17 using an ST Q3 system that provides data within 70 min at each patient's bedside. The patients were followed up for 12 months for the primary composite endpoint of cardiovascular death and the first occurrence of nonfatal myocardial infarction, nonfatal stroke, and major bleeding was defined according to Bleeding Academic Research Consortium type 3 to 5 criteria. The study was prematurely stopped at only 25% of prespecified enrollment, because of the lack of in vitro diagnosis certification of the genotyping instrument. However, despite only enrolling a fraction of the anticipated sample size, the primary endpoint occurred in 15.9% in the intervention arm and in 25.9% in the standard-of-care arm (HR: 0.58; 95% CI: 0.43 to 0.78; $p < 0.001$).

In the Netherlands, a multicenter trial named Cost-effectiveness of Genotype Guided Treatment With Antiplatelet Drugs in STEMI Patients: Optimization of Treatment (POPular Genetics, NCT01761786) started in 2011 to assess the efficacy, safety, and cost-effectiveness of the *CYP2C19* genotype-guided antiplatelet treatment strategy, using clopidogrel in non-carriers of the *CYP2C19**2 or *3 allele and ticagrelor or prasugrel in carriers of the *CYP2C19**2 or *3 allele in 2500 STEMI patients. [41]. Similarly, the Tailored Antiplatelet Therapy Following PCI (TAILOR-PCI) is a multi-site, open label, prospective, randomized trial, where 5000 patients with ACS or stable CAD who underwent PCI with stent will be recruited and randomized to receive a conventional therapy or a *CYP2C19* genotype-based anti-platelet therapy approach (NCT01742117).

2.1.5. Meta-Analyses

In 2018, a meta-analysis performed by Kheiri et al. [46] was published, including six RCTs with a total of 2371 patients. Of those studies, only three trials included ACS patients [39,40,47], Tuteja et al. [48] was not published and included CAD patients, Tomaniak et al. [49] included stable CAD patients, and Robert et al. [37] mainly included CAD (only 37% ACS). The results showed that the rate of MACEs was not significantly different between intervention groups and control groups (8.9% vs. 12.8%, RR0.67 IC 0.35–1.27, $p = 0.22$, $I^2 = 74\%$). The high heterogeneity was due to inconsistency in definitions of MACE among the trials, different follow-up times, different genotype testing systems with varied tested alleles, and a variety of dosing algorithms. Sensitivity analysis by excluding the unpublished trial [48] resulted in a significant reduction of MACE in favor to the genotype-guided group with almost no heterogeneity (RR 0.55, 95%CI 0.41–0.74, $p < 0.01$, I2 = 2%). Similarly, a sensitive analysis by including only the three trials that assessed genotype testing exclusively in ACS patients suggested a significant reduction of MACE.

2.1.6. Guidelines

Taking into account all the commented information, clopidogrel should be considered as an ideal target for pharmacogenetic intervention, at least in high-risk patients, due to the high level of evidence associated with the reduction of cardiovascular events rates and because there are other alternatives of antiplatelet drugs which are not affected by *CYP2C19* polymorphisms. This is supported by CIPC and DPGW guidelines, which have labelled the clopidogrel–CYP2C19 interaction as 1A. The CPIC and the DPWG recommend the use of genetic information to guide clopidogrel therapy, especially in ACS patients who have undergone PCI [50–53]. Both guidelines recommend considering an alternative drug for CYP2C19 poor or intermediate metabolizers due to increased risk for reduced response to clopidogrel.

In low-risk patients (no PCI–stent), no relationship was found between *CYP2C19**2 status and adverse outcomes [34,54]. Despite the evidence and the PGx guidelines, the current guidelines for the treatment of ACS by the American Heart Association/American College of Cardiology (AHA/ACC) and the guideline recommendations by European Society of Cardiology do not make references to the possibility of carrying out the pharmacogenetic test even in high-risk patients (ACS–PCI–stent) and, in consequence, they contradict the CPIC and DPGW guidelines and the FDA and EMA recommendations. A recent and very good review of the lack of updating of the American and European cardiology guidelines of ACS with respect to the clopidogrel test has been published by Luzum and Cheung [7]. The AHA/ACC recommends against routine pharmacogenetic testing for clopidogrel because no RCTs have demonstrated the testing improves patient's outcomes [55]. According to the authors of this article [7], the level of evidence supporting by *CYP2C19* genotype-guided clopidogrel therapy in patients that received PCI is at least as strong as the other genetic tests recommended by the AHA/ACC. Fortunately, several institutions have implemented pharmacogenetic testing for clopidogrel despite the negative recommendation by AHA/ACC [35,45,56,57] and they found improvement in the clinical results of patients [58,59].

2.1.7. Cost-Effectiveness Studies

There are different cost-effectiveness studies supporting that preventive genotyping test of *CYP2C19* is cost-effective and could be applicable in clinical practice [60–63]. In collaboration with The Golden Helix Foundation, in 2018 we performed a cost-effectiveness analysis of pharmacogenomic-guided antiplatelet treatment using the data published [60] by our team regarding Spanish ACS patients who underwent PCI [35]. This study is one of the very few that aims to compare the cost-effectiveness of antiplatelet treatment modalities retrospectively versus prospectively genotyped patients for the *CYP2C19**2, *CYP2C19**3, and *CYP2C19**17 alleles. Our analysis suggests that the prospective treatment strategy costs slightly less and has a marginally higher effectiveness compared to the retrospective group.

In 2015, Johnson et al. [64] estimated the financial impact of *CYP2C19* genotyping in a theoretical cohort of 1000 patients with ACS who received PCI–stent implantation and were treated with clopidogrel, prasugrel, or ticagrelor in a managed care setting. The budget-impact analysis used published event rates from primary literature to estimate costs of events analysis for three different scenarios: Scenario A, no *CYP2C19* genotyping; Scenario B, 50% of patients received *CYP2C19* genotyping with appropriate treatment based on genotype; and Scenario C, 100% of patients received *CYP2C19* genotyping with appropriate treatment based on genotype. They concluded that important financial benefits may be realized through use of genotype-guided antiplatelet therapy to reserve prasugrel or ticagrelor use for patients with reduced CYP2C19 activity to avoid costs associated with adverse cardiac events.

A systematic review of economic evaluation of pharmacogenetic testing for prevention of adverse drug reactions was published in 2016 [65]. There was evidence supporting the cost effectiveness of testing for different drugs, including clopidogrel.

2.2. *Warfarin*

Warfarin is an anticoagulant widely used for the prevention of thromboembolic and hemorrhagic episodes [66,67]. The drug decreases the activation of vitamin K-dependent coagulation factors by inhibiting the enzyme epoxide reductase [68]. Due to the great variability in the individual response and a narrow therapeutic window, there is a significant risk of thromboembolism if the doses are less than adequate, or of hemorrhage in case of overdose [69] for patients with the same International Normalized Ratio (INR) target [67].

Different algorithms based on clinical parameters such as age, weight, and height were published, but these are inaccurate and explain only 12–22% of the dose variation [70]. In recent years, different algorithms also including genetic polymorphisms that affect enzymes that mediate the metabolism of the drug were published. The most popular variants are the genes that encode CYP2C9 and the epoxide reductase of vitamin K in the *VKORC1* gene, which affect the properties pharmacokinetics and pharmacodynamics of warfarin [71].

The *CYP2C9* gene has many allelic variants. Individuals homozygous for the wild-type allele (*CYP2C9**1) have a "normal metabolism" of S-warfarin, the most potent form of this drug. The *2 (rs1799853) and *3 (rs1057910) alleles have a reduced enzymatic activity for the excretion of the drug, which entails a decrease of around 30% and 80%, respectively [67].

On the other hand, the enzyme encoded by *VKORC1* catalyzes the reduction of vitamin K, a necessary step to activate the coagulation factors. Its polymorphism, -1639G > A (rs9923231), is associated with an increased sensitivity to warfarin and the decrease in the amount required [67].

2.2.1. Genotype-Guided Algorithms

Gage et al. [72] published the first warfarin genotype-guided algorithm, including 369 patients who had a stable dose of warfarin. As genetic variants they only included *CYP2C9**2 and *3 and as demographic and clinical variants they included age, body surface area, gender race, target INR, and comedication (amiodarone and simvastatin). The algorithm presented a coefficient of determination (R^2) of 39%. In 2008, the same group published a new algorithm [70] which improved the $R^2 = 54\%$. They increased the number of patients to 1015 and included another genetic variant, *VKORC1* 1639G>A, smoking status, and the indication of the drug [70].

For these reasons, in 2007, the FDA approved the inclusion in the drug's data sheet of a dosage table that recommends taking into account polymorphisms -1639G>A in the *VKORC1* gene and *2 and *3 in the *CYP2C9* gene, to set the initial dose [73]. The decision was made because many studies showed that these polymorphisms were associated with great variability in the response to warfarin.

Other pharmacogenetic algorithms have been proposed that take into account both the genetic polymorphisms and the clinical variables of the patients to estimate the maintenance dose of warfarin [70,74–76], which seem to have greater accuracy than the tables in the technical data sheet [77]. However, they do not evaluate whether the pharmacogenetic algorithm can lead to the improvement of clinical results, such as % INR out of range, time to reach the INR, and frequency of appearance of thrombotic or hemorrhagic events. These algorithms explain about 50% of the dose variation [70,77], with greater benefit at the end of the dosage [74].

2.2.2. Clinical Trials

Different clinical trials have been published in recent years, measuring in these cases clinical outcomes such as thrombotic and hemorrhagic adverse events, time to reach the INR, and time in therapeutic range (Table 4). Among all of them we would like to highlight two pharmacogenetic trials of warfarin therapy, European Pharmacogenetics of Anticoagulant Therapy (EU-PACT), and Clarification of Optimal Anticoagulation through Genetics (COAG), reported by Pirmohamed et al. [3] and Kimmel et al. [78], respectively, that were published at the same time with contradictory messages. Pirmohamed et al. [3] recruited 455 patients with atrial fibrillation (AF) or venous thromboembolism. For patients assigned to the genotype-guided group, warfarin doses were prescribed according to a PGx algorithm for the first five days. Patients in the control group received a 3-day loading-dose regime (fixed-dose strategy). After the initiation period, the treatment of all patients was managed according to routine clinical practice. The primary outcome was the percentage of time in the therapeutic range (TTR) of 2.0 to 3.0 for the INR during the first 12 weeks after warfarin initiation. The mean percentage of time in the therapeutic range was 67.4% in the genotype group as compared with 60.3% in the control group ($p < 0.001$). The mean time to reach a therapeutic INR was 21 days in the genotype group as compared with 29 days in the control group ($p < 0.001$).

Kimmel et al. [78] recruited 1015 patients, 80% with AF or deep-vein thrombosis or pulmonary embolism. The dose of warfarin during the first five days of therapy was determined according to a dosing algorithm that included both clinical variables and genotype data, or to one that included clinical variables only. The primary outcome was the percentage of TTR from day 4 or 5 through day

28 of therapy. At 4 weeks, the mean percentage of TTR was 45.2% in the genotype group and 45% in the control group ($p = 0.91$). In North Africans patients, the mean percentage of time in the therapeutic range was less in the genotype group than in the control group.

One possible explanation could be the difference observed in the genotyping results [79], as the prevalence of homozygotes, who required the most significant dosing changes, was 17% in EU-PACT versus 11% in the COAG trial for the *VKORC1* variant and 3.4% in EU-PACT versus 1% in the COAG trial for the *CYP2C9**2 and *CYP2C9**3 variants. According to Shaw et al. [80] some key differences between the two studies were length of follow-up time (12 weeks for EU-PACT and 4 weeks for COAG), determination of dose in the non-genotype group (fixed dose in EUPACT and clinical dosing algorithm in COAG), patient ancestry (2% non-European in EU-PACT and 33% non-European in COAG), and the availability of genetic test results (EU-PACT genotype results were available in approximately 2 h, COAG genotype results were not available before the first dose for 55% of patients). Another possible explanation could be the different diseases affecting the patients which could also affect the warfarin dosing.

After these trials, others have been published in which it was demonstrated that the pharmacogenetic algorithm could reduce the time to reach the maintenance dose [81] or that a lower number of thrombotic or hemorrhagic events was achieved [82]. In 2017, the GIFT randomized clinical trial was published [82] to determine if genotype-guided dosing improves the safety of warfarin initiation among undergoing hip or knee arthroplasty. The results showed that genotype-guided warfarin dosing, compared with clinically guide dosing, reduced the combined risk of major bleeding, INR of 4 or greater, venous thromboembolism, and death. Further research is necessary to determine the cost-effectiveness of personalized warfarin dose.

Table 4. Main characteristics from the RCT about warfarin included in this review.

Ref	Year	Ethnic	Population Studied	*n*	Follow up	Endpoint	Polymorphisms	Homozygotes Action Required	Outcomes (Intervention Group vs. Control Group)	Availability Test	Dose in Non-Genotype Group
Pirmohamed (EU-PACT) [3]	2015	2% non-European	AF (72.1%) VT (27.9%)	455	12 weeks	%TTR	*CYP2C9*2,*3* *VKORC1*	*VKORC1*: 17% *CYP2C9*2* and *3: 3.4%	67.4% vs. 60.3%, $p < 0.001$	2h	Fixed-dose strategy
Kimel (COAG) [79]	2015	33% non-European	AF (23%) DVT or PE (56%)	1015	4 weeks	%TTR	*CYP2C9*2, *3* *VKORC1*	*VKORC1*: 11% *CYP2C9*2* and *3: 1%	45.2% vs. 45% $p = 0.91$	Not before the 1st dose for 55% of patients	Clinical dosing algorithm
Gage (GIFT) [82]	2017	91% European	Hip or knee arthroplasty	1650	30 and 60 days	Composite (major bleeding, INR ≥ 4, VT, death)	*CYP2C9*2,*3* *CYP4F2*	NA	RR 0.73 (0.56-0.95) $p = 0.02$	NA	NA

AF: atrial fibrillation, DVT: Deep-vein thrombosis, PE: pulmonary embolism. %TTR: percentage time in therapeutic range. NA: Not applicable.

2.2.3. Meta-Analyses

The efficacy of the different algorithms published has been analyzed in different meta-analyses. In 2014, Goulding et al. [83] performed a meta-analysis including nine RCTs which evaluated genotype-guided warfarin dosing. Analysis of the percentage of TTR showed a statistically significant benefit in favor of genotype-guided warfarin dosing (mean difference = 6.67; 95% CI 1.34, 12.0, $I^2 = 80\%$). Similarly, they found a statistically significant reduction in minor bleeding, major bleeding, and thromboembolism associated with genotype-guided warfarin dosing, RR 0.57 (95% CI 0.33, 0.99; $I^2 = 60\%$). As conclusion, they considered that the genotype-guided warfarin dosing algorithm could improve the clinical effectiveness.

In 2015, Liao et al. [84] performed a meta-analysis including seven trials. In total, 1910 patients were included, 960 patients who received genotype plus clinical algorithm of warfarin dosing and 950 patients who received clinical algorithm only. The results showed that the percentage of TTR in the genotype-guided group improved compared with the standard group in the RCTs when the initial standard dose was fixed (95% CI 0.09–0.40; $I^2 = 47.8\%$), but not when the studies were using no fixed initial doses. They did not find any difference in the incidences of adverse events (RR 0.94, 95% CI 0.84–1.04; $I^2 = 0\%$, $p = 0.647$) and death rates (RR 1.36, 95% CI 0.46–4.05; I2 = 10.4%, $p = 0.328$) between the two groups.

In 2014, Tang et al. [85] performed a systematic review and meta-analysis including ten studies with a total of 5299 patients. The control groups were treated with fixed dose or clinical algorithms. The results showed that patients in the genotype-guided group had higher percentage of TTR than the control group ($I^2 = 84\%$) and reduced risk for hemorrhagic complications ($I^2 = 0\%$).

In 2015, Belley-Cote et al. [86] performed a systematic review and a meta-analysis including 12 studies (3217 patients) (11 studies with warfarin and 1 study with acenocoumarol and phenprocoumon). The control group was treated with fixed dose or clinical algorithms. They concluded that the genotype-guide approach compared to the non-genotype guide was not found to decrease a composite of death, thromboembolism, and major bleeding ($I^2 = 10\%$), but the results improved the TTR ($I^2 = 79\%$) in comparison with fixed vitamin K-antagonist dosing, but not with the clinical algorithms.

In 2015, Li et al. [87] conducted a meta-analysis of the published RCTs comparing PGx algorithm-based warfarin dosing with clinical variants or standard protocols (control group). A total of ten RCTs were retrieved for the meta-analysis, including 2601 participants. No heterogeneity was found for the primary or subgroup analyses of major bleeding and thromboembolic events ($I^2 \leq 25\%$). The results showed that major bleeding and thromboembolic events were significantly lower in the PGx group than in the control group. Similarly, there was a trend towards increased percentage of TTR ($p = 0.05$) in the PGx group, but no difference was observed for over-anticoagulation (INR > 4).

In 2015, Dahal et al. [88] performed a meta-analysis including ten RCTs, which included 2505 patients, and compared PGx algorithm-based warfarin dosing with clinical variants or standard protocols (control group). After one month, improved percentage of TTR and major bleeding incidence ($I^2 = 26\%$) was observed, making this a cost-effective strategy in patients requiring longer anticoagulation therapy.

In 2015, Shi et al. [89] included 11 trials involving 2678 patients in a meta-analysis. The results showed that the PGx approach did not improve the TTR compared to control group ($I^2 = 82\%$), although it significantly shortened the time to maintenance dose and the time to first therapeutic INR. Moreover, the PGx approach significantly reduced the risk of adverse events and major bleeding ($I^2 = 15\%$).

2.2.4. Guidelines

In 2017 an update of the CPIC guidelines for pharmacogenetics-guided warfarin dosing was published [90]. Evidence from the literature has permitted including another variant (*CYP4F2* rs12777823), related to the limitation of the excessive accumulation of vitamin K that improves the accuracy of dose prediction [91]. Similarly, the CPNDS clinical recommendation group has published guidelines for the use of pharmacogenetic testing for variants in *VKORC1* and *CYP2C9* in adult and pediatric patients with an indication for warfarin [80]. They recommend testing for the *VKORC1* SNP (Single nucleotide polymorphism) -1639G>A (rs9923231) and the *CYP2C9* alleles *2 and *3 in order to better guide warfarin dosage.

2.2.5. Cost-Effectiveness Studies

Similar to clopidogrel, there are different cost-effectiveness studies supporting that preventive genotype testing for warfarin is cost-effective. Most of the studies have demonstrated that the genotype-guided dosing approach can lead to reduced bleeding and improve quality-adjusted life-years (QALYs) gained. In 2009, Eckman et al. [92] examined the cost-effectiveness of genotype-guided dosing (*CYP2C9**2, *CYP2C9**3, and/or *VKORC1*) versus standard induction of warfarin therapy for patients with nonvalvular AF using the Markov decision model. Effectiveness was measured in QALYs. They concluded that warfarin-related genotyping is unlikely to be cost-effective for typical patients with nonvalvular AF, but may be cost-effective in patients at high risk for hemorrhage who are starting warfarin therapy.

In 2009, Leey et al. [93] evaluated the potential clinical and economic outcomes of genotype-guided warfarin therapy in elderly patients newly diagnosed with AF. A decision tree was designed to represent the medical decision (pharmacogenetic testing or not) and the main clinical outcomes (embolic stroke, bleeding). They found that any reduction in major bleeding as a result of pharmacogenetic testing would lead to improved utility.

In 2013, Pink et al. [94] compared the cost-effectiveness of a variety of clinical dosing algorithms, pharmacogenetic dosing algorithms, and new anticoagulant-based therapies. Warfarin pharmacogenetic algorithms were more cost-effective than clinical-based dosing algorithms. Neither dabigatran nor rivaroxaban were cost-effective options, but apixaban appeared to be the most cost-effective treatment when warfarin therapy was poorly controlled.

2.3. Acenocumarol

Acenocoumarol is a vitamin K epoxide reductase inhibitor. The drug inhibits recycling of the inactive oxidized to the active reduced form of vitamin K. It is used for the prevention of thromboembolic and hemorrhagic episodes [95]. As with warfarin, different polymorphisms in *CYP2C9* and *VKORC1* genes have been associated with the efficacy of the drug.

2.3.1. Pharmacogenetics Algorithms

In the last years, several pharmacogenetics algorithms have also been published for acenocoumarol in diverse populations. Verde et al. constructed an "acenocoumarol-dose genotype score" based on the number of alleles associated with a higher acenocoumarol dosage carried by each participant for each polymorphism [96]. They concluded that this approach could discriminate patients requiring high acenocoumarol doses to achieve the target. Rathore et al. [97] and Krishna et al. [98] published two algorithms for Indian populations, including demographic, clinical, and genetic variants, and the coefficients of determinations obtained were 41% and 61.5%, respectively [97,98]. Four algorithms were developed for European populations. In 2011, the European Pharmacogenetics of Anticoagulant Therapy (EU-PACT) study group published an algorithm including *CYP2C9* and *VKORC1* variants and clinical variables (age, sex, weight, height, and amiodarone use). The PGx algorithm explained 52.6% of the dosage variance, whereas the non-genotype algorithm explained 23.7% [99]. Borobia et al. [100] developed an algorithm for a cohort of 147 patients with thromboembolic venous disease who were on stable doses including clinical variables (age, body mass index (BMI), amiodarone use, and enzyme-inducer use) and genetic variations of *CYP2C9*, *VKORC1*, *CYP4F2*, and *APOE*. The clinical factors explained 22% of the dose variability, which increased to 60.6% when pharmacogenetic information was included ($p < 0.001$) [100]. Cerezo-Manchado et al. [101] published an algorithm including 973 patients undergoing anticoagulation therapy. The algorithm was composite of clinical factors (age and BMI) and genetic variants (*VKORC1*, *CYP2C9*, and *CYP4F2* variants). The algorithm explained 50% of the variance in the acenocoumarol dosage, whereas the clinical algorithm explained 16% [101].

In 2016, a new algorithm including clinical (age, weight, amiodarone use, enzyme inducer status, international normalized ratio target range) and genetic variables (*CYP2C9*2* (rs1799853), *CYP2C9*3* (rs1057910), *VKORC1* (rs9923231), and *CYP4F2* (rs2108622)) to predict the most appropriate acenocoumarol dosage for stable anticoagulation in a cohort of 685 Spanish patients was published by our team in collaboration with Hospital de la Paz [102]. The R^2 explained by the algorithm was 52.8% in the generation cohort and 64% in the validation cohort. When the patients were classified into three dosage groups according to the stable dosage (<11 mg/week, 11–21 mg/week, >21 mg/week), the percentage of correctly classified patients was higher in the intermediate group, whereas differences between pharmacogenetic and clinical algorithms increased in the extreme dosage groups.

The utility of PGx-guided acenocoumarol and phenprocoumon prescribing during therapy initiation was investigated in a prospective trial: EU-PACT [2]. The genotype-guided dosing algorithm included clinical variables and genotyping for *CYP2C9* and *VKORC1* and the control-dosing algorithm included only clinical variables for the initiation of acenocoumarol or phenprocoumon treatment in patients with AF or venous thromboembolism. The primary outcome was the percentage of TTR in the 12-week period after the initiation of therapy. The intervention arm showed no statistically significant difference in the mean percentage of time in the therapeutic INR range compared with the control group. ($p = 0.52$). Some years later, to explore the potential reasons for these findings, the same team performed subanalyses stratifying the data by the *VKORC1* and *CYP2C9* genotypes [103]. They realized that the EU-PACT genetic-guided dose initiation algorithms for acenocoumarol and phenprocumon could have predicted the dose overcautiously in the *VKORC1* AA-*CYP2C9**1/*1 subgroup.

2.3.2. Meta-Analyses

Recently, a meta-analysis has been published [104] including 15,754 patients. The *CYP4F2**3 polymorphism was consistently associated with an increase in mean coumarin dose (+9% (95% CI 7–10%), with a larger effect in females, in patients taking acenocoumarol, and in Europeans. The inclusion of the *CYP4F2**3 in dosing algorithms slightly improved the prediction of stable coumarin dose. New pharmacogenetic equations potentially useful for clinical practice were derived [104].

2.3.3. Guidelines

The DPWG recommends checking INR more frequently after initiating or discontinuing NSAIDs in individuals taking acenocoumarol with at least one *CYP2C9**2 or *3 allele. While *VKORC1* genotype has been found to contribute to acenocoumarol dose variability, there are no dosing recommendations at this time because of strict INR monitoring by the Dutch Thrombosis Service. They recommend checking INR more frequently in patients with the AA genotype [52,53].

2.4. Simvastatin

Simvastatin is a lipid-modifying agent used in the treatment of different kinds of hypercholesterolemia, one of the most significant risk factors in cardiovascular disease. Furthermore, it has shown a decrease of morbimortality in atherosclerotic cardiovascular disease patients, even those with normal cholesterol levels.

Simvastatin has been significantly associated with skeletal muscle toxicity (myalgia, myopathy, and rhabdomyolysis) [105], especially a high risk of myopathy with a dose of 80 mg daily [106].

Simvastatin inhibits the cholesterol production by competitive inhibition of HMG-CoA reductase, increasing the number of LDL receptors on liver cells. Its metabolism is mediated by many CYP isoenzymes (CYP3A4, CYP3A5, CYP2C9, CYP2C19, etc.) and its movement depends on SLCO1B1 and ABCB isoforms [12]. The FDA approved a drug label for simvastatin indicating that simvastatin is a substrate for the transport protein SLCO1B1. Genetic variants contained in genes encoding these transporters and metabolic enzymes expression may affect a patient's simvastatin response.

2.4.1. Observational Studies

The SLCO1B1 enzyme, encoded by the *SLCO1B1* gene, is involved in the simvastatin carriage from intestinal to liver cells [12]. In this gene, there may be a variant, the *c.521T>C* (rs4149056), considered in *SLCO1B1*5, *15,* and *17 haplotypes, which is the only one which has reached the highest level of evidence about its association with interindividual differences in simvastatin patients' responses [107].

Among healthy individuals, the *SLCO1B1 521 CC* genotype has been associated with higher plasma concentration of simvastatin [108,109]. This genotype has been also significantly related to an increased likelihood of muscular disease in patients treated with simvastatin after ACS (OR = 16.9; 95%CI = 4.7–61.1; p = 6.0E-4) and with a higher risk of muscular disease in occlusive vascular disease or diabetes patients (RR = 2.6; 95%CI = 1.3–5; p = 0.004) [110] when compared with *CT* or *TT* genotypes. Furthermore, *CC* compared to *CT* genotype confirmed these results, with *SLCO1B1*5 CC* individuals showing a higher risk of muscular disease.

2.4.2. Clinical Trials

The STRENGTH study was a pharmacogenetics study of statin efficacy and safety. 509 patients were randomized to atorvastatin, simvastatin, or pravastatin. The composite adverse event (discontinuation for any side effect, myalgia, or CK > 3× baseline during follow-up) occurred in 99 subjects. *SLCO1B1*5* genotype and female sex were associated with mild statin-induced side effects. In patients with hypercholesterolemia, the C allele was associated with increased risk of adverse drug events when treated with atorvastatin, pravastatin, or simvastatin (OR = 1.7; 95%CI = 1.04–2.08; p = 0.03) [111]. Furthermore, regarding patients with hyperlipidemia treated with simvastatin only, carrying the *SLCO1B1*5 (CC/CT* vs. *TT*) allele was associated with higher risk of muscular diseases [112].

2.4.3. Guidelines

The FDA recommends against 80 mg daily simvastatin dosage. In patients with the *C* allele at *SLCO1B1* rs4149056, there are modest increases in myopathy risk even at lower simvastatin doses (40 mg daily); if optimal efficacy is not achieved with a lower dose, alternate agents should be considered. This annotation is based on the CPIC guideline for simvastatin and *SLCO1B1* [107].

3. Discussion

There are many barriers that hinder the implementation of PGx in daily clinical practice. In our opinion, once the regulatory agencies recommend doing the pharmacogenetic test, their implementation should not be delayed. However, as we have shown in this review, it is not performing at the expected rate as there is a disconnection between drug labels and the standard of care in daily clinical practice.

Regulators are often confronted with challenges involved in translating data from pharmacogenomic studies into clinically relevant and meaningful product information, starting with the level of scientific evidence required to justify the inclusion of PGx data in the product information [11]. In case of the new drugs, there are two guidelines on pharmacogenomics during drug development and the post-authorization phase, respectively [113].

With them, the EMA intends further to enable the potential of PGx during drug development and surveillance and to gain insight into the associated scientific challenges and discuss potential solutions. The guidelines are expected to improve genomic data-informed drug development and clinical experience, thereby promoting understanding of interindividual drug response variations and, consequently, providing guidance towards more personalized treatments in the interest of patients and the public.

However, older drugs, such as warfarin, acenocoumarol, simvastatin, and clopidogrel, have been subject to pharmacogenomic scrutiny by the EMA after their authorization [11]. So, the implementation of the PGx test should be easy.

Knowing the evidence commented above for clopidogrel, it would appear therefore that genotype-directed therapy with clopidogrel would more likely benefit a population with the greatest risk (PCI–stent). Administration of stronger antiplatelet drugs in low-risk patients would probably not reduce the thrombotic risk, but would increase the risk of bleedings [114]. However, prescribing stronger antiplatelet drugs only to the high-risk patients resistant to clopidogrel could add to a new era of personalized medicine. The old "one size fits all" regime should come to an end; tailored antiplatelet therapy is taking over, based on the patient's individual risk factors for atherothrombotic events such as HPR (High platelet reactivity), diabetes, ACS, and genetic polymorphisms.

The AHA/ACC guidelines recommend against routine pharmacogenetic testing because there are no clinical trials published yet [14,55], but, before the no recommendation to do the PGx test of clopidogrel by the AHA/ACC due to the lack of RCT, there was already one published by Xie et al. [39], in which it was shown that the incidence of secondary cardiovascular events was lower in the intervention group with respect to the control group, as we have commented in this review. It is probably necessary to wait for the clinical results of the rest of RCTs discussed in this review and wait for the next update of the AHA/ACC.

In our opinion, the level of evidence supporting *CYP2C19* genotype-guided clopidogrel therapy in patients undergoing PCI is high enough and endorsed by the regulatory agencies for the AHA/ACC guide to include it, given that the AHA/ACC recommends other PGx tests in absence of prospective clinical trials. The evidence showed by large-scale observational studies in high-risk patients suggests that the *CYP2C19* LOF alleles are associated with MACE. The meta-analysis published by Osnabrugge et al. [44] showed that there is high heterogeneity between studies and publication bias and since the validity of the overall conclusion of a meta-analysis depends, to a large extent, on the homogeneity of the studies included, in our opinion this should be considered as an important limitation of the meta-analysis [115]. Regarding clinical trials, one non-RCT [35] and five RCTs [36,37,39–41] (and TAILOR-PCI) show that PGx tests can improve results in the health of patients. Similarly, the meta-analysis including these RCTs [46] showed high heterogeneity due to inconsistency in definitions of MACE, different follow-up time, different genotype systems, etc. Despite this, when an unpublished article [48] was excluded from the meta-analysis, there was almost no heterogeneity and the results showed that the intervention group reduced MACE and was statistically significant. Moreover, several studies have shown that the application of PGx to clopidogrel is cost-effective.

Regarding warfarin, several PGx algorithms, including clinical variables, have been published and considered efficient methods for determining individual stable warfarin dose. Although there is enough information to show the association between genetic variants and warfarin dose, the results published in RCTs are controversial, mainly because of the complexity, the important differences in the design, the differences observed in the prevalence of the genotyping results [79], and the different diseases included, all of which could affect warfarin dosing. In spite of this, most of the meta-analyses of RCTs show at least an improvement of percentage of TTR when using the pharmacogenetic algorithm compared with the standard protocol.

Sample size in genotyping trials (e.g., Tailored Antiplatelet Initiation to Lessen Outcomes Due to Decreased Clopidogrel Response after Percutaneous Coronary Intervention [TAILOR-PCI trial, ClinicalTrials.gov number, NCT01742117) should probably be calculated on the basis of the prevalence of reduced-function or loss-of-function alleles that affect the phenotype, since we do not anticipate a difference in outcomes in patients without such mutations [116].

In our opinion, the greatest benefit of the implementation of the PGx test for warfarin would be in those patients who initiate the treatment; then we could anticipate if the drug is going to work or if it is better to prescribe a new oral anticoagulant drug and in those patients who, after a reasonable period, do not manage to maintain the INR in order to justify that it is due to poor metabolism of the drug.

Observational evidence suggests that the use of a genotype-guided dosing algorithm may increase the effectiveness and safety of acenocoumarol therapy. Although it's important to note that the published algorithms differ in the kind of patients and diseases, the clinical and genetic included variables, and the methods used to develop the predictive models.

However, the only clinical trial achieved reported initially that genotype-guided dosing of acenocoumarol (and phenprocoumon) did not improve the percentage of time in the therapeutic INR range during the 12 weeks after the initiation of therapy. After performing subanalyses stratifying the data by the *VKORC1* and *CYP2C9* genotypes [103], they realized that the EU-PACT genetic-guided dose initiation algorithms for acenocoumarol (and phenprocumon) could have predicted the dose overcautiously in the *VKORC1* AA-*CYP2C9**1/*1 subgroup.

This trial had limitations that could have influenced the final result; on the one hand, it is important to know that the CYP2C9 enzyme has much less influence on the pharmacokinetics of phenprocoumon than on the pharmacokinetics of warfarin [117], but on the other hand, the number of patients included was lower than the number required according to the power calculation.

In our opinion, those patients who fail to reach or maintain the INR after a period of treatment could benefit from the PGx test. More studies are necessary to implement the PGx test before the prescription for guiding the dose of acenocoumarol.

Regarding simvastatin, an RCT showed that *SLCO1B1**5 genotype and female sex were associated mild statin-induced side effects. As the FDA and CPIC guidelines recommend the PGx test, this should at least be used when symptomatology of myopathy starts.

In conclusion, PGx tests for clopidogrel in high-risk patients and warfarin in patients including all indications could begin to be implemented in daily clinical practice, similar to simvastatin tests. Acenocoumarol should be limited to patients who do not reach the INR after a certain time of treatment. The algorithm could improve acenocoumarol dosage selection for patients who will begin treatment with this drug, especially in extreme-dosage patients. Further studies are necessary to confirm that the PGx test for acenocoumarol is ready for use.

References

1. Mallal, S.; Phillips, E.; Carosi, G.; Molina, J.M.; Workman, C.; Tomazic, J.; Jagel-Guedes, E.; Rugina, S.; Kozyrev, O.; Cid, J.F.; et al. Hla-b*5701 screening for hypersensitivity to abacavir. *N. Engl. J. Med.* **2008**, *358*, 568–579. [CrossRef]
2. Verhoef, T.I.; Ragia, G.; de Boer, A.; Barallon, R.; Kolovou, G.; Kolovou, V.; Konstantinides, S.; Le Cessie, S.; Maltezos, E.; van der Meer, F.J.; et al. A randomized trial of genotype-guided dosing of acenocoumarol and phenprocoumon. *N. Engl. J. Med.* **2013**, *369*, 2304–2312. [CrossRef] [PubMed]
3. Pirmohamed, M.; Burnside, G.; Eriksson, N.; Jorgensen, A.L.; Toh, C.H.; Nicholson, T.; Kesteven, P.; Christersson, C.; Wahlstrom, B.; Stafberg, C.; et al. A randomized trial of genotype-guided dosing of warfarin. *N. Engl. J. Med.* **2013**, *369*, 2294–2303. [CrossRef] [PubMed]
4. Wu, A.H. Pharmacogenomic testing and response to warfarin. *Lancet* **2015**, *385*, 2231–2232. [CrossRef]
5. Coenen, M.J.; de Jong, D.J.; van Marrewijk, C.J.; Derijks, L.J.; Vermeulen, S.H.; Wong, D.R.; Klungel, O.H.; Verbeek, A.L.; Hooymans, P.M.; Peters, W.H.; et al. Identification of patients with variants in tpmt and dose reduction reduces hematologic events during thiopurine treatment of inflammatory bowel disease. *Gastroenterology* **2015**, *149*, 907–917. [CrossRef] [PubMed]
6. Bank, P.C.D.; Swen, J.J.; Guchelaar, H.J. Implementation of pharmacogenomics in everyday clinical settings. *Adv. Pharmacol.* **2018**, *83*, 219–246.
7. Luzum, J.A.; Cheung, J.C. Does cardiology hold pharmacogenetics to an inconsistent standard? A comparison of evidence among recommendations. *Pharmacogenomics* **2018**, *19*, 1203–1216. [CrossRef]
8. Van der Wouden, C.H.; Cambon-Thomsen, A.; Cecchin, E.; Cheung, K.C.; Davila-Fajardo, C.L.; Deneer, V.H.; Dolzan, V.; Ingelman-Sundberg, M.; Jonsson, S.; Karlsson, M.O.; et al. Implementing pharmacogenomics in europe: Design and implementation strategy of the ubiquitous pharmacogenomics consortium. *Clin. Pharmacol. Ther.* **2017**, *101*, 341–358. [CrossRef]

9. Van der Wouden, C.H.; Cambon-Thomsen, A.; Cecchin, E.; Cheung, K.C.; Davila-Fajardo, C.L.; Deneer, V.H.; Dolzan, V.; Ingelman-Sundberg, M.; Jonsson, S.; Karlsson, M.O.; et al. Corrigendum: Implementing pharmacogenomics in europe: Design and implementation strategy of the ubiquitous pharmacogenomics consortium. *Clin. Pharmacol. Ther.* **2017**, *102*, 152. [CrossRef] [PubMed]
10. Bank, P.C.D.; Caudle, K.E.; Swen, J.J.; Gammal, R.S.; Whirl-Carrillo, M.; Klein, T.E.; Relling, M.V.; Guchelaar, H.J. Comparison of the guidelines of the clinical pharmacogenetics implementation consortium and the dutch pharmacogenetics working group. *Clin. Pharmacol. Ther.* **2018**, *103*, 599–618. [CrossRef] [PubMed]
11. Ehmann, F.; Caneva, L.; Papaluca, M. European medicines agency initiatives and perspectives on pharmacogenomics. *Br. J. Clin. Pharmacol.* **2014**, *77*, 612–617. [CrossRef]
12. Whirl-Carrillo, M.; McDonagh, E.M.; Hebert, J.M.; Gong, L.; Sangkuhl, K.; Thorn, C.F.; Altman, R.B.; Klein, T.E. Pharmacogenomics knowledge for personalized medicine. *Clin. Pharmacol. Ther.* **2012**, *92*, 414–417. [CrossRef]
13. King, S.B., 3rd; Smith, S.C., Jr.; Hirshfeld, J.W., Jr.; Jacobs, A.K.; Morrison, D.A.; Williams, D.O.; Feldman, T.E.; Kern, M.J.; O'Neill, W.W.; Schaff, H.V.; et al. 2007 focused update of the acc/aha/scai 2005 guideline update for percutaneous coronary intervention: A report of the american college of cardiology/american heart association task force on practice guidelines. *J. Am. Coll. Cardiol.* **2008**, *51*, 172–209. [CrossRef]
14. Kushner, F.G.; Hand, M.; Smith, S.C., Jr.; King, S.B., 3rd; Anderson, J.L.; Antman, E.M.; Bailey, S.R.; Bates, E.R.; Blankenship, J.C.; Casey, D.E., Jr.; et al. 2009 focused updates: ACC/AHA guidelines for the management of patients with ST-elevation myocardial infarction (updating the 2004 guideline and 2007 focused update) and ACC/AHA/SCAI guidelines on percutaneous coronary intervention (updating the 2005 guideline and 2007 focused update): A report of the American College of Cardiology Foundation/American Heart Association Task Force on Practice Guidelines. *J. Am. Coll. Cardiol.* **2009**, 2205–2241.
15. Snoep, J.D.; Hovens, M.M.; Eikenboom, J.C.; van der Bom, J.G.; Jukema, J.W.; Huisman, M.V. Clopidogrel nonresponsiveness in patients undergoing percutaneous coronary intervention with stenting: A systematic review and meta-analysis. *Am. Heart J.* **2007**, *154*, 221–231. [CrossRef]
16. Giusti, B.; Gori, A.M.; Marcucci, R.; Saracini, C.; Vestrini, A.; Abbate, R. Determinants to optimize response to clopidogrel in acute coronary syndrome. *Pharmgenomics Pers. Med.* **2010**, *3*, 33–50. [CrossRef]
17. Mega, J.L.; Close, S.L.; Wiviott, S.D.; Shen, L.; Walker, J.R.; Simon, T.; Antman, E.M.; Braunwald, E.; Sabatine, M.S. Genetic variants in abcb1 and CYP2C19 and cardiovascular outcomes after treatment with clopidogrel and prasugrel in the triton-timi 38 trial: A pharmacogenetic analysis. *Lancet* **2010**, *376*, 1312–1319. [CrossRef]
18. Fuster, V.; Sweeny, J.M. Clopidogrel and the reduced-function CYP2C19 genetic variant: A limited piece of the overall therapeutic puzzle. *JAMA* **2010**, *304*, 1839–1840. [CrossRef]
19. Giusti, B.; Gori, A.M.; Marcucci, R.; Abbate, R. Current status of clopidogrel pharmacogenomics. *Pharmacogenomics* **2012**, *13*, 1671–1674. [CrossRef]
20. Wang, X.Q.; Shen, C.L.; Wang, B.N.; Huang, X.H.; Hu, Z. Genetic polymorphisms of CYP2C19*2 and abcb1 c3435t affect the pharmacokinetic and pharmacodynamic responses to clopidogrel in 401 patients with acute coronary syndrome. *Gene* **2015**, *558*, 200–207. [CrossRef]
21. Su, J.; Xu, J.; Li, X.; Zhang, H.; Hu, J.; Fang, R.; Chen, X. Abcb1 c3435t polymorphism and response to clopidogrel treatment in coronary artery disease (cad) patients: A meta-analysis. *PLoS ONE* **2012**, *7*, e46366. [CrossRef]
22. Mega, J.L.; Close, S.L.; Wiviott, S.D.; Shen, L.; Hockett, R.D.; Brandt, J.T.; Walker, J.R.; Antman, E.M.; Macias, W.; Braunwald, E.; et al. Cytochrome p-450 polymorphisms and response to clopidogrel. *N. Engl. J. Med.* **2009**, *360*, 354–362. [CrossRef]
23. Sibbing, D.; Koch, W.; Gebhard, D.; Schuster, T.; Braun, S.; Stegherr, J.; Morath, T.; Schomig, A.; von Beckerath, N.; Kastrati, A. Cytochrome 2c19*17 allelic variant, platelet aggregation, bleeding events, and stent thrombosis in clopidogrel-treated patients with coronary stent placement. *Circulation* **2010**, *121*, 512–518. [CrossRef]
24. Sibbing, D.; Gebhard, D.; Koch, W.; Braun, S.; Stegherr, J.; Morath, T.; Von Beckerath, N.; Mehilli, J.; Schomig, A.; Schuster, T.; et al. Isolated and interactive impact of common CYP2C19 genetic variants on the antiplatelet effect of chronic clopidogrel therapy. *J. Thromb. Haemost.* **2010**, *8*, 1685–1693. [CrossRef]

25. Frere, C.; Cuisset, T.; Gaborit, B.; Alessi, M.C.; Hulot, J.S. The CYP2C19*17 allele is associated with better platelet response to clopidogrel in patients admitted for non-st acute coronary syndrome. *J. Thromb. Haemost.* **2009**, *7*, 1409–1411. [CrossRef]
26. Tiroch, K.A.; Sibbing, D.; Koch, W.; Roosen-Runge, T.; Mehilli, J.; Schomig, A.; Kastrati, A. Protective effect of the CYP2C19 *17 polymorphism with increased activation of clopidogrel on cardiovascular events. *Am. Heart J.* **2010**, *160*, 506–512. [CrossRef]
27. Harmsze, A.M.; van Werkum, J.W.; Hackeng, C.M.; Ruven, H.J.; Kelder, J.C.; Bouman, H.J.; Breet, N.J.; Ten Berg, J.M.; Klungel, O.H.; de Boer, A.; et al. The influence of CYP2C19*2 and *17 on on-treatment platelet reactivity and bleeding events in patients undergoing elective coronary stenting. *Pharmacogenet. Genomics* **2012**, *22*, 169–175. [CrossRef]
28. US Department of Health and Human Services. *FDA Drug Safety Communication: Reduced Effectiveness of Plavix (Clopidogrel) in Patients Who Are Poor Metabolizers of the Drug*; US Food and Drug Administration: Silver Spring, MD, USA, 2010.
29. Collet, J.P.; Hulot, J.S.; Pena, A.; Villard, E.; Esteve, J.B.; Silvain, J.; Payot, L.; Brugier, D.; Cayla, G.; Beygui, F.; et al. Cytochrome p450 2c19 polymorphism in young patients treated with clopidogrel after myocardial infarction: A cohort study. *Lancet* **2009**, *373*, 309–317. [CrossRef]
30. Simon, T.; Verstuyft, C.; Mary-Krause, M.; Quteineh, L.; Drouet, E.; Meneveau, N.; Steg, P.G.; Ferrieres, J.; Danchin, N.; Becquemont, L.; et al. Genetic determinants of response to clopidogrel and cardiovascular events. *N. Engl. J. Med.* **2009**, *360*, 363–375. [CrossRef]
31. Sorich, M.J.; Vitry, A.; Ward, M.B.; Horowitz, J.D.; McKinnon, R.A. Prasugrel vs. Clopidogrel for cytochrome p450 2c19-genotyped subgroups: Integration of the triton-timi 38 trial data. *J. Thromb. Haemost.* **2010**, *8*, 1678–1684. [CrossRef]
32. Shuldiner, A.R.; O'Connell, J.R.; Bliden, K.P.; Gandhi, A.; Ryan, K.; Horenstein, R.B.; Damcott, C.M.; Pakyz, R.; Tantry, U.S.; Gibson, Q.; et al. Association of cytochrome p450 2c19 genotype with the antiplatelet effect and clinical efficacy of clopidogrel therapy. *JAMA* **2009**, *302*, 849–857. [CrossRef]
33. Wallentin, L.; James, S.; Storey, R.F.; Armstrong, M.; Barratt, B.J.; Horrow, J.; Husted, S.; Katus, H.; Steg, P.G.; Shah, S.H.; et al. Effect of CYP2C19 and abcb1 single nucleotide polymorphisms on outcomes of treatment with ticagrelor versus clopidogrel for acute coronary syndromes: A genetic substudy of the plato trial. *Lancet* **2010**, *376*, 1320–1328. [CrossRef]
34. Pare, G.; Mehta, S.R.; Yusuf, S.; Anand, S.S.; Connolly, S.J.; Hirsh, J.; Simonsen, K.; Bhatt, D.L.; Fox, K.A.; Eikelboom, J.W. Effects of CYP2C19 genotype on outcomes of clopidogrel treatment. *N. Engl. J. Med.* **2010**, *363*, 1704–1714. [CrossRef]
35. Sanchez-Ramos, J.; Davila-Fajardo, C.L.; Toledo Frias, P.; Diaz Villamarin, X.; Martinez-Gonzalez, L.J.; Martinez Huertas, S.; Burillo Gomez, F.; Caballero Borrego, J.; Bautista Paves, A.; Marin Guzman, M.C.; et al. Results of genotype-guided antiplatelet therapy in patients who undergone percutaneous coronary intervention with stent. *Int. J. Cardiol.* **2016**, *225*, 289–295. [CrossRef]
36. Shen, D.L.; Wang, B.; Bai, J.; Han, Q.; Liu, C.; Huang, X.H.; Zhang, J.Y. Clinical value of CYP2C19 genetic testing for guiding the antiplatelet therapy in a chinese population. *J. Cardiovasc. Pharmacol.* **2016**, *67*, 232–236. [CrossRef]
37. Roberts, J.D.; Wells, G.A.; Le May, M.R.; Labinaz, M.; Glover, C.; Froeschl, M.; Dick, A.; Marquis, J.F.; O'Brien, E.; Goncalves, S.; et al. Point-of-care genetic testing for personalisation of antiplatelet treatment (rapid gene): A prospective, randomised, proof-of-concept trial. *Lancet* **2012**, *379*, 1705–1711. [CrossRef]
38. So, D.Y.; Wells, G.A.; McPherson, R.; Labinaz, M.; Le May, M.R.; Glover, C.; Dick, A.J.; Froeschl, M.; Marquis, J.F.; Gollob, M.H.; et al. A prospective randomized evaluation of a pharmacogenomic approach to antiplatelet therapy among patients with st-elevation myocardial infarction: The rapid stemi study. *Pharmacogenomics J.* **2016**, *16*, 71–78. [CrossRef]
39. Xie, X.; Ma, Y.T.; Yang, Y.N.; Li, X.M.; Zheng, Y.Y.; Ma, X.; Fu, Z.Y.; Ba, B.; Li, Y.; Yu, Z.X.; et al. Personalized antiplatelet therapy according to CYP2C19 genotype after percutaneous coronary intervention: A randomized control trial. *Int. J. Cardiol.* **2013**, *168*, 3736–3740. [CrossRef]
40. Notarangelo, F.M.; Maglietta, G.; Bevilacqua, P.; Cereda, M.; Merlini, P.A.; Villani, G.Q.; Moruzzi, P.; Patrizi, G.; Malagoli Tagliazucchi, G.; Crocamo, A.; et al. Pharmacogenomic approach to selecting antiplatelet therapy in patients with acute coronary syndromes: The pharmclo trial. *J. Am. Coll. Cardiol.* **2018**, *71*, 1869–1877. [CrossRef]

41. Bergmeijer, T.O.; Janssen, P.W.; Schipper, J.C.; Qaderdan, K.; Ishak, M.; Ruitenbeek, R.S.; Asselbergs, F.W.; van't Hof, A.W.; Dewilde, W.J.; Spano, F.; et al. CYP2C19 genotype-guided antiplatelet therapy in st-segment elevation myocardial infarction patients-rationale and design of the patient outcome after primary pci (popular) genetics study. *Am. Heart J.* **2014**, *168*, 16-22.e1. [CrossRef]

42. Wiviott, S.D.; Braunwald, E.; McCabe, C.H.; Montalescot, G.; Ruzyllo, W.; Gottlieb, S.; Neumann, F.J.; Ardissino, D.; De Servi, S.; Murphy, S.A.; et al. Prasugrel versus clopidogrel in patients with acute coronary syndromes. *N. Engl. J. Med.* **2007**, *357*, 2001–2015. [CrossRef]

43. Wallentin, L.; Becker, R.C.; Budaj, A.; Cannon, C.P.; Emanuelsson, H.; Held, C.; Horrow, J.; Husted, S.; James, S.; Katus, H.; et al. Ticagrelor versus clopidogrel in patients with acute coronary syndromes. *N. Engl. J. Med.* **2009**, *361*, 1045–1057. [CrossRef]

44. Osnabrugge, R.L.; Head, S.J.; Zijlstra, F.; ten Berg, J.M.; Hunink, M.G.; Kappetein, A.P.; Janssens, A.C. A systematic review and critical assessment of 11 discordant meta-analyses on reduced-function CYP2C19 genotype and risk of adverse clinical outcomes in clopidogrel users. *Genet. Med.* **2015**, *17*, 3–11. [CrossRef]

45. Davila-Fajardo, C.L.; Sanchez-Ramos, J.; Villamarin, X.D.; Martinez-Gonzalez, L.J.; Frias, P.T.; Huertas, S.M.; Gomez, F.B.; Borrego, J.C.; Paves, A.B.; Guzman, M.C.; et al. The study protocol for a non-randomized controlled clinical trial using a genotype-guided strategy in a dataset of patients who undergone percutaneous coronary intervention with stent. *Data Brief.* **2017**, *10*, 518–524. [CrossRef] [PubMed]

46. Kheiri, B.; Osman, M.; Abdalla, A.; Haykal, T.; Pandrangi, P.V.; Chahine, A.; Ahmed, S.; Osman, K.; Bachuwa, G.; Hassan, M.; et al. CYP2C19 pharmacogenetics versus standard of care dosing for selecting antiplatelet therapy in patients with coronary artery disease: A meta-analysis of randomized clinical trials. *Catheter. Cardiovasc. Interv.* **2018**. [CrossRef] [PubMed]

47. Tam, C.C.; Kwok, J.; Wong, A.; Yung, A.; Shea, C.; Kong, S.L.; Tang, W.H.; Siu, D.; Chan, R.; Lee, S. Genotyping-guided approach versus the conventional approach in selection of oral p2y12 receptor blockers in chinese patients suffering from acute coronary syndrome. *J. Int. Med. Res.* **2017**, *45*, 134–146. [CrossRef] [PubMed]

48. American College of Cardiology Annual Scientific Session. *Assessment of Prospective CYP2C19 Genotype Guided Dosing of Anti-Platelet Therapy in Percutaneous Coronary Intervention (Adapt)*; American College of Cardiology Annual Scientific Session (ACC 2018): Orlando, FL, USA, 2018.

49. Tomaniak, M.; Koltowski, L.; Kochman, J.; Huczek, Z.; Rdzanek, A.; Pietrasik, A.; Gasecka, A.; Gajda, S.; Opolski, G.; Filipiak, K.J. Can prasugrel decrease the extent of periprocedural myocardial injury during elective percutaneous coronary intervention? *Pol. Arch. Intern. Med.* **2017**, *127*, 730–740.

50. Scott, S.A.; Sangkuhl, K.; Gardner, E.E.; Stein, C.M.; Hulot, J.S.; Johnson, J.A.; Roden, D.M.; Klein, T.E.; Shuldiner, A.R.; Clinical Pharmacogenetics Implementation Consortium. Clinical pharmacogenetics implementation consortium guidelines for cytochrome p450-2c19 (CYP2C19) genotype and clopidogrel therapy. *Clin. Pharmacol. Ther.* **2011**, *90*, 328–332. [CrossRef]

51. Scott, S.A.; Sangkuhl, K.; Stein, C.M.; Hulot, J.S.; Mega, J.L.; Roden, D.M.; Klein, T.E.; Sabatine, M.S.; Johnson, J.A.; Shuldiner, A.R.; et al. Clinical pharmacogenetics implementation consortium guidelines for CYP2C19 genotype and clopidogrel therapy: 2013 update. *Clin. Pharmacol. Ther.* **2013**, *94*, 317–323. [CrossRef]

52. Swen, J.J.; Wilting, I.; de Goede, A.L.; Grandia, L.; Mulder, H.; Touw, D.J.; de Boer, A.; Conemans, J.M.; Egberts, T.C.; Klungel, O.H.; et al. Pharmacogenetics: From bench to byte. *Clin. Pharmacol. Ther.* **2008**, *83*, 781–787. [CrossRef]

53. Swen, J.J.; Nijenhuis, M.; de Boer, A.; Grandia, L.; Maitland-van der Zee, A.H.; Mulder, H.; Rongen, G.A.; van Schaik, R.H.; Schalekamp, T.; Touw, D.J.; et al. Pharmacogenetics: From bench to byte—An update of guidelines. *Clin. Pharmacol. Ther.* **2011**, *89*, 662–673. [CrossRef] [PubMed]

54. Bhatt, D.L.; Pare, G.; Eikelboom, J.W.; Simonsen, K.L.; Emison, E.S.; Fox, K.A.; Steg, P.G.; Montalescot, G.; Bhakta, N.; Hacke, W.; et al. The relationship between CYP2C19 polymorphisms and ischaemic and bleeding outcomes in stable outpatients: The charisma genetics study. *Eur. Heart J.* **2012**, *33*, 2143–2150. [CrossRef] [PubMed]

55. Levine, G.N.; Bates, E.R.; Bittl, J.A.; Brindis, R.G.; Fihn, S.D.; Fleisher, L.A.; Granger, C.B.; Lange, R.A.; Mack, M.J.; Mauri, L.; et al. 2016 ACC/AHA guideline focused update on duration of dual antiplatelet therapy in patients with coronary artery disease: A report of the american college of cardiology/american heart association task force on clinical practice guidelines. *J. Am. Coll. Cardiol.* **2016**, *68*, 1082–1115. [CrossRef]
56. Weitzel, K.W.; Elsey, A.R.; Langaee, T.Y.; Burkley, B.; Nessl, D.R.; Obeng, A.O.; Staley, B.J.; Dong, H.J.; Allan, R.W.; Liu, J.F.; et al. Clinical pharmacogenetics implementation: Approaches, successes, and challenges. *Am. J. Med. Genet. C Semin. Med. Genet.* **2014**, *166C*, 56–67. [CrossRef] [PubMed]
57. Pulley, J.M.; Denny, J.C.; Peterson, J.F.; Bernard, G.R.; Vnencak-Jones, C.L.; Ramirez, A.H.; Delaney, J.T.; Bowton, E.; Brothers, K.; Johnson, K.; et al. Operational implementation of prospective genotyping for personalized medicine: The design of the vanderbilt predict project. *Clin. Pharmacol. Ther.* **2012**, *92*, 87–95. [CrossRef]
58. Cavallari, L.H.; Franchi, F.; Rollini, F.; Been, L.; Rivas, A.; Agarwal, M.; Smith, D.M.; Newsom, K.; Gong, Y.; Elsey, A.R.; et al. Clinical implementation of rapid CYP2C19 genotyping to guide antiplatelet therapy after percutaneous coronary intervention. *J. Transl. Med.* **2018**, *16*, 92. [CrossRef]
59. Lee, C.R.; Sriramoju, V.B.; Cervantes, A.; Howell, L.A.; Varunok, N.; Madan, S.; Hamrick, K.; Polasek, M.J.; Lee, J.A.; Clarke, M.; et al. Clinical outcomes and sustainability of using CYP2C19 genotype-guided antiplatelet therapy after percutaneous coronary intervention. *Circ. Genom. Precis. Med.* **2018**, *11*, e002069. [CrossRef]
60. Fragoulakis, V.; Bartsakoulia, M.; Diaz-Villamarin, X.; Chalikiopoulou, K.; Kehagia, K.; Ramos, J.G.S.; Martinez-Gonzalez, L.J.; Gkotsi, M.; Katrali, E.; Skoufas, E.; et al. Cost-effectiveness analysis of pharmacogenomics-guided clopidogrel treatment in spanish patients undergoing percutaneous coronary intervention. *Pharmacogenomics J.* **2019**. [CrossRef]
61. Reese, E.S.; Daniel Mullins, C.; Beitelshees, A.L.; Onukwugha, E. Cost-effectiveness of cytochrome p450 2c19 genotype screening for selection of antiplatelet therapy with clopidogrel or prasugrel. *Pharmacotherapy* **2012**, *32*, 323–332. [CrossRef]
62. Kazi, D.S.; Garber, A.M.; Shah, R.U.; Dudley, R.A.; Mell, M.W.; Rhee, C.; Moshkevich, S.; Boothroyd, D.B.; Owens, D.K.; Hlatky, M.A. Cost-effectiveness of genotype-guided and dual antiplatelet therapies in acute coronary syndrome. *Ann. Intern. Med.* **2014**, *160*, 221–232. [CrossRef]
63. Jiang, M.; You, J.H. Cost-effectiveness analysis of personalized antiplatelet therapy in patients with acute coronary syndrome. *Pharmacogenomics* **2016**, *17*, 701–713. [CrossRef]
64. Johnson, S.G.; Gruntowicz, D.; Chua, T.; Morlock, R.J. Financial analysis of CYP2C19 genotyping in patients receiving dual antiplatelet therapy following acute coronary syndrome and percutaneous coronary intervention. *J. Manag. Care Spec. Pharm.* **2015**, *21*, 552–557. [CrossRef]
65. Plumpton, C.O.; Roberts, D.; Pirmohamed, M.; Hughes, D.A. A systematic review of economic evaluations of pharmacogenetic testing for prevention of adverse drug reactions. *Pharmacoeconomics* **2016**, *34*, 771–793. [CrossRef]
66. Carlquist, J.F.; Horne, B.D.; Muhlestein, J.B.; Lappe, D.L.; Whiting, B.M.; Kolek, M.J.; Clarke, J.L.; James, B.C.; Anderson, J.L. Genotypes of the cytochrome p450 isoform, cyp2c9, and the vitamin k epoxide reductase complex subunit 1 conjointly determine stable warfarin dose: A prospective study. *J. Thromb. Thrombolysis* **2006**, *22*, 191–197. [CrossRef]
67. Johnson, J.A.; Gong, L.; Whirl-Carrillo, M.; Gage, B.F.; Scott, S.A.; Stein, C.M.; Anderson, J.L.; Kimmel, S.E.; Lee, M.T.; Pirmohamed, M.; et al. Clinical pharmacogenetics implementation consortium guidelines for cyp2c9 and vkorc1 genotypes and warfarin dosing. *Clin. Pharmacol. Ther.* **2011**, *90*, 625–629. [CrossRef]
68. Stehle, S.; Kirchheiner, J.; Lazar, A.; Fuhr, U. Pharmacogenetics of oral anticoagulants: A basis for dose individualization. *Clin. Pharmacokinet.* **2008**, *47*, 565–594. [CrossRef]
69. Kamali, F.; Wynne, H. Pharmacogenetics of warfarin. *Annu. Rev. Med.* **2010**, *61*, 63–75. [CrossRef]
70. Gage, B.F.; Eby, C.; Johnson, J.A.; Deych, E.; Rieder, M.J.; Ridker, P.M.; Milligan, P.E.; Grice, G.; Lenzini, P.; Rettie, A.E.; et al. Use of pharmacogenetic and clinical factors to predict the therapeutic dose of warfarin. *Clin. Pharmacol. Ther.* **2008**, *84*, 326–331. [CrossRef]
71. Wadelius, M.; Pirmohamed, M. Pharmacogenetics of warfarin: Current status and future challenges. *Pharm. J.* **2007**, *7*, 99–111. [CrossRef]

72. Gage, B.F.; Eby, C.; Milligan, P.E.; Banet, G.A.; Duncan, J.R.; McLeod, H.L. Use of pharmacogenetics and clinical factors to predict the maintenance dose of warfarin. *Thromb. Haemost.* **2004**, *91*, 87–94.
73. *Coumadin- (Warfarin Sodium) Tablet [Package Insert]*; Bristol-Myers Squibb Pharma Company: Princeton, NJ, USA, 2015.
74. International Warfarin Pharmacogenetics Consortium; Klein, T.E.; Altman, R.B.; Eriksson, N.; Gage, B.F.; Kimmel, S.E.; Lee, M.T.; Limdi, N.A.; Page, D.; Roden, D.M.; et al. Estimation of the warfarin dose with clinical and pharmacogenetic data. *N. Engl. J. Med.* **2009**, *360*, 753–764.
75. Santos, P.C.; Marcatto, L.R.; Duarte, N.E.; Gadi Soares, R.A.; Cassaro Strunz, C.M.; Scanavacca, M.; Krieger, J.E.; Pereira, A.C. Development of a pharmacogenetic-based warfarin dosing algorithm and its performance in brazilian patients: Highlighting the importance of population-specific calibration. *Pharmacogenomics* **2015**, *16*, 865–876. [CrossRef]
76. Wei, M.; Ye, F.; Xie, D.; Zhu, Y.; Zhu, J.; Tao, Y.; Yu, F. A new algorithm to predict warfarin dose from polymorphisms of cyp4f2, cyp2c9 and vkorc1 and clinical variables: Derivation in han chinese patients with non valvular atrial fibrillation. *Thromb. Haemost.* **2012**, *107*, 1083–1091. [CrossRef]
77. Finkelman, B.S.; Gage, B.F.; Johnson, J.A.; Brensinger, C.M.; Kimmel, S.E. Genetic warfarin dosing: Tables versus algorithms. *J. Am. Coll. Cardiol.* **2011**, *57*, 612–618. [CrossRef]
78. Kimmel, S.E.; French, B.; Kasner, S.E.; Johnson, J.A.; Anderson, J.L.; Gage, B.F.; Rosenberg, Y.D.; Eby, C.S.; Madigan, R.A.; McBane, R.B.; et al. A pharmacogenetic versus a clinical algorithm for warfarin dosing. *N. Engl. J. Med.* **2013**, *369*, 2283–2293. [CrossRef] [PubMed]
79. Kimmel, S.E.; French, B.; Geller, N.L.; Investigators, C. Genotype-guided dosing of vitamin k antagonists. *N. Engl. J. Med.* **2014**, *370*, 1763–1764.
80. Shaw, K.; Amstutz, U.; Kim, R.B.; Lesko, L.J.; Turgeon, J.; Michaud, V.; Hwang, S.; Ito, S.; Ross, C.; Carleton, B.C.; et al. Clinical practice recommendations on genetic testing of cyp2c9 and vkorc1 variants in warfarin therapy. *Ther. Drug Monit.* **2015**, *37*, 428–436. [CrossRef] [PubMed]
81. Jiang, N.X.; Ge, J.W.; Xian, Y.Q.; Huang, S.Y.; Li, Y.S. Clinical application of a new warfarin-dosing regimen based on the cyp2c9 and vkorc1 genotypes in atrial fibrillation patients. *Biomed. Rep.* **2016**, *4*, 453–458. [CrossRef]
82. Gage, B.F.; Bass, A.R.; Lin, H.; Woller, S.C.; Stevens, S.M.; Al-Hammadi, N.; Li, J.; Rodriguez, T., Jr.; Miller, J.P.; McMillin, G.A.; et al. Effect of genotype-guided warfarin dosing on clinical events and anticoagulation control among patients undergoing hip or knee arthroplasty: The gift randomized clinical trial. *JAMA* **2017**, *318*, 1115–1124. [CrossRef] [PubMed]
83. Goulding, R.; Dawes, D.; Price, M.; Wilkie, S.; Dawes, M. Genotype-guided drug prescribing: A systematic review and meta-analysis of randomized control trials. *Br. J. Clin. Pharmacol.* **2015**, *80*, 868–877. [CrossRef] [PubMed]
84. Liao, Z.; Feng, S.; Ling, P.; Zhang, G. Meta-analysis of randomized controlled trials reveals an improved clinical outcome of using genotype plus clinical algorithm for warfarin dosing. *J. Thromb. Thrombolysis* **2015**, *39*, 228–234. [CrossRef]
85. Tang, Q.; Zou, H.; Guo, C.; Liu, Z. Outcomes of pharmacogenetics-guided dosing of warfarin: A systematic review and meta-analysis. *Int. J. Cardiol.* **2014**, *175*, 587–591. [CrossRef]
86. Belley-Cote, E.P.; Hanif, H.; D'Aragon, F.; Eikelboom, J.W.; Anderson, J.L.; Borgman, M.; Jonas, D.E.; Kimmel, S.E.; Manolopoulos, V.G.; Baranova, E.; et al. Genotype-guided versus standard vitamin k antagonist dosing algorithms in patients initiating anticoagulation. A systematic review and meta-analysis. *Thromb. Haemost.* **2015**, *114*, 768–777. [CrossRef] [PubMed]
87. Li, X.; Yang, J.; Wang, X.; Xu, Q.; Zhang, Y.; Yin, T. Clinical benefits of pharmacogenetic algorithm-based warfarin dosing: Meta-analysis of randomized controlled trials. *Thromb. Res.* **2015**, *135*, 621–629. [CrossRef] [PubMed]
88. Dahal, K.; Sharma, S.P.; Fung, E.; Lee, J.; Moore, J.H.; Unterborn, J.N.; Williams, S.M. Meta-analysis of randomized controlled trials of genotype-guided vs standard dosing of warfarin. *Chest* **2015**, *148*, 701–710. [CrossRef]
89. Shi, C.; Yan, W.; Wang, G.; Wang, F.; Li, Q.; Lin, N. Pharmacogenetics-based versus conventional dosing of warfarin: A meta-analysis of randomized controlled trials. *PLoS ONE* **2015**, *10*, e0144511. [CrossRef] [PubMed]

90. Johnson, J.A.; Caudle, K.E.; Gong, L.; Whirl-Carrillo, M.; Stein, C.M.; Scott, S.A.; Lee, M.T.; Gage, B.F.; Kimmel, S.E.; Perera, M.A.; et al. Clinical pharmacogenetics implementation consortium (cpic) guideline for pharmacogenetics-guided warfarin dosing: 2017 update. *Clin. Pharmacol. Ther.* **2017**, *102*, 397–404. [CrossRef] [PubMed]

91. Borgiani, P.; Ciccacci, C.; Forte, V.; Sirianni, E.; Novelli, L.; Bramanti, P.; Novelli, G. Cyp4f2 genetic variant (rs2108622) significantly contributes to warfarin dosing variability in the italian population. *Pharmacogenomics* **2009**, *10*, 261–266. [CrossRef]

92. Eckman, M.H.; Rosand, J.; Greenberg, S.M.; Gage, B.F. Cost-effectiveness of using pharmacogenetic information in warfarin dosing for patients with nonvalvular atrial fibrillation. *Ann. Intern. Med.* **2009**, *150*, 73–83. [CrossRef]

93. Leey, J.A.; McCabe, S.; Koch, J.A.; Miles, T.P. Cost-effectiveness of genotype-guided warfarin therapy for anticoagulation in elderly patients with atrial fibrillation. *Am. J. Geriatr. Pharmacother.* **2009**, *7*, 197–203. [CrossRef]

94. Pink, J.; Pirmohamed, M.; Lane, S.; Hughes, D.A. Cost-effectiveness of pharmacogenetics-guided warfarin therapy vs. Alternative anticoagulation in atrial fibrillation. *Clin. Pharmacol. Ther.* **2014**, *95*, 199–207. [CrossRef]

95. Trailokya, A.; Hiremath, J.S.; Sawhney, J.; Mishra, Y.K.; Kanhere, V.; Srinivasa, R.; Tiwaskar, M. Acenocoumarol: A review of anticoagulant efficacy and safety. *J. Assoc. Physicians India* **2016**, *64*, 88–93.

96. Verde, Z.; Ruiz, J.R.; Santiago, C.; Valle, B.; Bandres, F.; Calvo, E.; Lucia, A.; Gomez Gallego, F. A novel, single algorithm approach to predict acenocoumarol dose based on cyp2c9 and vkorc1 allele variants. *PLoS ONE* **2010**, *5*, e11210. [CrossRef]

97. Rathore, S.S.; Agarwal, S.K.; Pande, S.; Singh, S.K.; Mittal, T.; Mittal, B. Therapeutic dosing of acenocoumarol: Proposal of a population specific pharmacogenetic dosing algorithm and its validation in north indians. *PLoS ONE* **2012**, *7*, e37844. [CrossRef]

98. Krishna Kumar, D.; Shewade, D.G.; Loriot, M.A.; Beaune, P.; Sai Chandran, B.V.; Balachander, J.; Adithan, C. An acenocoumarol dosing algorithm exploiting clinical and genetic factors in south indian (dravidian) population. *Eur. J. Clin. Pharmacol.* **2015**, *71*, 173–181. [CrossRef]

99. Van Schie, R.M.; Wessels, J.A.; le Cessie, S.; de Boer, A.; Schalekamp, T.; van der Meer, F.J.; Verhoef, T.I.; van Meegen, E.; Rosendaal, F.R.; Maitland-van der Zee, A.H.; et al. Loading and maintenance dose algorithms for phenprocoumon and acenocoumarol using patient characteristics and pharmacogenetic data. *Eur. Heart J.* **2011**, *32*, 1909–1917. [CrossRef]

100. Borobia, A.M.; Lubomirov, R.; Ramirez, E.; Lorenzo, A.; Campos, A.; Munoz-Romo, R.; Fernandez-Capitan, C.; Frias, J.; Carcas, A.J. An acenocoumarol dosing algorithm using clinical and pharmacogenetic data in spanish patients with thromboembolic disease. *PLoS ONE* **2012**, *7*, e41360. [CrossRef]

101. Cerezo-Manchado, J.J.; Rosafalco, M.; Anton, A.I.; Perez-Andreu, V.; Garcia-Barbera, N.; Martinez, A.B.; Corral, J.; Vicente, V.; Gonzalez-Conejero, R.; Roldan, V. Creating a genotype-based dosing algorithm for acenocoumarol steady dose. *Thromb. Haemost.* **2013**, *109*, 146–153. [CrossRef]

102. Tong, H.Y.; Davila-Fajardo, C.L.; Borobia, A.M.; Martinez-Gonzalez, L.J.; Lubomirov, R.; Perea Leon, L.M.; Blanco Banares, M.J.; Diaz-Villamarin, X.; Fernandez-Capitan, C.; Cabeza Barrera, J.; et al. A new pharmacogenetic algorithm to predict the most appropriate dosage of acenocoumarol for stable anticoagulation in a mixed spanish population. *PLoS ONE* **2016**, *11*, e0150456. [CrossRef]

103. Baranova, E.V.; Verhoef, T.I.; Ragia, G.; le Cessie, S.; Asselbergs, F.W.; de Boer, A.; Manolopoulos, V.G.; Maitland-van der Zee, A.H.; EU-PACT group. Dosing algorithms for vitamin k antagonists across vkorc1 and cyp2c9 genotypes. *J. Thromb. Haemost.* **2017**, *15*, 465–472. [CrossRef]

104. Danese, E.; Raimondi, S.; Montagnana, M.; Tagetti, A.; Langaee, T.; Borgiani, P.; Ciccacci, C.; Carcas, A.J.; Borobia, A.M.; Tong, H.Y.; et al. The effect of CYP4F2, VKORC1 and CYP2C9 in influencing coumarin dose. A single patient data meta-analysis in more than 15,000 individuals. *Clin. Pharmacol. Ther.* **2018**. [CrossRef]

105. Wilke, R.A.; Lin, D.W.; Roden, D.M.; Watkins, P.B.; Flockhart, D.; Zineh, I.; Giacomini, K.M.; Krauss, R.M. Identifying genetic risk factors for serious adverse drug reactions: Current progress and challenges. *Nat. Rev. Drug Discov.* **2007**, *6*, 904–916. [CrossRef]

106. Group, S.S.C.; Bowman, L.; Armitage, J.; Bulbulia, R.; Parish, S.; Collins, R. Study of the effectiveness of additional reductions in cholesterol and homocysteine (search): Characteristics of a randomized trial among 12064 myocardial infarction survivors. *Am. Heart J.* **2007**, *154*, 815–823, 823.e1–823.e6.
107. Ramsey, L.B.; Johnson, S.G.; Caudle, K.E.; Haidar, C.E.; Voora, D.; Wilke, R.A.; Maxwell, W.D.; McLeod, H.L.; Krauss, R.M.; Roden, D.M.; et al. The clinical pharmacogenetics implementation consortium guideline for slco1b1 and simvastatin-induced myopathy: 2014 update. *Clin. Pharmacol. Ther.* **2014**, *96*, 423–428. [CrossRef]
108. Tsamandouras, N.; Dickinson, G.; Guo, Y.; Hall, S.; Rostami-Hodjegan, A.; Galetin, A.; Aarons, L. Development and application of a mechanistic pharmacokinetic model for simvastatin and its active metabolite simvastatin acid using an integrated population pbpk approach. *Pharm. Res.* **2015**, *32*, 1864–1883. [CrossRef]
109. Pasanen, M.K.; Neuvonen, M.; Neuvonen, P.J.; Niemi, M. Slco1b1 polymorphism markedly affects the pharmacokinetics of simvastatin acid. *Pharmacogenet. Genomics* **2006**, *16*, 873–879. [CrossRef]
110. Group, S.C.; Link, E.; Parish, S.; Armitage, J.; Bowman, L.; Heath, S.; Matsuda, F.; Gut, I.; Lathrop, M.; Collins, R. Slco1b1 variants and statin-induced myopathy—A genomewide study. *N. Engl. J. Med.* **2008**, *359*, 789–799.
111. Voora, D.; Shah, S.H.; Spasojevic, I.; Ali, S.; Reed, C.R.; Salisbury, B.A.; Ginsburg, G.S. The slco1b1*5 genetic variant is associated with statin-induced side effects. *J. Am. Coll. Cardiol.* **2009**, *54*, 1609–1616. [CrossRef]
112. Brunham, L.R.; Lansberg, P.J.; Zhang, L.; Miao, F.; Carter, C.; Hovingh, G.K.; Visscher, H.; Jukema, J.W.; Stalenhoef, A.F.; Ross, C.J.; et al. Differential effect of the rs4149056 variant in slco1b1 on myopathy associated with simvastatin and atorvastatin. *Pharmacogenomics J.* **2012**, *12*, 233–237. [CrossRef]
113. EMA: Guideline on the Use of Pharmacogenetic Methodologies in the Pharmacokinetic Evaluation of Medical Products. Available online: https://www.ema.europa.eu/en/use-pharmacogenetic-methodologies-pharmacokinetic-evaluation-medicinal-products (accessed on 2 February 2012).
114. Bergmeijer, T.O.; ten Berg, J.M. Value of CYP2C19 *2 and *17 genotyping in clinical practice. Promising but not ready yet. *Rev. Esp. Cardiol. (Engl. Ed.)* **2012**, *65*, 205–207. [CrossRef]
115. Higgins, J.P.; Thompson, S.G.; Deeks, J.J.; Altman, D.G. Measuring inconsistency in meta-analyses. *BMJ* **2003**, *327*, 557–560. [CrossRef]
116. Koller, E.A.; Roche, J.C.; Rollins, J.A. Genotype-guided dosing of vitamin k antagonists. *N. Engl. J. Med.* **2014**, *370*, 1761.
117. Kirchheiner, J.; Ufer, M.; Walter, E.C.; Kammerer, B.; Kahlich, R.; Meisel, C.; Schwab, M.; Gleiter, C.H.; Rane, A.; Roots, I.; et al. Effects of CYP2C9 polymorphisms on the pharmacokinetics of r- and s-phenprocoumon in healthy volunteers. *Pharmacogenetics* **2004**, *14*, 19–26. [CrossRef]

12

Quantifying Risk Pathway Crosstalk Mediated by miRNA to Screen Precision drugs for Breast Cancer Patients

Yingqi Xu [1], Shuting Lin [1], Hongying Zhao [1], Jingwen Wang [1], Chunlong Zhang [1], Qun Dong [1], Congxue Hu [1], Desi Shang [1], Li Wang [1] and Yanjun Xu [1,*]

College of Bioinformatics Science and Technology, Harbin Medical University, Harbin 150081, China
* Correspondence: xuyanjun@hrbmu.edu.cn

Abstract: Breast cancer has become the most common cancer that leads to women's death. Breast cancer is a complex, highly heterogeneous disease classified into various subtypes based on histological features, which determines the therapeutic options. System identification of effective drugs for each subtype remains challenging. In this work, we present a computational network biology approach to screen precision drugs for different breast cancer subtypes by considering the impact intensity of candidate drugs on the pathway crosstalk mediated by miRNAs. Firstly, we constructed and analyzed the subtype-specific risk pathway crosstalk networks mediated by miRNAs. Then, we evaluated 36 Food and Drug Administration (FDA)-approved anticancer drugs by quantifying their effects on these subtype-specific pathway crosstalk networks and combining with survival analysis. Finally, some first-line treatments of breast cancer, such as Paclitaxel and Vincristine, were optimized for each subtype. In particular, we performed precision screening of subtype-specific therapeutic drugs and also confirmed some novel drugs suitable for breast cancer treatment. For example, Sorafenib was applicable for the basal subtype treatment, Irinotecan was optimum for Her2 subtype treatment, Vemurafenib was suitable for the LumA subtype treatment, and Vorinostat could apply to LumB subtype treatment. In addition, the mechanism of these optimal therapeutic drugs in each subtype of breast cancer was further dissected. In summary, our study offers an effective way to screen precision drugs for various breast cancer subtype treatments. We also dissected the mechanism of optimal therapeutic drugs, which may provide novel insight into the precise treatment of cancer and promote researches on the mechanisms of action of drugs.

Keywords: breast cancer subtype; miRNA; pathway; crosstalk network; precision drugs

---

1. Introduction

Breast cancer is the most common cancer type that leads to women's death, especially in China. The high heterogeneity of breast cancer makes it a great challenge to adopt therapeutic options [1], because a heterogeneous group of diseases may exhibit distinct features in terms of histological, prognostic, and clinical outcomes [2]. At present, breast cancer can mainly be classified into four primary subtypes, including her2-enriched, luminal A, luminal B, and basal-like [3,4], distinguished by the expression of some signature genes such as the estrogen receptor (ER), progesterone receptor (PR), and HER2. Different subtypes have distinct biological behaviors and prognosis, and also exhibit various responses to drug therapy [5,6]. Thus, further research on the biological heterogeneity of each subtype of breast cancer will be an effective way to improve the therapeutic efficacy and prognosis of breast cancer [7].

The oncogenesis processes may result from the dysregulations of a series of important biological pathways [8]. Some studies have shown that the pathway crosstalk exists extensively in the processes of development and cell fate [9–11]. Cancer cells have been found to be able to establish alternative signaling pathways through crosstalk to adapt to drug treatment. In addition, crosstalk can also promote cancer therapy by inhibiting the main oncogenic pathways. The inhibition of functional redundancy and pathway crosstalk that promotes the survival of cancer cells can prevent the resistance in tumor treatment [12]. Therefore, it is essential to dissect the crosstalk of dysfunctional pathways and further capture the key molecules that mediate this functional crosstalk in breast cancer.

MicroRNAs are endogenous, non-coding RNA molecules that have been widely regarded as important post-transcriptional regulators by damping the expression level of their target genes. In recent years, studies have indicated that miRNAs are important component elements of biological pathways [13]. They regulate the function of biological pathways through target genes, and then work together with them to disrupt the pathways of diseases. According to estimates, many microRNAs play vital roles by regulating processes that are implicated with the development of cancer [14], such as proliferation, apoptosis, cell cycle, angiogenesis, etc. Some studies suggest that the crosstalk between miRNAs and the Wnt pathway may impact oncogenesis, cancer metastasis, and even drug-resistance processes [15]. Furthermore, miRNAs can also mediate the functional crosstalk of pathways related with oncogenic processes by targeting their shared or interacted genes, thus promoting the initiation and progression of tumors.

In recent years, miRNAs have shown great promise to serve as a target for drug therapy of cancer. More importantly, some studies have nominated miRNA-based therapy as a promising strategy for the treatment of breast cancer [16]. Some evidence demonstrates that drugs could modulate the expression of miRNAs in various diseases as well. For example, an experiment has validated that simvastatin could lead to cell death of breast cancer by up-regulating miR-140-5p [17]. Triiodothyronine has been demonstrated to modulate miR-204 and thus facilitate the proliferation process in breast cancer [18]. Especially, Shenoda et al. have also demonstrated that miRNA could mediate the expression of genes related with drug metabolism [19]. Furthermore, Liu et al. have established a database SM2miR [20], which provides a comprehensive resource about the influences of drugs on miRNA expression and offers unprecedented opportunities for researchers on the screening and action mechanism of drugs for disease treatment. In addition, our previous research also displays that miRNA participates in the crosstalk among pathways that play important roles in cancer development [21], indicating that it might be more effective for screening cancer treatment to evaluate the effects of drugs on the miRNA-mediated crosstalk between pathways.

In order to match the best treatment for breast cancer, in the present study, we firstly integrated the disease high-throughput molecular profiles, miRNA regulation data, and pathway and drug data to construct and analyze the miRNA-mediated pathway crosstalk network for various breast cancer subtypes. Then, we derived a novel computational method to screen precision drugs for different breast cancer subtypes by quantifying the impact intensity of candidate drugs on the pathway crosstalk mediated by miRNAs. Finally, survival analysis was combined for further screening and optimization of the drugs for breast cancer treatment (Figure 1). In summary, our study proposes an effective method to screen precision drugs for various breast cancer subtype treatments. We also dissected the mechanism of optimal therapeutic drugs, which may promote the shift from inexact medicine to precision life science.

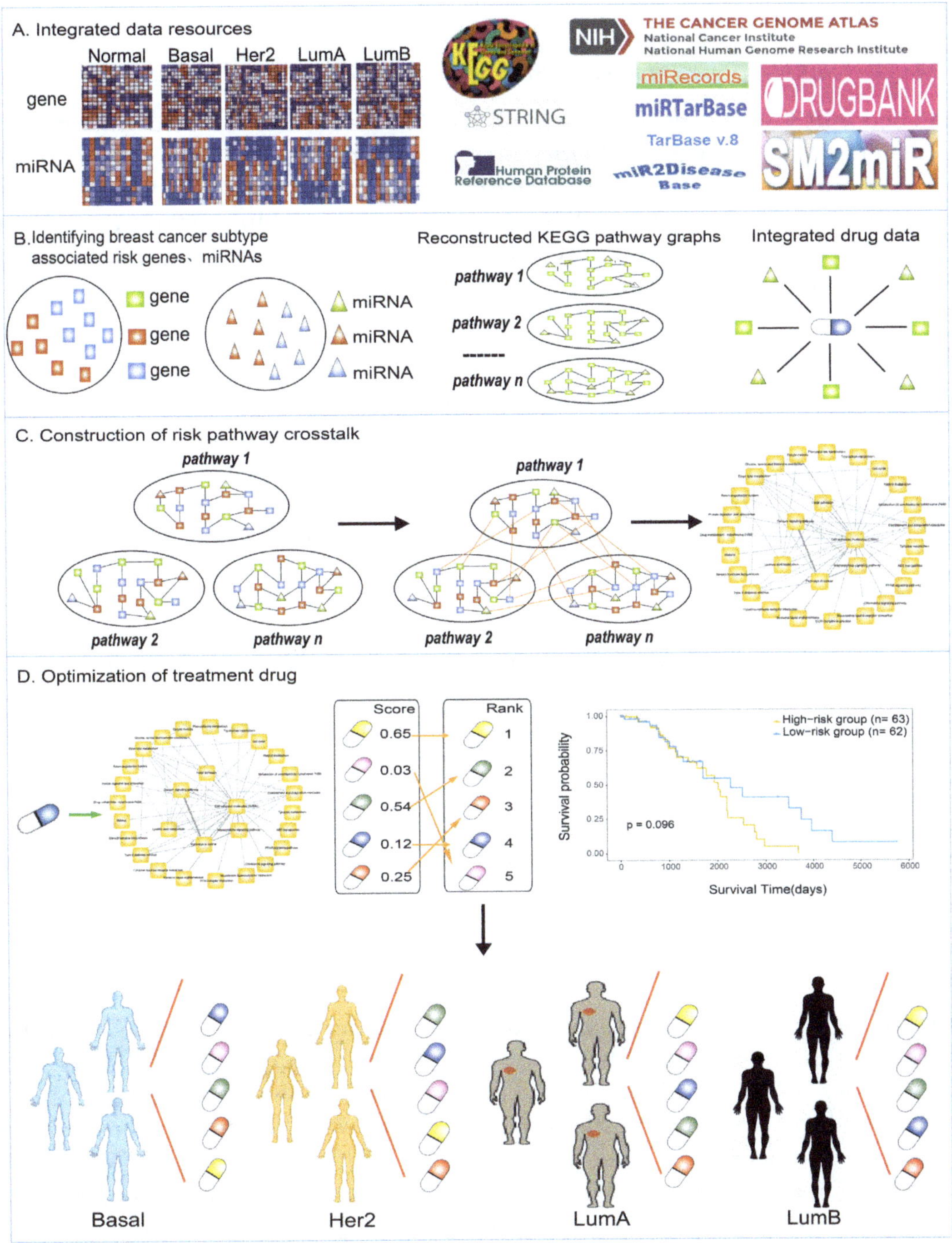

Figure 1. The workflow of optimizing drugs for different subtypes of breast cancer. (**A**) In this work, breast cancer was taken as the research model. Firstly, we integrated related data resources, including gene/miRNA expression profile of each breast cancer subtype and matching patients' survival information, miRNA-target relationship data, PPI network and pathway data, and drug and drug target data. (**B**) We identified the differential genes/miRNAs of each breast cancer subtype, and then reconstructed KEGG pathway based on miRNA-target interactions, which contained both genes and miRNAs. We also screened the target genes and target miRNAs of Food and Drug Administration (FDA)-approved anticancer drugs. (**C**) Identification of breast cancer subtype-associated risk pathways based on the differential genes/miRNAs, and calculated crosstalk for any two interrelated risk pathways. Furthermore we constructed miRNA-mediated specific pathway crosstalk networks in different subtypes of breast cancer, respectively. (**D**) The effectiveness assessment of drugs on dysfunction crosstalk network to screen candidate drugs, combined with survival analysis to optimize drugs for each breast cancer subtype. (See Methods section for details.)

2. Material and Methods

2.1. Sample Matched miRNA/Gene Expression Profiles and Clinical Data

The matched miRNA and gene expression data of breast cancer were downloaded from TCGA (The Cancer Genome Atlas) database (http://tcga-data.nci.nih.gov/), including 553 human breast cancer samples and 87 normal samples. These breast cancer samples were divided into four subtypes, including basal-like (n= 97), Her2 (n = 47), luminal A (n = 291) and luminal B (n = 118) according to the guidelines in Cirielloet et al. [22]. All selected expression datasets were log2-transformed, then standardized. Furthermore, clinical survival data of these samples in each subtype were also obtained.

2.1.1. miRNA-Target Relationship Data

In this study, we collected experimentally verified miRNA-target interactions data from four well-known data resources: miRTarBase [23], mir2Disease [24], miRecords (V4.0) [25], and TarBase (V6.0) [26]. MiRNA-target relationships in homo species were extracted and combined together to obtain a more comprehensive dataset. In total, 57,863 miRNA-target relationships involving 579 miRNAs and 14,652 target genes were collected and used for further analysis.

2.1.2. PPI Network and Pathway Data

The protein–protein interaction (PPI) network data used in this study were integrated from two databases, HPRD (Human Protein Reference Database) and STRING (Search Tool for the Retrieval of Interacting Genes/Proteins) [27,28]. The interactions stored in HPRD were mainly from experimental validation and text mining. For each recorded entry in the STRING database, a weighted score was given to measure their confidence of interaction by considering multiple factors. To collect high-quality interaction data, we only extracted interactions with a confidence score ≥900. Then, we combined interactions from the HPRD and STRING databases. The pathway data used in this study for functional analysis were obtained from the KEGG (Kyoto Encyclopedia of Genes and Genomes) database [29].

2.1.3. Drug and Drug Target Data

In this study, according to our research purpose, in order to improve the practicability of our study, the candidate drugs need to satisfy two requirements simultaneously. Firstly, existing gene targets and regulatory effects on miRNA have to be confirmed. Secondly, the drugs have to have been approved by US Food and Drug Administration (FDA, https://www.fda.gov/), which are prescribed for cancer treatment. We extracted drugs and drug targets from DrugBank [30] and SM2miR [20]. Finally, a total of 36 anticancer drugs were used in this study. The complete information of the 36 anticancer drugs can be found in Supplementary Table S1, including drug ID and drug targets.

2.2. Reconstructed KEGG Pathway Graphs

The reconstructed KEGG (Kyoto Encyclopedia of Genes and Genomes) pathway graphs contained both genes and miRNAs, replicating real biological pathways. We firstly collected 220 KEGG pathway data and converted them into undirected graphs with genes as nodes and their interactions as edges by using our previously developed R package "iSubpathway Miner" [31]. Then, we reconstructed these pathways by wiring miRNAs into these pathways through integrating miRNA-target relations and pathway data. More details, if target genes of a specific miRNA were over-represented within a pathway, the miRNA was wired into the pathway by connecting with target genes within the pathway. The hypergeometric test was used to evaluate the significance of enrichment. The formulas is as follows:

$$P = 1 - \sum_{t=0}^{q-1} \frac{\binom{l}{t}\binom{n-l}{m-t}}{\binom{n}{m}}$$

where n represents the number of background genes (all genome-wide genes), m is the number of genes involved in a given pathway, l is the number of target genes for a specific miRNA, and q is the number of miRNA target genes annotated in the given pathway.

2.3. Identification of Risk Genes and miRNAs Related to Breast Cancer Subtypes

For each breast cancer subtype, we identified significant differentially expressed genes/miRNAs by comparing the tumor with normal samples in each subtype. The unpaired Student's t-test and fold-change methods were simultaneously used to evaluate differentially expressed genes/miRNAs. Then, the significance p-values from the t-test were calibrated by Benjamini-Hochberg multiple tests to obtain the false discovery rate (FDR) values. Finally, we applied $p < 0.01$ and $|\log_2 \text{FC}| > 2$ as thresholds to identify differentially expressed genes/miRNAs. These significant differentially expressed genes/miRNAs were regarded as breast cancer subtype-associated genes, which were also defined by us as risk genes and miRNAs, respectively.

2.4. Mining Risk Pathways Associated with Breast Cancer Subtypes

In order to explore the roles of these risk genes and miRNAs in the occurrence and development of breast cancer, we performed them to conduct pathway enrichment analysis to dig out the pathways closely related to breast cancer. We identified pathways with significant enrichment results as risk pathways for each subtype based on risk genes and miRNAs. The cumulative hypergeometric test was used to calculate the significance of each pathway that enriched by risk genes and miRNAs. The formula of the cumulative hypergeometric test is as follows:

$$P = 1 - \sum_{k=0}^{m} \frac{\binom{n}{k}\binom{N-n}{M-k}}{\binom{N}{M}}$$

where N represents the number of background genes (all genome-wide genes), M is the number of a given pathway's genes and miRNAs that are annotated in the N genes, n is total number of the risk genes and miRNAs of a given subtype of breast cancer, and m is the number of risk genes and miRNAs in the given pathway.

2.5. Establishing the Risk Pathways' Crosstalk of Breast Cancer

In each breast cancer subtype, we calculated the crosstalk of each pair of risk pathways based on the correlation strength of genes and miRNAs between them according to previous studies [21]. The Pearson's product moment correlation coefficient and unpaired Student's t-test were performed to measure correlation strength for any two interrelated pathways. As for genes and miRNAs presenting both in pathway i and j, we reckoned their correlation strength only if they interact with other genes or miRNAs in the PPI network. Then, we used correlation strength to construct and assess risk pathways' crosstalk. The formula of calculating correlation strength is as follows:

$$CS(i,j) = F\big(P(i), P(j)\big|Exp_i, Exp_j\big) = -2 * (log_e P(i) + log_e P(j) + log_e P(i,j))$$

where i is the gene that is annotated in pathway a is the gene that is annotated in pathway b; Exp_i and Exp_j are the expression values of genes i and j in samples, respectively; $P(i)$ and $P(j)$ are the differential significance p-values of genes i and j calculated using the unpaired Student's t-test, respectively; and $P(i, j)$ is the significant p-value of expression correlation coefficient between a and b genes/miRNAs based on the Pearson's product moment correlation coefficient.

The crosstalk of any pair of risk pathways was gained by adding up all the correlation strengths between them, and crosstalk of risk pathways i and j was developed based on formula as follows:

$$Crosstalk_{(a,b)} = \sum_{a}^{n} CS$$

where n presents the number of all gene–gene, gene–miRNA, and miRNA–miRNA interactions between any two pathways.

In order to strengthen the differences of risk pathways in different subtypes, we constructed specific dysfunctional crosstalk networks based on the specific crosstalk relationship in each subtype for subsequent calculation and research, which means that when a pair of crosstalk pathways only exist in a certain subtype, they will be selected to construct the subtype crosstalk network.

2.6. Evaluating the Impacts of Drugs on Crosstalk

We integrated the drug information from the DrugBank and SM2miR databases and screened them for Food and Drug Administration (FDA)-approved anticancer drugs that contain both target genes and target miRNAs, and a total of 36 anticancer drugs were screened. Research has shown that the crosstalk among the signaling pathways plays a key role in the occurrence and development of breast cancer. Thus, evaluating the impact of drugs on pathway crosstalk based on the expression of drug targets could help to optimize the treatment of various subtypes of breast cancer. From this standpoint, in order to assess the impacts of drug on dysfunction crosstalk network, for each drug, we first removed its target genes and miRNAs from the specific risk pathway crosstalk of a given subtype. Next, we recalculated the crosstalk to quantify the destructive effects of drugs on different subtypes. At the same time, a formula was designed and developed. The destructive score (DS) of drug to crosstalk was gained using the following formula:

$$DS(d) = \frac{\sum_{i}^{k} \left| 1 - \frac{Crosstalk_d}{Crosstalk} \right|}{k}$$

where $Crosstalk_d$ is the crosstalk after drug action, and k presents the number of all specific crosstalks in the subtype.

We determined the destructive score (DS) of all anticancer drugs to specific crosstalk networks in each subtype to assess the impacts of drugs on pathway crosstalk of the drugs. A higher DS score indicates the greater effects of the drug on crosstalk between risk pathways. In each subtype, we only screened anticancer drugs that could impact the crosstalk between dysregulated pathways (DS score greater than zero) as candidate drugs, and we ranked candidate drugs of each subtype by DS score from high to low in various subtypes of breast cancer.

2.7. Survival Analysis

We performed survival analysis based on the targets of candidate drugs that were implicated in the specific pathway crosstalk of each subtypes of breast cancer to evaluate the effects for patient survival of candidate drugs. For a given drug, we extracted its target genes and miRNAs that target a specific crosstalk network as drug target signatures. Each candidate drug target signature was performed for survival analysis in patients of each subtype separately, and we used the K-mean clustering method to stratify patients into shorter survival time and longer survival time groups based on the level of these drug target molecules' expression. In this project, we used 100 as the maximum number of iterations of k means algorithm, and randomly started k means algorithm 20 times to return the best result. Then Kaplan–Meier estimate method was used to evaluate the survival difference of these two classified groups in each subtype, respectively. Finally, the significance p-value of survival difference was estimated using the log-rank test.

3. Results

3.1. Identifying Breast Cancer Subtype-Associated Risk Pathways

We identified the risk miRNAs and genes by comparing tumor samples in each subtype with normal controls, respectively. The differentially expressed genes and miRNAs were detected using t-test and fold-change methods, and then multiple testing correction by the Benjamini–Hochberg procedure was used. Genes/miRNAs with adjusted p-values < 0.01and |log_2 FC| > 2 were identified as differential expression (risk genes/miRNAs). In total, we obtained 4096 risk genes (2284 from basal-like subtype, 2192 from her2-enriched subtype, 1831 from luminal A subtype, and 2487 from luminal B subtype) and 223 risk miRNAs (148 from basal-like subtype, 72 from her2-enriched subtype, 76 from luminal A subtype, and 116 from luminal B subtype). Unsupervised hierarchical clustering analysis was performed to observe discrepancy of the expression of risk genes and miRNAs between case samples and normal samples, as shown in Figure 2A. We also performed the degree of overlap of risk genes and miRNAs between subtypes, displayed in Figure 2B. These results indicate that genes and miRNAs exhibit widespread expression disorder in the various breast cancer subtypes.

Breast cancer is affected by multiple factors and pathways. In order to veritably and accurately reflect the changes of the pathways of breast cancer, we used the methods that we developed previously to reconstruct all biological pathways among KEGG, and miRNAs were added into the signaling pathway to form a more abundant signaling pathway. To discover the biological function of these risk genes and miRNAs, we used pathway enrichment analysis to identify risk pathways in each subtype. A pathway is identified as a risk pathway only if risk genes and miRNAs are enriched in it under the significance level $p < 0.05$. In total, there were 32 risk pathways in basal-like subtype, 29 risk pathways in her2-enriched subtype, 21 risk pathways in luminal A subtype, and 26 risk pathways in luminal B subtype. We show the top ten pathways of each breast cancer subtype in Figure 2C. We found that some risk pathways such as the Chemokine signaling pathway, ECM–receptor interaction, the PPAR signaling pathway, and Tyrosine metabolism were simultaneously identified in different breast cancer subtypes. Furthermore, we found some subtype-specific risk pathways in each subtype of breast cancer. Amoebiasis, drug metabolism–other enzymes, fatty acid metabolism, the p53 signaling pathway, and salivary secretion were found in basal-like, cell adhesion molecules (CAMs) in her2-enriched, histidine metabolism in Luminal A, and glycerolipid metabolism and TGF-beta signaling pathway in Luminal B subtypes. These subtype-specific risk pathways may be one of the reasons that resulted in distinct molecular mechanisms and clinical outcomes of breast cancer subtypes.

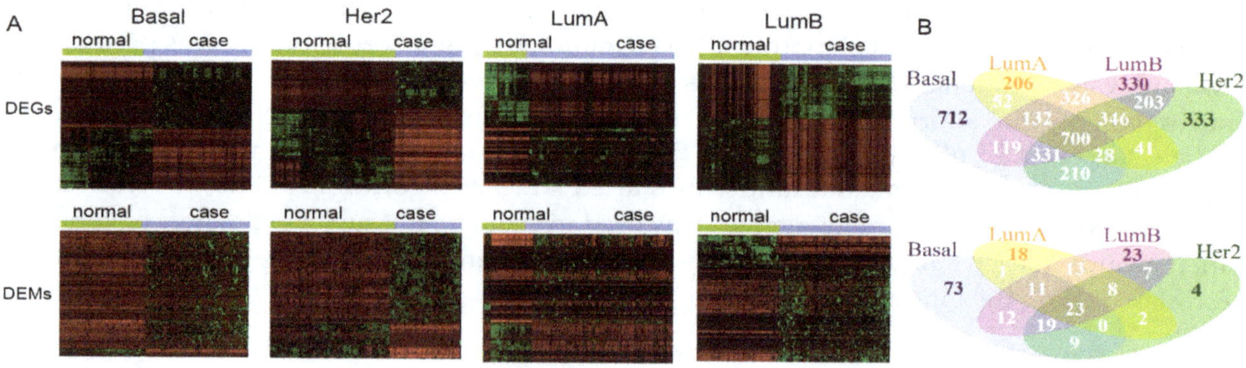

C

Basal		
Pathway ID	Pathway Name	P value
path:04080	Neuroactive ligand-receptor interaction	1.29E-13
path:05322	Systemic lupus erythematosus	2.49E-11
path:04060	Cytokine-cytokine receptor interaction	1.76E-06
path:00830	Retinol metabolism	1.35E-05
path:04110	Cell cycle	5.07E-05
path:04114	Oocyte meiosis	7.82E-05
path:03320	PPAR signaling pathway	0.00021066
path:04974	Protein digestion and absorption	0.00024571
path:02010	ABC transporters	0.00027692
path:00350	Tyrosine metabolism	0.00040658

Her2		
Pathway ID	Pathway Name	P value
path:05322	Systemic lupus erythematosus	1.59E-12
path:04080	Neuroactive ligand-receptor interaction	2.52E-12
path:00350	Tyrosine metabolism	2.89E-06
path:04512	ECM-receptor interaction	2.70E-05
path:00360	Phenylalanine metabolism	3.12E-05
path:03320	PPAR signaling pathway	6.72E-05
path:00830	Retinol metabolism	0.00016989
path:04610	Complement and coagulation cascades	0.00076731
path:04114	Oocyte meiosis	0.00094046
path:04060	Cytokine-cytokine receptor interaction	0.00106473

LumA		
Pathway ID	Pathway Name	P value
path:04080	Neuroactive ligand-receptor interaction	3.67E-09
path:05322	Systemic lupus erythematosus	9.65E-07
path:00830	Retinol metabolism	4.24E-06
path:03320	PPAR signaling pathway	1.17E-05
path:00980	Metabolism of xenobiotics by cytochrome P450	2.72E-05
path:00982	Drug metabolism - cytochrome P450	0.00010736
path:00350	Tyrosine metabolism	0.00116789
path:00380	Tryptophan metabolism	0.0013381
path:00591	Linoleic acid metabolism	0.00138696
path:04512	ECM-receptor interaction	0.00148693

LumB		
Pathway ID	Pathway Name	P value
path:05322	Systemic lupus erythematosus	3.01E-11
path:04080	Neuroactive ligand-receptor interaction	4.77E-08
path:03320	PPAR signaling pathway	1.33E-06
path:00350	Tyrosine metabolism	0.00027541
path:00360	Phenylalanine metabolism	0.00060702
path:00830	Retinol metabolism	0.00099021
path:04512	ECM-receptor interaction	0.00158489
path:00980	Metabolism of xenobiotics by cytochrome P450	0.0017189
path:04610	Complement and coagulation cascades	0.00176985
path:00140	Steroid hormone biosynthesis	0.00271651

Figure 2. Global view of risk genes and miRNAs in each subtype of breast cancer. (**A**) Heat maps show risk genes and miRNAs in four breast cancer subtypes. Unsupervised hierarchical clustering analysis is used, which divided genes and miRNAs into two clusters, the lower and higher expression values are represented by green and the red colors, respectively. (**B**) Venn plots of risk genes and miRNAs associated with breast cancer subtypes separately. (**C**) Results of top 10 pathways with significant enrichment result of each subtype. Note: Basal, basal-like subtype; Her2, her2-enriched subtype; LumA, luminal A subtype; LumB, luminal B subtype.

3.2. Constructing Risk Pathway Crosstalk Networks for Various Subtypes of Breast Cancer

The occurrence of breast cancer is complex and there is crosstalk between different functional biological pathways in the process of cancer development. Thus, it is necessary to dissect the crosstalk of dysfunctional pathways related to breast cancer. To elucidate the molecular mechanism of various breast cancer subtypes, we analyzed the crosstalk between dysfunctional pathways that are related to breast cancer. In our study, the risk pathway crosstalk networks for each breast cancer subtype were constructed. The quantification of crosstalk was conducted by calculating both the correlation strength and the dysfunction degree of genes and miRNAs in any two risk pathways of each breast cancer subtype, and the expression correlation coefficient between genes and miRNAs and the unpaired Student's t-test of genes and miRNAs were used for assessment of crosstalk.

Our results showed that there were crosstalks with significant differences in the extent of crosstalk between risk pathways in each subtype (Figure 3). For example, 'calcium signaling pathway' and 'focal adhesion' have more crosstalk relationships with other pathways in basal-like subtype. 'Pathways in cancer' and 'focal adhesion' crosstalk more with other pathways in her2-enriched subtype. In luminal A subtype, 'Jak–STAT signaling pathway' has the greatest crosstalk with 'cytokine–cytokine receptor interaction'. In luminal B subtype, 'pathways in cancer' and 'cytokine–cytokine receptor interaction' possess larger crosstalk values with other pathways.

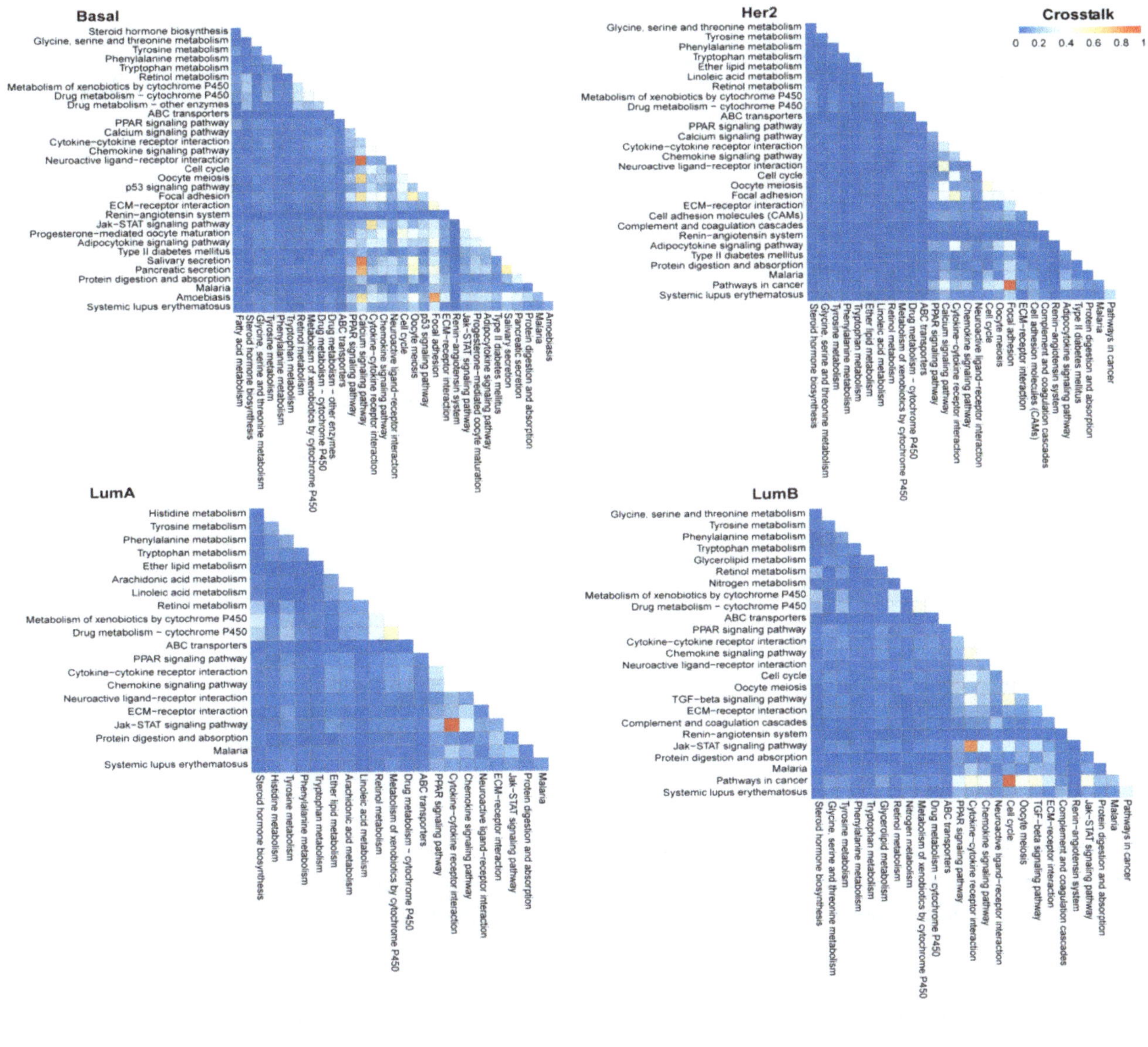

Figure 3. The crosstalk for each two interrelated risk pathways in breast cancer subtypes. Heat maps of crosstalk between risk pathways for comparing the heterogeneity of crosstalk across different subtypes of breast cancer. The color of the box represents the crosstalk between the two pathways, the lower and higher crosstalk are represented by blue and the red colors, respectively.

Moreover, we found some subtype-specific crosstalk of pathways in breast cancer. We extracted the specific crosstalk risk pathways of each subtype and used them to construct the specific crosstalk network of the risk pathway in four subtypes (Figure 4). There are 197 specific crosstalk relationships in basal-like, 56 specific crosstalk relationships in her2-enriched, 41 specific crosstalk relationships in luminal A, and 74 specific crosstalk relationships in luminal B subtypes. The above results indicate that these subtype-specific crosstalks of risk pathways may be one of the molecular mechanisms that lead to distinct clinical outcomes of breast cancer patients, which will help us to understand the discrepancy between subtypes and points a new way to optimize the treatment of breast cancer patients.

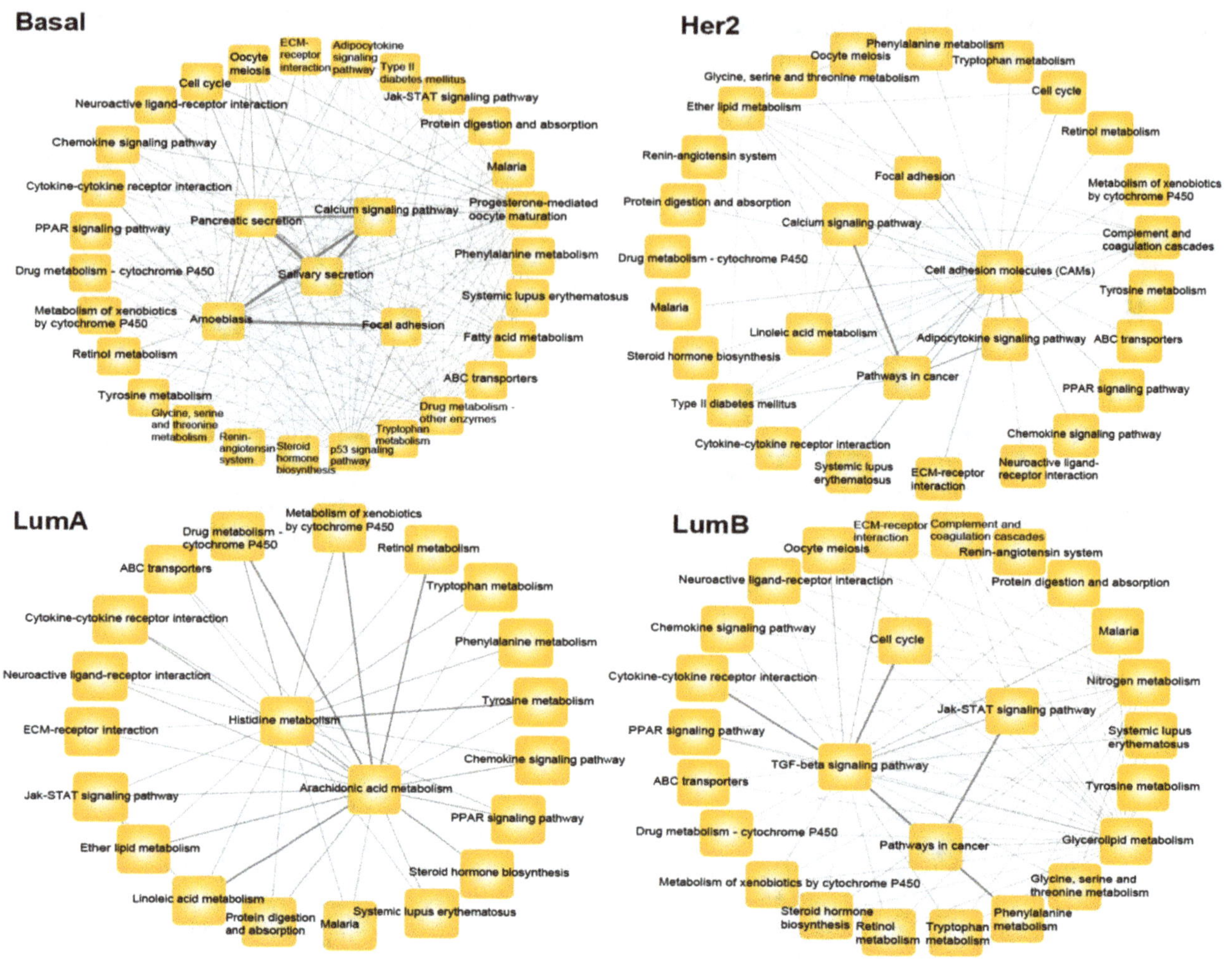

Figure 4. The specific crosstalk network of each breast cancer subtype. The yellow rectangle represents the pathways of the specific crosstalk network. The thickness of edges represents the intensity of crosstalk between pathways; the larger the crosstalk value, the thicker the edge.

3.3. Screening Candidate Therapeutic Drugs for Each Subtype of Breast Cancer Based on DS Score

Previous experimental studies have demonstrated that cancer cells could adapt signaling pathway circuits under drug treatment by establishing alternative signaling routes through crosstalk [32,33]. Based on this point of view, we developed an evaluation method to optimize the therapeutic drugs for each subtype of breast cancer by assessing the impact of drugs on crosstalk among risk pathways. The drug targets of each drug were removed from risk pathways and we reconstructed crosstalk networks targeted by drugs to evaluate the perturbance effects of those drugs. Next, we recalculated the crosstalk to measure the perturbance effects of drugs on different subtypes and optimize the drug use for each subtype of breast cancer. We obtained 36 anticancer drugs that target both genes and miRNAs, and the results of evaluation of anticancer drugs are shown in Table 1. We only screened anticancer drugs of each subtype with a *DS* score greater than zero as candidate drugs, and ranked candidate drugs of each subtype by *DS* score from high to low. A higher DS score indicates the greater effects of the drug on crosstalk between risk pathways. In total, there are 33 drugs in basal-like, 32 drugs in her2-enriched, 22 drugs in luminal A, and 30 drugs in luminal B subtypes.

Table 1. Screened candidate drugs for various subtypes of breast cancer based on *DS* score.

DS Score Ranking	Basal	Her2	LumA	LumB
1	5-Fluorouracil	Arsenic trioxide	Arsenic trioxide	Arsenic trioxide
2	Arsenic trioxide	Adriamycin	5-Fluorouracil	Adriamycin
3	Tamoxifen	5-Fluorouracil	Adriamycin	5-Fluorouracil
4	Trastuzumab	Trastuzumab	Trastuzumab	Trastuzumab
5	Etoposide	Paclitaxel	Etoposide	Etoposide
6	Cisplatin	Temozolomide	Tamoxifen	Cisplatin
7	Paclitaxel	Etoposide	Vorinostat	Topotecan
8	Vorinostat	Gemcitabine	Bicalutamide	Irinotecan
9	Gemcitabine	Everolimus	Cisplatin	Paclitaxel
10	Adriamycin	Sunitinib	Vemurafenib	Tamoxifen
11	Temozolomide	Tamoxifen	Medroxyprogesterone acetate	Vemurafenib
12	Cyclophosphamide	Vorinostat	Gemcitabine	Gemcitabine
13	Bicalutamide	Cisplatin	Temozolomide	Sunitinib
14	Sunitinib	Sorafenib	Everolimus	Vorinostat
15	Vemurafenib	Cyclophosphamide	Sunitinib	Temozolomide
16	Medroxyprogesterone acetate	Goserelin	Paclitaxel	Everolimus
17	Everolimus	Vemurafenib	Oxaliplatin	Lenalidomide
18	Vinblastine	Bicalutamide	Cyclophosphamide	Cyclophosphamide
19	Lenalidomide	Vinblastine	Sorafenib	Bicalutamide
20	Oxaliplatin	Lenalidomide	Irinotecan	Goserelin
21	Sorafenib	Imatinib mesylate	Topotecan	Rapamycin
22	Goserelin	Bortezomib	Lenalidomide	Oxaliplatin
23	Irinotecan	Oxaliplatin		Vinblastine
24	Mitoxantrone	Medroxyprogesterone acetate		Sorafenib
25	Topotecan	Melphalan		Vincristine
26	Imatinib mesylate	Gefitinib		Medroxyprogesterone acetate
27	Vincristine	Rapamycin		Bortezomib
28	Gefitinib	Vincristine		Imatinib mesylate
29	Docetaxel	Irinotecan		Mitoxantrone
30	Bortezomib	Topotecan		Melphalan
31	Melphalan	Mitoxantrone		
32	Rapamycin	Docetaxel		
33	Epirubicin			

3.4. Dissecting the Effects of Candidate Therapeutic Drugs for Patient Survival in Each Subtype of Breast Cancer

A drug could specifically interact with a target molecule to modulate a physiological process and further impact the progression of a disease [34]. In order to further screen drugs for breast cancer patients, we got the patients' clinical survival information in each breast cancer subtype. For each candidate therapeutic drug that was screened based on DS score in different subtypes, we evaluated the drug target signature's influence on patient survival. Patients from each subtype of breast cancer were divided into two groups (shorter survival time group and longer survival time group) based on the expression of drug target signatures. As shown in Figure 5, we found that there were, in total, six candidate therapeutic drugs screened based on DS score (DS score greater than zero) that significantly correlated with overall survival (OS) in the different subtypes of breast cancer patients. Paclitaxel, Vincristine, and Sorafenib in basal-like, Irinotecan in her2-enriched, Vemurafenib in luminal A, and Vorinostat in luminal B subtypes. These six dugs not only impacted the crosstalk of risk pathways, but they also had an effect on the patients' survival in their corresponding subtypes. This indicates that they may be more suitable treatment candidates for the corresponding subtypes of breast cancer. More details, according to drug target signatures of Paclitaxel and Sorafenib in the basal-like subtype, these 97 patients were divided into a shorter survival group (n = 5) and a longer survival group (n = 92), respectively. Vincristine drug target signatures divided 97 patients in the basal-like subtype into a shorter survival group (n = 63) and a longer survival group (n = 55). The 47 patients in the her2-enriched subtype were separated into a shorter survival group (n = 10) and a longer survival group (n = 37) by Irinotecan drug target signatures. Based on the drug target signatures of Vemurafenib in luminal A subtype, the 287 patients (survival information was missing in four patients) were stratified into a shorter survival group (n = 78) and a longer survival group (n = 209), and Vorinostat drug target signatures stratified 118 luminal B subtype patients into a shorter survival group (n = 63) and a longer survival group (n = 55). Here, drugs' signatures stratified the patients into two groups in a statistically significant manner and their expression direction were not considered.

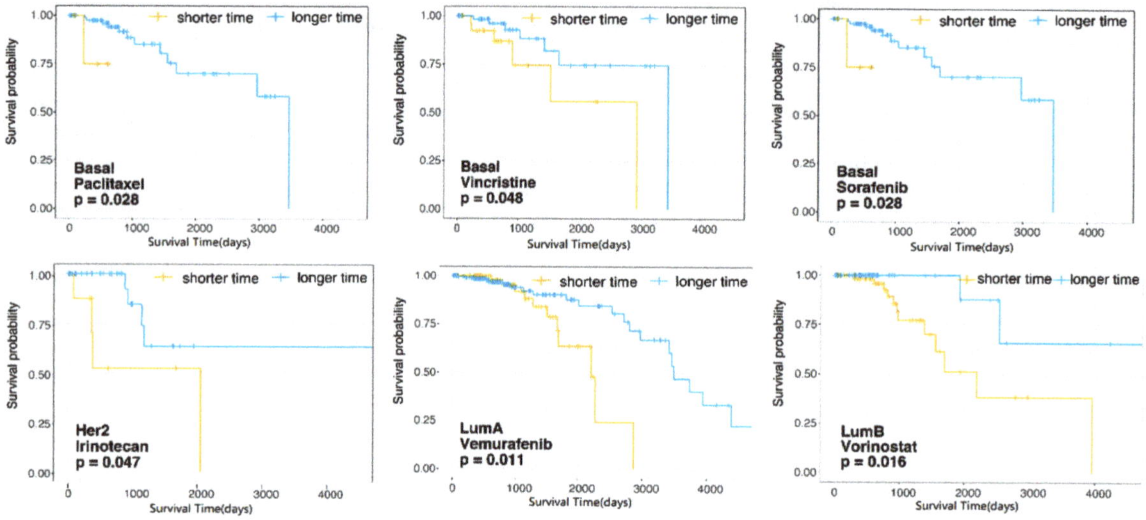

Figure 5. Kaplan-Meier survival curves of patients at shorter survival time group or longer survival time group stratified by drug target signatures of candidate drugs of each breast cancer subtype.

3.5. Dissecting the Mechanism of Candidate Drugs for Each Subtype

In our drugs' optimization results, Paclitaxel, Sorafenib, and Vincristine were found to have potential therapy effect in the basal-like subtype of breast cancer. Consistent with clinical findings, Paclitaxel and Vincristine were the optimal adjuvant therapy for triple-negative breast cancer [35,36]. Sorafenib is a multiple targeted agent which can inhibit tumor cell proliferation and angiogenesis by inhibiting the activation of multiple different kinases [37], and our results indicate that Sorafenib plays a therapeutic role in the basal-like subtype of breast cancer mainly through affecting specific risk pathway crosstalk mediated by hsa-miR-30a, hsa-miR-222, and hsa-miR-193a. Some studies have confirmed that hsa-miR-30a, hsa-miR-222, and hsa-miR-193a play key roles in breast cancer [38–40]. Irinotecan, an antitumor enzyme inhibitor mainly used for the treatment of colorectal cancer [41], is suitable for the her2-enriched subtype, which mediates the specific crosstalk among the risk pathways of the her2-enriched subtype through regulating hsa-miR-23a and hsa-miR-324. In accordance with the result of WT Kuo and Eissa [42,43], hsa-miR-324 and hsa-miR-23a have distinct biological functions in breast cancer. Vemurafenib has long been approved for the treatment of metastatic melanoma with BRAF mutation [44], and our results showed that this drug had a damaging effect on the specific crosstalk of risk pathway of the luminal A subtype through action on hsa-miR-145. Just as some researches have shown that miR-145 is a potential cancer biomarker and serves as a novel target for cancer therapy, including breast cancer [45]. Vorinostat as an anticancer agent that inhibits histone deacetylases, approved for cutaneous T-cell lymphoma [46], and plays a key role in the epigenetic regulation of gene expression. Vorinostat could act on the specific risk pathways crosstalk of the luminal B subtype via 14 miRNAs (Figure 6), which have been found to play important roles in the occurrence and development of breast cancer, such as hsa-miR-155, hsa-miR-34a, hsa-miR-17, hsa-miR-22, and hsa-miR-140 [47–51].

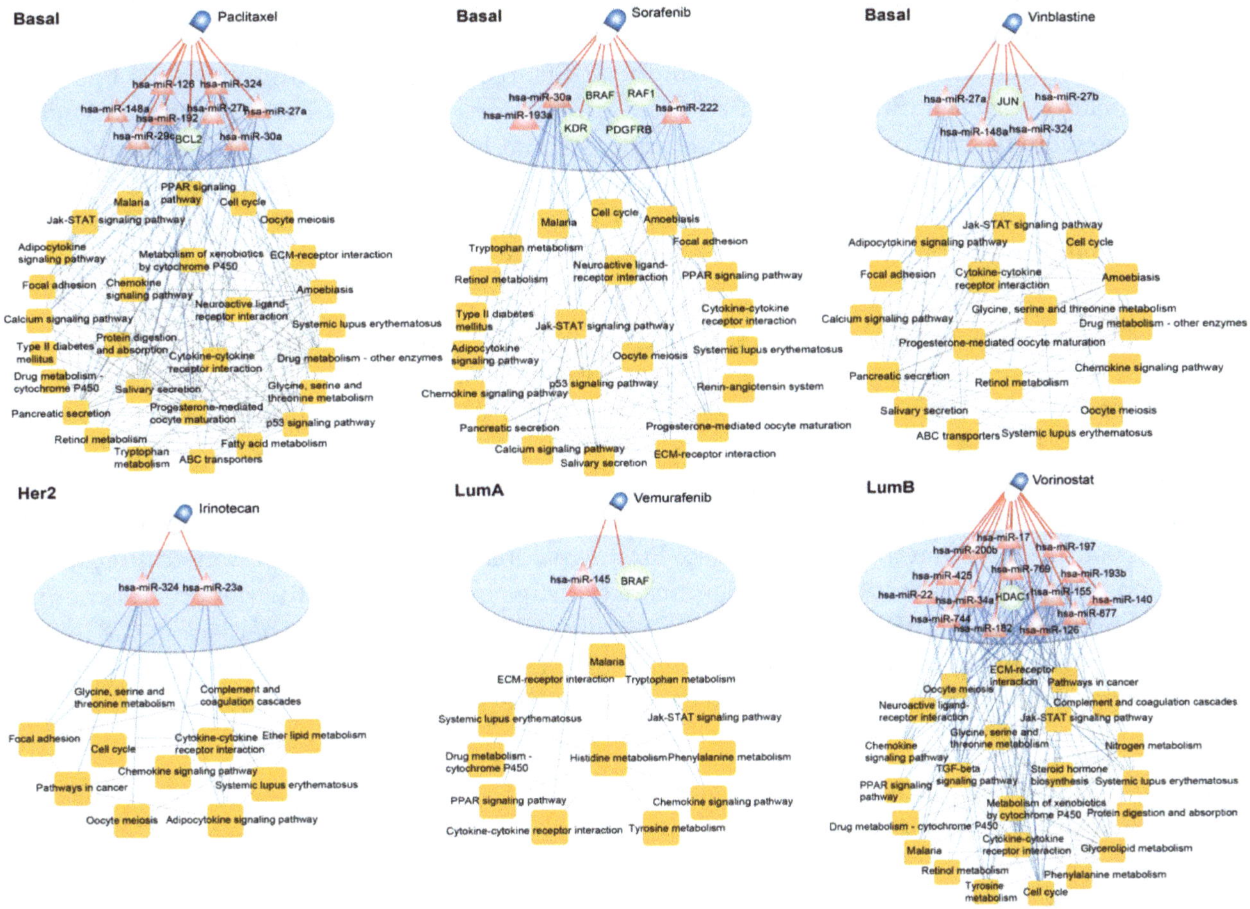

Figure 6. The mechanism of optimal therapeutic drugs in each subtype of breast cancer. Sorafenib, Paclitaxel, and Vincristine were applicable for the basal-like subtype treatment, Irinotecan was optimum for the her2-enriched subtype treatment, Vemurafenib was suitable for the luminal A subtype treatment, and Vorinostat was applied to the luminal B subtype treatment.

4. Discussion

Breast cancer is a complex disease with high heterogeneity in terms of the underlying molecular alterations, the cellular composition of tumors, and even the clinical outcomes. Different subtypes exhibit distinct biological behavior, prognosis, and usually different responses to drug treatment [52], yet identifing applicable drugs for each subtype still largely remains limited. Therefore, it is urgently needed to develop a systematic pipeline to identify medications for different subtypes of breast cancer.

The occurrence and development of tumors is a complex process involving many steps, links, and factors. It is mostly the action of a single molecule (gene or miRNA) that leads to poor therapeutic effect among many chemotherapeutic regimens [53]. In recent years, many researches have revealed that the occurrence of tumors is closely related to the abnormality of biological pathways, and crosstalk of abnormal pathways is one of the prime reasons for the poor outcomes of tumor treatment [54]. Studies have shown that regulatory molecules such as non-coding RNA participate in the anomaly of biological pathways through the regulation of genes, adding to the difficulty of cancer treatment [55]. In order to actually reflect the intricate crosstalk of pathways, we have developed a new method based on biological pathways—that is, reconstruction of biological pathways which include both genes and miRNAs. We have also identified the optimal drugs by quantifying the effect of candidate drugs on miRNA-mediated crosstalk of pathways. We have successfully identified the specific crosstalk of pathways in each subtype of breast cancer and revealed their pathogenesis respectively by applying this method. Moreover, we also screened applicable drugs for each subtype of breast cancer. We successfully screened the most suitable drugs for each subtype of breast cancer, including Paclitaxel and Vincristine, which are breast cancer treatment drugs in clinical application. On the basis of the original application, we accurately identified their applications in each subtype, such that Paclitaxel and Vincristine were best for basal-like, Irinotecan was suitable for her2-enriched, and Vorinostat was the optimal drug for luminal B subtypes. We also identified other anticancer drugs application in each subtypes of breast cancer. The results show that our approach could help doctors to further improve treatment strategies with the current menu of chemotherapy options.

Currently, several methods have been proposed to optimize drugs for human cancers. For example, Lamb et al. provided a computational method to connect diseases and their potential therapeutic small molecules based on gene expression profiles form disease and cultured human cells treated with bioactive small molecules respectively [56]. Gottlieb et al. predicted novel drug indications based on multiple drug–drug and disease–disease similarity measures [57]. Furthermore, Malas et al. prioritized drugs using the semantic information between drug and disease concepts [58]. Comparing with these methods, our study has some unique features. First, we considered the role of non-coding RNAs in our approach. Second, our study optimized anticancer drugs by measuring their effects for mediating the crosstalk between risk pathways, which was an important molecular mechanism in the initiation and progression of human cancers. Finally, we optimized candidate drugs for different breast cancer subtypes, which may further promote the precise use of drugs for human cancer.

There are also several limitations in our study. First of all, drugs targeting miRNAs for therapeutic purposes are limited, and there are many drugs without miRNA targets. Secondly, miRNAs affected by the drugs are required for further study. We believe that more and more drugs that regulate miRNAs and drug-regulated miRNAs will be discovered with the development of in-depth study on the interaction of drugs and miRNAs, and our method can identify the optimal therapeutic agent for complex diseases more accurately and comprehensively. In summary, the results in this study highlight that dissecting subtype-specific risk pathway crosstalk could provide novel insights into the underlying molecular mechanisms and thus promote the drug discovery for various breast cancer subtype. Moreover, we focused on breast cancer in this study, but the method proposed here could also be applied to many other complex diseases, as pathway crosstalk is widespread in biological systems and the dysregulation of which play a critical role in the occurrence of disease.

Author Contributions: Conceptualization, Y.X. and Y.X.; data curation, J.W. and C.Z.; formal analysis, Y.X., H.Z., and C.H.; investigation, S.L., H.Z., and J.W.; methodology, Y.X.; supervision, Y.X. and L.W.; validation, H.Z. and Q.W.; visualization, S.L. and C.H.; writing—original draft, Y.X. and S.L; writing—review and editing, C.Z., Q.D., D.S., Y.X., and L.W.

Acknowledgments: Not applicable.

References

1. Holm, J.; Eriksson, L.; Ploner, A.; Eriksson, M.; Rantalainen, M.; Li, J.; Hall, P.; Czene, K. Assessment of breast cancer risk factors reveals subtype heterogeneity. *Cancer Res.* **2017**, *77*, 3708–3717. [CrossRef] [PubMed]
2. Zardavas, D.; Irrthum, A.; Swanton, C.; Piccart, M. Clinical management of breast cancer heterogeneity. *Nat. Rev. Clin. Oncol.* **2015**, *12*, 381–394. [CrossRef] [PubMed]

3. Goldhirsch, A.; Wood, W.C.; Coates, A.S.; Gelber, R.D.; Thurlimann, B.; Senn, H.J.; Panel Members. Strategies for subtypes—Dealing with the diversity of breast cancer: Highlights of the st. Gallen international expert consensus on the primary therapy of early breast cancer 2011. *Ann. Oncol. Off. J. Eur. Soc. Med. Oncol.* **2011**, *22*, 1736–1747. [CrossRef] [PubMed]
4. Onitilo, A.A.; Engel, J.M.; Greenlee, R.T.; Mukesh, B.N. Breast cancer subtypes based on er/pr and her2 expression: Comparison of clinicopathologic features and survival. *Clin. Med. Res.* **2009**, *7*, 4–13. [CrossRef] [PubMed]
5. Cancer Genome Atlas Network. Comprehensive molecular portraits of human breast tumours. *Nature* **2012**, *490*, 61–70. [CrossRef]
6. Sorlie, T.; Perou, C.M.; Tibshirani, R.; Aas, T.; Geisler, S.; Johnsen, H.; Hastie, T.; Eisen, M.B.; van de Rijn, M.; Jeffrey, S.S.; et al. Gene expression patterns of breast carcinomas distinguish tumor subclasses with clinical implications. *Proc. Natl. Acad. Sci. USA* **2001**, *98*, 10869–10874. [CrossRef] [PubMed]
7. Cheung, P.S. Recent advances in breast cancer treatment. *Hong Kong Med. J. Xianggang Yi Xue Za Zhi* **2018**, *24*, 6–8. [CrossRef]
8. Wang, L.; Li, J.; Zhao, H.; Hu, J.; Ping, Y.; Li, F.; Lan, Y.; Xu, C.; Xiao, Y.; Li, X. Identifying the crosstalk of dysfunctional pathways mediated by lncRNAs in breast cancer subtypes. *Mol. BioSyst.* **2016**, *12*, 711–720. [CrossRef]
9. Restelli, M.; Magni, M.; Ruscica, V.; Pinciroli, P.; De Cecco, L.; Buscemi, G.; Delia, D.; Zannini, L. A novel crosstalk between ccar2 and akt pathway in the regulation of cancer cell proliferation. *Cell Death Dis.* **2016**, *7*, e2453. [CrossRef]
10. Brechbiel, J.M.-M.K.; Adjei, A.A. Crosstalk between hedgehog and other signaling pathways as a basis for combination therapies in cancer. *Cancer Treat. Rev.* **2014**, *40*, 750–759. [CrossRef]
11. Aksamitiene, E.; Kiyatkin, A.; Kholodenko, B.N. Cross-talk between mitogenic ras/mapk and survival pi3k/akt pathways: A fine balance. *Biochem. Soc. Focus. Meet.* **2012**, *40*, 139–146. [CrossRef] [PubMed]
12. Jaeger, S.; Igea, A.; Arroyo, R.; Alcalde, V.; Canovas, B.; Orozco, M.; Nebreda, A.R.; Aloy, P. Quantification of pathway cross-talk reveals novel synergistic drug combinations for breast cancer. *Cancer Res.* **2017**, *77*, 459–469. [CrossRef] [PubMed]
13. Godard, P.; van Eyll, J. Pathway analysis from lists of microRNAs: Common pitfalls and alternative strategy. *Nucleic Acids Res.* **2015**, *43*, 3490–3497. [CrossRef] [PubMed]
14. Mulrane, L.; McGee, S.F.; Gallagher, W.M.; O'Connor, D.P. miRNA dysregulation in breast cancer. *Cancer Res.* **2013**, *73*, 6554–6562. [CrossRef] [PubMed]
15. Anton, R.; Chatterjee, S.S.; Simundza, J.; Cowin, P.; Dasgupta, R. A systematic screen for micro-RNAs regulating the canonical wnt pathway. *PLoS ONE* **2011**, *6*, e26257. [CrossRef] [PubMed]
16. Kaboli, P.J.; Rahmat, A.; Ismail, P.; Ling, K.H. MicroRNA-based therapy and breast cancer: A comprehensive review of novel therapeutic strategies from diagnosis to treatment. *Pharmacol. Res.* **2015**, *97*, 104–121. [CrossRef] [PubMed]
17. Bai, F.; Yu, Z.; Gao, X.; Gong, J.; Fan, L.; Liu, F. Simvastatin induces breast cancer cell death through oxidative stress up-regulating mir-140-5p. *Aging (Albany NY)* **2019**, *11*, 3198–3219. [CrossRef]
18. Zhang, L.; Zhang, F.; Li, Y.; Qi, X.; Guo, Y. Triiodothyronine promotes cell proliferation of breast cancer via modulating mir-204/amphiregulin. *Pathol. Oncol. Res. POR* **2019**, *25*, 653–658. [CrossRef]
19. Shenoda, B.B.; Ramanathan, S.; Ajit, S.K. In vitro validation of miRNA-mediated gene expression linked to drug metabolism. *Curr. Protoc. Pharmacol.* **2017**, *79*, 9.26.1–9.26.15.
20. Liu, X.; Wang, S.; Meng, F.; Wang, J.; Zhang, Y.; Dai, E.; Yu, X.; Li, X.; Jiang, W. Sm2mir: A database of the experimentally validated small molecules' effects on microRNA expression. *Bioinformatics* **2013**, *29*, 409–411. [CrossRef]
21. Zhang, Y.; Xu, Y.; Li, F.; Li, X.; Feng, L.; Shi, X.; Wang, L.; Li, X. Dissecting dysfunctional crosstalk pathways regulated by miRNAs during glioma progression. *Oncotarget* **2016**, *7*, 25769–25782. [CrossRef] [PubMed]
22. Ciriello, G.; Gatza, M.L.; Beck, A.H.; Wilkerson, M.D.; Rhie, S.K.; Pastore, A.; Zhang, H.; McLellan, M.; Yau, C.; Kandoth, C.; et al. Comprehensive molecular portraits of invasive lobular breast cancer. *Cell* **2015**, *163*, 506–519. [CrossRef] [PubMed]
23. Hsu, S.D.; Lin, F.M.; Wu, W.Y.; Liang, C.; Huang, W.C.; Chan, W.L.; Tsai, W.T.; Chen, G.Z.; Lee, C.J.; Chiu, C.M.; et al. Mirtarbase: A database curates experimentally validated microRNA-target interactions. *Nucleic Acids Res.* **2011**, *39*, D163–D169. [CrossRef] [PubMed]

24. Jiang, Q.; Wang, Y.; Hao, Y.; Juan, L.; Teng, M.; Zhang, X.; Li, M.; Wang, G.; Liu, Y. Mir2disease: A manually curated database for microRNA deregulation in human disease. *Nucleic Acids Res.* **2009**, *37*, D98–D104. [CrossRef] [PubMed]
25. Xiao, F.; Zuo, Z.; Cai, G.; Kang, S.; Gao, X.; Li, T. Mirecords: An integrated resource for microRNA-target interactions. *Nucleic Acids Res.* **2009**, *37*, D105–D110. [CrossRef] [PubMed]
26. Vergoulis, T.; Vlachos, I.S.; Alexiou, P.; Georgakilas, G.; Maragkakis, M.; Reczko, M.; Gerangelos, S.; Koziris, N.; Dalamagas, T.; Hatzigeorgiou, A.G. Tarbase 6.0: Capturing the exponential growth of miRNA targets with experimental support. *Nucleic Acids Res.* **2012**, *40*, D222–D229. [CrossRef] [PubMed]
27. Keshava Prasad, T.S.; Goel, R.; Kandasamy, K.; Keerthikumar, S.; Kumar, S.; Mathivanan, S.; Telikicherla, D.; Raju, R.; Shafreen, B.; Venugopal, A.; et al. Human protein reference database—2009 update. *Nucleic Acids Res.* **2009**, *37*, D767–D772. [CrossRef] [PubMed]
28. Szklarczyk, D.; Franceschini, A.; Wyder, S.; Forslund, K.; Heller, D.; Huerta-Cepas, J.; Simonovic, M.; Roth, A.; Santos, A.; Tsafou, K.P.; et al. String v10: Protein-protein interaction networks, integrated over the tree of life. *Nucleic Acids Res.* **2015**, *43*, D447–D452. [CrossRef]
29. Kanehisa, M.; Goto, S.; Hattori, M.; Aoki-Kinoshita, K.F.; Itoh, M.; Kawashima, S.; Katayama, T.; Araki, M.; Hirakawa, M. From genomics to chemical genomics: New developments in kegg. *Nucleic Acids Res.* **2006**, *34*, D354–D357. [CrossRef]
30. Wishart, D.S.; Feunang, Y.D.; Guo, A.C.; Lo, E.J.; Marcu, A.; Grant, J.R.; Sajed, T.; Johnson, D.; Li, C.; Sayeeda, Z.; et al. Drugbank 5.0: A major update to the drugbank database for 2018. *Nucleic Acids Res.* **2018**, *46*, D1074–D1082. [CrossRef]
31. Li, C.; Li, X.; Miao, Y.; Wang, Q.; Jiang, W.; Xu, C.; Li, J.; Han, J.; Zhang, F.; Gong, B.; et al. Subpathwayminer: A software package for flexible identification of pathways. *Nucleic Acids Res.* **2009**, *37*, e131. [CrossRef] [PubMed]
32. Bernards, R. A missing link in genotype-directed cancer therapy. *Cell* **2012**, *151*, 465–468. [CrossRef] [PubMed]
33. Yamaguchi, H.; Chang, S.S.; Hsu, J.L.; Hung, M.C. Signaling cross-talk in the resistance to her family receptor targeted therapy. *Oncogene* **2014**, *33*, 1073–1081. [CrossRef] [PubMed]
34. Koscielny, G.; An, P.; Carvalho-Silva, D.; Cham, J.A.; Fumis, L.; Gasparyan, R.; Hasan, S.; Karamanis, N.; Maguire, M.; Papa, E.; et al. Open targets: A platform for therapeutic target identification and validation. *Nucleic Acids Res.* **2017**, *45*, D985–D994. [CrossRef] [PubMed]
35. Zeng, F.; Ju, R.J.; Liu, L.; Xie, H.J.; Mu, L.M.; Zhao, Y.; Yan, Y.; Hu, Y.J.; Wu, J.S.; Lu, W.L. Application of functional vincristine plus dasatinib liposomes to deletion of vasculogenic mimicry channels in triple-negative breast cancer. *Oncotarget* **2015**, *6*, 36625–36642. [CrossRef] [PubMed]
36. Wahba, H.A.; El-Hadaad, H.A. Current approaches in treatment of triple-negative breast cancer. *Cancer Biol. Med.* **2015**, *12*, 106–116. [PubMed]
37. Wilhelm, S.; Carter, C.; Lynch, M.; Lowinger, T.; Dumas, J.; Smith, R.A.; Schwartz, B.; Simantov, R.; Kelley, S. Discovery and development of sorafenib: A multikinase inhibitor for treating cancer. *Nat. Rev. Drug Discov.* **2006**, *5*, 835–844. [CrossRef]
38. Zhang, N.; Wang, X.; Huo, Q.; Sun, M.; Cai, C.; Liu, Z.; Hu, G.; Yang, Q. MicroRNA-30a suppresses breast tumor growth and metastasis by targeting metadherin. *Oncogene* **2014**, *33*, 3119–3128. [CrossRef]
39. Shah, M.Y.; Calin, G.A. MicroRNAs mir-221 and mir-222: A new level of regulation in aggressive breast cancer. *Genome Med.* **2011**, *3*, 56. [CrossRef]
40. Tsai, K.W.; Leung, C.M.; Lo, Y.H.; Chen, T.W.; Chan, W.C.; Yu, S.Y.; Tu, Y.T.; Lam, H.C.; Li, S.C.; Ger, L.P.; et al. Arm selection preference of microRNA-193a varies in breast cancer. *Sci. Rep.* **2016**, *6*, 28176. [CrossRef]
41. Vanhoefer, U.; Harstrick, A.; Achterrath, W.; Cao, S.; Seeber, S.; Rustum, Y.M. Irinotecan in the treatment of colorectal cancer: Clinical overview. *J. Clin. Oncol. Off. J. Am. Soc. Clin. Oncol.* **2001**, *19*, 1501–1518. [CrossRef] [PubMed]
42. Kuo, W.T.; Yu, S.Y.; Li, S.C.; Lam, H.C.; Chang, H.T.; Chen, W.S.; Yu, C.C. MicroRNA-324 in human cancer: Mir-324-5p and mir-324-3p have distinct biological functions in human cancer. *Anticancer Res.* **2016**, *36*, 5189–5196. [CrossRef] [PubMed]
43. Eissa, S.; Matboli, M.; Shehata, H.H. Breast tissue–based microRNA panel highlights microRNA-23a and selected target genes as putative biomarkers for breast cancer. *Transl. Res.* **2015**, *165*, 417–427. [CrossRef] [PubMed]

44. Bollag, G.; Tsai, J.; Zhang, J.; Zhang, C.; Ibrahim, P.; Nolop, K.; Hirth, P. Vemurafenib: The first drug approved for braf-mutant cancer. *Nat. Rev. Drug Discov.* **2012**, *11*, 873–886. [CrossRef] [PubMed]
45. Sachdeva, M.; Mo, Y.Y. Mir-145-mediated suppression of cell growth, invasion and metastasis. *Am. J. Transl. Res.* **2010**, *2*, 170–180. [PubMed]
46. Mann, B.S.; Johnson, J.R.; He, K.; Sridhara, R.; Abraham, S.; Booth, B.P.; Verbois, L.; Morse, D.E.; Jee, J.M.; Pope, S.; et al. Vorinostat for treatment of cutaneous manifestations of advanced primary cutaneous t-cell lymphoma. *Clin. Cancer Res. Off. J. Am. Assoc. Cancer Res.* **2007**, *13*, 2318–2322. [CrossRef]
47. Li, L.; Xie, X.; Luo, J.; Liu, M.; Xi, S.; Guo, J.; Tang, J. Targeted expression of mir-34a using the t-visa system suppresses breast cancer cell growth and invasion. *Mol. Ther.* **2012**, *20*, 2326–2334. [CrossRef]
48. Mattiske, S.; Suetani, R.J.; Neilsen, P.M.; Callen, D.F. The oncogenic role of mir-155 in breast cancer. *Cancer Epidemiol. Biomark. Prev. Publ. Am. Assoc. Cancer Res. Cosponsored Am. Soc. Prev. Oncol.* **2012**, *21*, 1236–1243. [CrossRef]
49. Hossain, A.; Kuo, M.T.; Saunders, G.F. Mir-17-5p regulates breast cancer cell proliferation by inhibiting translation of aib1 mRNA. *Mol. Cell. Biol.* **2006**, *26*, 8191–8201. [CrossRef]
50. Chen, B.; Tang, H.; Liu, X.; Liu, P.; Yang, L.; Xie, X.; Wei, W. Mir-22 as a prognostic factor targets glucose transporter protein type 1 in breast cancer. *Cancer Lett.* **2015**, *356*, 410–417. [CrossRef]
51. Li, Q.; Yao, Y.; Eades, G.; Liu, Z.; Zhang, Y.; Zhou, Q. Downregulation of mir-140 promotes cancer stem cell formation in basal-like early stage breast cancer. *Oncogene* **2014**, *33*, 2589–2600. [CrossRef] [PubMed]
52. DeSantis, C.E.; Ma, J.; Goding Sauer, A.; Newman, L.A.; Jemal, A. Breast cancer statistics, 2017, racial disparity in mortality by state. *CA Cancer J. Clin.* **2017**, *67*, 439–448. [CrossRef] [PubMed]
53. Ayers, D.; Vandesompele, J. Influence of microRNAs and long non-coding RNAs in cancer chemoresistance. *Genes* **2017**, *8*, 95. [CrossRef] [PubMed]
54. Burrell, R.A.; McGranahan, N.; Bartek, J.; Swanton, C. The causes and consequences of genetic heterogeneity in cancer evolution. *Nature* **2013**, *501*, 338–345. [CrossRef] [PubMed]
55. Zuzic, M.; Rojo Arias, J.E.; Wohl, S.G.; Busskamp, V. Retinal miRNA functions in health and disease. *Genes* **2019**, *10*, 377. [CrossRef] [PubMed]
56. Lamb, J.; Crawford, E.D.; Peck, D.; Modell, J.W.; Blat, I.C.; Wrobel, M.J.; Reich, M. The Connectivity Map: Using gene-expression signatures to connect small molecules, genes, and disease. *Science* **2006**, *313*, 1929–1935. [CrossRef] [PubMed]
57. Gottlieb, A.; Stein, G.Y.; Ruppin, E.; Sharan, R. PREDICT: A method for inferring novel drug indications with application to personalized medicine. *Mol. Syst. Biol.* **2011**, *7*, 496. [CrossRef] [PubMed]
58. Malas, T.B.; Vlietstra, W.J.; Kudrin, R.; Starikov, S.; Charrout, M.; Roos, M.; van Mulligen, E.M. Drug prioritization using the semantic properties of a knowledge graph. *Sci. Rep.* **2019**, *9*, 6281. [CrossRef] [PubMed]

13

Azathioprine Biotransformation in Young Patients with Inflammatory Bowel Disease: Contribution of Glutathione-S Transferase M1 and A1 Variants

Marianna Lucafò [1,2], Gabriele Stocco [3,*], Stefano Martelossi [2], Diego Favretto [2], Raffaella Franca [4], Noelia Malusà [5], Angela Lora [2,4], Matteo Bramuzzo [2], Samuele Naviglio [2], Erika Cecchin [1], Giuseppe Toffoli [1], Alessandro Ventura [2,4] and Giuliana Decorti [2,4]

1 Centro di Riferimento Oncologico, IRCCS, 33081 Aviano, Italy; mlucafo@units.it (M.L.); ececchin@cro.it (E.C.); gtoffoli@cro.it (G.T.)
2 Institute for Maternal and Child Health IRCCS Burlo Garofolo, 34137 Trieste, Italy; stefano.martelossi@aulss2.veneto.it (S.M.); dieg.o@libero.it (D.F.); angelalora86@gmail.com (A.L.); matteo.bramuzzo@burlo.trieste.it (M.B.); samuele.naviglio@burlo.trieste.it (S.N.); alessandro.ventura@burlo.trieste.it (A.V.); decorti@units.it (G.D.)
3 Department of Life Sciences, University of Trieste, 34127 Trieste, Italy
4 Department of Medical, Surgical and Health Sciences, University of Trieste, 34149 Trieste, Italy; rfranca@units.it
5 Sanitary Services Agency 1, 34129 Trieste, Italy; tossicologia.forense@asuits.sanita.fvg.it
* Correspondence: stoccog@units.it

Abstract: The contribution of candidate genetic variants involved in azathioprine biotransformation on azathioprine efficacy and pharmacokinetics in 111 young patients with inflammatory bowel disease was evaluated. Azathioprine doses, metabolites thioguanine-nucleotides (TGN) and methylmercaptopurine-nucleotides (MMPN) and clinical effects were assessed after at least 3 months of therapy. Clinical efficacy was defined as disease activity score below 10. Candidate genetic variants (*TPMT* rs1142345, rs1800460, rs1800462, *GSTA1* rs3957357, *GSTM1*, and *GSTT1* deletion) were determined by polymerase chain reaction (PCR) assays and pyrosequencing. Statistical analysis was performed using linear mixed effects models for the association between the candidate variants and the pharmacological variables (azathioprine doses and metabolites). Azathioprine metabolites were measured in 257 samples (median 2 per patient, inter-quartile range IQR 1-3). Clinical efficacy at the first evaluation available resulted better in ulcerative colitis than in Crohn's disease patients (88.0% versus 52.5% responders, $p = 0.0003$, linear mixed effect model, LME). TGN concentration and the ratio TGN/dose at the first evaluation were significantly higher in responder. *TPMT* rs1142345 variant (4.8% of patients) was associated with increased TGN (LME $p = 0.0042$), TGN/dose ratio (LME $p < 0.0001$), decreased azathioprine dose (LME $p = 0.0087$), and MMPN (LME $p = 0.0011$). *GSTM1* deletion (58.1% of patients) was associated with a 18.5% decrease in TGN/dose ratio (LME $p = 0.041$) and 30% decrease in clinical efficacy (LME $p = 0.0031$). *GSTA1* variant (12.8% of patients) showed a trend ($p = 0.046$, LME) for an association with decreased clinical efficacy; however, no significant effect on azathioprine pharmacokinetics could be detected. In conclusion, GSTs variants are associated with azathioprine efficacy and pharmacokinetics.

Keywords: azathioprine; inflammatory bowel disease; glutathione-S transferase; pharmacogenetics; pharmacokinetics

1. Introduction

Inflammatory bowel disease (IBD) is a chronic, relapsing and remitting disease of the gastrointestinal tract that comprises two main entities, Crohn's disease (CD) and ulcerative colitis (UC). The disease has a peak onset in subjects 15 to 30 years old, and its incidence is rising in the pediatric population [1]. Despite the recent introduction in therapy of biologicals, thiopurines continue to be widely used in this disease; indeed, these are cheap drugs, and maintain at least 20% of patients in a state of stable long term steroid free clinical remission [2]. Among thiopurines, azathioprine is mainly used as an immunosuppressant in IBD, and, although it has a well described risk benefit profile, adverse drug reactions are relatively common, occurring in 15–18% of patients, and can be severe enough to require the withdrawal of therapy [3,4] In addition, a significant proportion of patients does not respond to therapy with this agent [5–7]. The reasons of this high heterogeneity in clinical response is not clear yet [8]; however, variability in azathioprine metabolism can be important; indeed, azathioprine is a prodrug that requires metabolic conversion to its active form. The first step in this metabolic conversion is mediated by conjugation with glutathione, resulting in the formation of mercaptopurine. This reaction is in part nonenzymatic but it is even controlled, as demonstrated by recent publications, by the enzyme glutathione S-transferase (GST in particular by the isoforms A and M [9]. The latter is also inactive and is converted by the enzymes of the purine salvage pathway to the active thioguanine nucleotides, which are responsible of the cytotoxic and apoptotic effect of these drugs [10]. Mercaptopurine is metabolized by the enzyme xanthine oxidase in the liver, and by thiopurine methyltransferase (TPMT) and inosine triphosphatase (ITPA), mainly in extra hepatic tissues [10]. Polymorphisms in genes involved in azathioprine metabolism can hence influence the efficacy and toxicity of this drug [6].

In this study, we aimed to evaluate the contribution of candidate genetic variants involved in azathioprine biotransformation on azathioprine efficacy and pharmacokinetics in young patients with IBD.

2. Materials and Methods

2.1. Patient Characteristics

111 patients with IBD were enrolled by the Gastroenterology Unit of the Pediatric Hospital "Burlo Garofolo" in Trieste, Italy between March 2004 and February 2015. The study was conducted in accordance with the Declaration of Helsinki, and the protocol was approved by the Institutional Ethics Committee (Projects RC 23/2005 and 12/2013). All subjects and parents gave their informed consent for inclusion before they participated in the study. The inclusion criteria were age less than 30 years, previous diagnosis of IBD and treatment with azathioprine for at least 3 months. The patients enrolled are all the patients taking azathioprine at "Burlo Garofolo" in Trieste in the time-frame of the study. Blood samples for azathioprine metabolites measurement and for genotyping were taken at the appropriate clinic visit. Timing of metabolite level measurement was determined by the clinical setting of azathioprine administration at the hospital: generally, azathioprine metabolites levels were measured after 3, 6, and 12 months of treatment and then every year. Patients were treated with a dose-escalating strategy to reduce the risk of adverse events starting, however, from a relatively high dose (median of 2 mg/kg). At subsequent follow-up visits (every 3 months), the dose was increased or reduced so as to obtain the optimal clinical response; the criteria used to increase or reduce the dose of azathioprine were the level of disease activity and laboratory parameters used to monitor azathioprine toxicity (in particular leukocyte, erythrocyte and platelet counts, hemoglobin concentration, mean corpuscular volume, liver enzymes alanine aminotransferase, aspartate aminotransferase and γ-glutamyltransferase, and amylase levels). According to current guidelines, genotyping information was shared with the clinicians only for patients presenting *TPMT* variant alleles, in order to allow increased monitoring of adverse events.

Clinical response was assessed using Pediatric Crohn's Disease Activity Index and Pediatric Ulcerative Colitis Activity Index, respectively [11], for CD and UC patients at the time of blood sample collection for the first metabolites' measurement, which occurred at least 3 months since the beginning of therapy. The disease was considered inactive if the disease activity index was <10 at the time of sample collection.

2.2. Measurement of Azathioprine Metabolites

Metabolites (TGN and MMPN) were measured in patients' erythrocytes using the high performance liquid chromatography assay by Dervieux and Boulieu [12]. The ratio between TGN and the dose of azathioprine was calculated considering, for each individual measurement of the metabolites, the dose the patients took the day the blood sample was recorded.

2.3. Genotypes

Genomic DNA was extracted from peripheral blood samples using a commercial kit (Sigma, Milan, Italy), to characterize genetic polymorphisms in the candidate genes *TPMT* (rs1142345, rs1800460 and rs1800462), *GSTA1* (rs3957357), *GSTM1* (deletion), and *GSTT1* (deletion). The considered genotypes and method of analysis are described in Table 1. Genotypes for *TPMT* rs1800462 was determined by polymerase chain reaction (PCR) with allele specific oligonucleotides (ASO). Primers used were, for the wild-type allele, as forward P2W 5′-GTATGATTTTATGCAGGTTTG-3′ and as reverse P2C 5′-TAAATAGGAACCATCGGACAC-3′; primers. For the variant allele, a second tube was used with P2M 5′-GTATGATTTTATGCAGGTTTC-3′ as forward primer and the above-mentioned P2C 5′-TAAATAGGAACCATCGGACAC-3′ as reverse. PCR protocol for these primers were: initial denaturation 5 min at 94 °C, followed by 37 cycles with 30 s at 94 °C, 30 s at 57 °C, and 2 min at 72 °C, with a final extension for 10 min at 72 °C. PCR product was visualized on a 2% agarose gel. In case of a patient carrying the wild type allele, the product (254 bp) was present with the P2W and P2C primers; in case of patients carrying the variant allele, with the P2M and P2C primers for *TPMT* rs1800460 and rs1142345, PCR- restriction fragment length polymorphism (RFLP) was used. For rs1800460, primers used were: forward 5′-AGGCAGCTAGGGAAAAAGAAAGGTG-3′ and reverse 5′-CAAGCCTTATAGCCTTACACCCAGG-3′. PCR protocol for these primers was: initial denaturation 5 min at 94 °C, followed by 37 cycles with 30 s at 94 °C, 30 s at 55 °C, and 2 min at 72 °C, with a final extension for 10 min at 72 °C. The DNA amplification produces an amplicon of 694 bp, which is subsequently digested enzymatically with the enzyme Mwol (concentration of 1 U/10 μl) incubated for 90 min at 60 °C. The enzyme recognizes the wild-type site and cuts the DNA strand into two fragments of 443 bp and 251 bp, while it does not cut the variant fragment. A 2% agarose gel was prepared for visualization. For rs1142345, primers used were forward 5′-AATCCCTGCTGTCATTCTTCATAGTATTT-3′ and reverse 5′-CACATCATAATCTCCTCTCC-3′. PCR protocol was the same as *TPMT* rs1800460. PCR produces a 401 bp amplicon, which is subsequently digested enzymatically with the Accl enzyme (concentration 1 U/10 μl) and incubated for 90 min at 37 °C. The enzyme recognizes the variant site and cuts the DNA strand into two 252 pb and 149 pb fragments while the wild-type strand is not cut. A 2% agarose gel was prepared for visualization. *GSTM1* and *GSTT1* genotypes were determined by MULTIPLEX-PCR-ASO as previously described [13], in which three pairs of primers were used simultaneously: a specific pair for the T isoform, one for the M isoform and one for the β-globin gene, which acts as an internal positive control in order to verify the amplification. The three pairs of primers lead to three fragments of different sizes: 480 bp (*GSTT*), 286 bp (β-globin), and 219 bp (*GSTM*). The primers used have the following sequence: *GSTM* Forward: 5′-GAACTCCCTGAAAAGCTAAAGC-3′; *GSTM* Reverse: 5′-GTTGGGCTCAAATATACGGTGC-3′; *β-Globin*Forward: 5′-GAAGAGCCAAGGACAGGT-3′; *β-Globin* Reverse: 5′-CAACTTCATCCACGTTCACC-3′; *GSTT* Forward: 5′-TTCCTTACTGGTCCTCACATCTC-3′; *GSTT* Reverse: 5′-TCACCGGATCATGGCCAGCA-3′. PCR protocol for these primers were: initial denaturation 5 min at 94 °C, followed by 37 cycles with 30 s at 94 °C, 30 s at 57 °C, and 2 min at 72 °C, with a final extension for 7 min at 72 °C. All PCR reactions described were carried out using RedTaq polymerase (Sigma, Milan, Italy), with the addition of dNTPs 0,25 nM and with a primer concentration of 1 mM.

Table 1. Assay used for genotyping of the considered variants.

Gene	Polymorphism		
	rs Number	**Primary Locus Alleles [14]**	**Genotyping Method**
TPMT	rs1800462	C > G missense	PCR-ASO [13]
	rs1800460	C > T missense	PCR-RFLP [13]
	rs1142345	T > C missense	PCR-RFLP [13]
GSTM1	No rs number	Deletion	MULTIPLEX-PCR-ASO [13]
GSTT1	No rs number	Deletion	MULTIPLEX-PCR-ASO [13]
GSTA1	rs3957357	A > G (5′-UTR)	Pyrosequencing [15]

ASO: allele specific oligonucleotides; *GST*: glutathione-S-transferase, *TPMT*: thiopurine-S-methyl transferase; RFLP: restriction fragment length polymorphism. PCR: polymerase chain reaction.

For *GSTA1*, pyrosequencing was employed (Table 1), since this genotyping method was already validated in the laboratory. The primers used for the pyrosequencing were: forward 5′-ATCCAGTAGGTGGCCCCTTG-3′, reverse 5′-ACCGTCCTGGCTCGACAA-3′ (biotinylated). Sequencing primer was: 5′-GCTTTTCCCTAACTTGAC-3′. PCR protocol for these primers were: initial denaturation 10 min at 95 °C, followed by 40 cycles with 30 s at 95 °C, 30 s at 66 °C, and 30 s at 72 °C and with a final extension for 10 min at 72 °C. PCR produces a 148 bp amplicon. For pyrosequencing, we used PSQ96MA (Qiagen, Hilden, Germany). PCR amplifications were performed in an Eppendorf Mastercycler gradient, with TaqGold DNA Polymerase (AB Applied Biosystems, Foster City, CA, USA).

2.4. Statistical Analysis

Statistical analysis was performed using the software R (version 2.15). The association between pharmacological phenotypes of interest (i.e., clinical efficacy of treatment, dose of azathioprine, TGN metabolites concentrations, MMPN metabolites concentrations, ratio TGN/dose) and the considered demographic variables, IBD type, cotreatment or genotypes in a univariate analysis, was evaluated using linear mixed effects model built using the phenotype as the dependent variable, each covariate as the fixed effect and the patients as the random effect in the model. For clinical efficacy, the first available measurement was used, while for other pharmacological variables, all available measurements were used.

Multivariate analysis was carried out to test the independence of the effects of the genotypes significant in the univariate analysis on the phenotypes considered (i.e., TGN or MMPN concentrations, dose of azathioprine, ratio TGN/dose); for this multivariate analysis generalized linear models of the Gaussian family were used considering individually each phenotype from the univariate analysis as the dependent variable and the covariates significant in the univariate analysis as the independent variables. Normality of the phenotype was tested by the Shapiro test and log10 transformation was applied if needed, in order to adjust the normality of the distribution.

3. Results

3.1. Patients Enrolled and Samples Collected

111 patients were enrolled from March 2004 to February 2015; median age was 15.05 years (IQR 12.28–16-82), 52 (46.8%) were females. Clinical and demographic characteristics of the enrolled patients are reported in Table 2.

Table 2. Demographic and clinical characteristics of the patients enrolled in the study.

		All Patients (n = 111)
Age (Years) at Time of Sample Collection		**15.1, 12.3–16.8**
Gender	Female (%)	52 (46.8%)
	Male (%)	59 (53.2%)
Type of IBD	Crohn's disease (%)	61 (55.0%)
	Ulcerative colitis (%)	50 (45.0%)
Length (days) of treatment with azathioprine		533, 245–917

For continuous variables, median, 1st–3rd quartiles values are reported. To report age and length of treatment median and interquartile range are provided; for patients with more than one measurement of azathioprine metabolites, median age and length of treatment were used.

Azathioprine metabolites were measured in 257 samples (median 2 per patient, IQR 1-3). Among these, 89 were obtained during treatment with azathioprine alone and 161 during treatment with azathioprine and other medications and in particular: 93 with an aminosalicylate, 18 with an aminosalicylate and a glucocorticoid, 15 with infliximab, 10 with an antibiotic, 4 with an aminosalicylate and an antibiotic, 4 with an antibiotic and a glucocorticoid, 3 with an aminosalicylate, an antibiotic and a glucocorticoid, 2 with an infliximab and a glucocorticoid, and 1 with an aminosalicylate and infliximab; for 7 patients, information about concomitant treatment could not be retrieved.

3.2. Measurement of Azathioprine Metabolites: Association with Demographic and Clinical Covariates

Results of measurements together with azathioprine dose are shown in Table 3.

Table 3. Summary of azathioprine's dose and metabolites' concentrations.

	TGN (pmol/8 × 10^8 Erythrocytes)	MMPN (pmol/8 × 10^8 Erythrocytes)	Dose (mg/kg)	TGN/Dose ((pmol/8 × 10^8 Erythrocytes)/(mg/kg))
Mean	361.6	1698.1	2.0	192.8
Median	345.0	1044.0	2.1	179.4
Interquartile range	240.1–465.1	431.2–2079.7	1.7–2.3	120.1–227.9

MMPN indicated methylated nucleotides, TGN indicates thioguanine nucleotides.

Concentration of TGN metabolites were associated with IBD type, with UC patients showing slightly increased concentrations (Supplementary Figure S1, LME $p = 0.047$), but not with gender or treatment length. Azathioprine dose was strongly associated with age, with younger patients taking higher doses (Supplementary Figure S2, LME $p = 0.0001$), but not with gender, IBD type or treatment length. Concentration of MMPN metabolites or the ratio between TGN concentration and azathioprine dose were not associated with IBD type, gender, or treatment length. Interestingly, the ratio between TGN concentration and azathioprine dose was strongly associated with azathioprine dose when the analysis was limited to pediatric patients (i.e., with age less than 18, Supplementary Figure S3, LME $p = 0.0043$). Clinical efficacy, defined as disease activity score below 10 at the time of first sample collection for measurement of azathioprine metabolites, was assessed in all patients. Azathioprine was more effective in UC than in CD patients (88.0% versus 52.5% responders, LME $p = 0.0003$), while gender, age, and duration of azathioprine treatment were not associated with azathioprine efficacy. A higher concentration of TGN metabolites at the first evaluation was observed in patients in remission (Figure 1, LME $p = 0.0099$), similarly a positive correlation was observed with TGN/dose ratio (Figure 1, LME $p = 0.0023$).

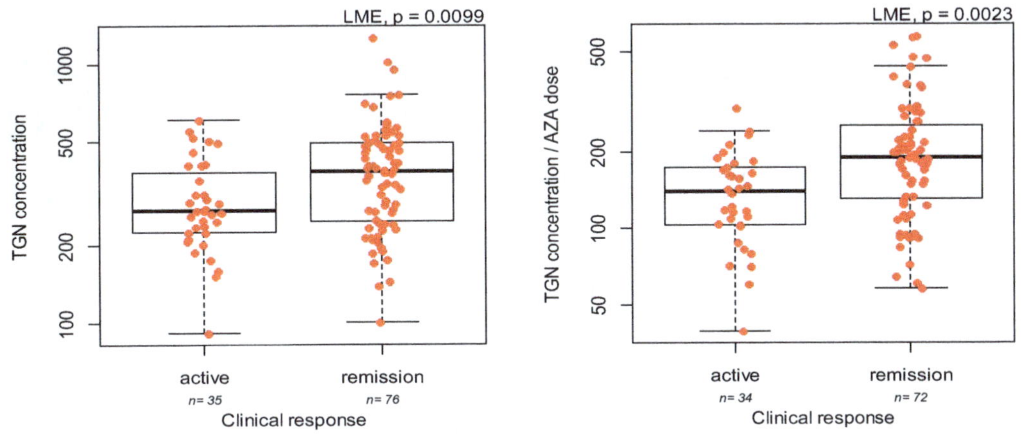

Figure 1. Response to azathioprine (AZA) and thioguanine nucleotides (TGN) concentration, as pmol/8 × 10^8 erythrocytes (left panel) or ratio between TGN concentration/daily azathioprine dose as pmol/8 × 10^8 erythrocytes/mg/kg/day (right panel). p-values are from linear mixed effect model (LME).

On the contrary, azathioprine dose and the concentration of MMPN metabolites were not associated with a clinical response (data not shown).

3.3. Genotyping

Results of genotyping are reported in Table 4.

Table 4. Genotype distribution in the 111 patients enrolled in the study.

Gene	Polymorphism	Genotyping Result				
	rs Number	**Wild-Type**	**Hetero-zygous**	**Homozygous Variant**	**Not Available**	***p*-value Hardy Weinberg**
TPMT	rs1800462	105 (100%)	0	0	6	NA
TPMT	rs1800460	101 (97.1%)	3 (2.9%)	0	7	0.88
TPMT	rs1142345	100 (95.2%)	5 (4.8%)	0	6	0.81
GSTA1	rs3957357	38 (44.2%)	37 (43.0%)	11 (12.8%)	25	0.77
Gene	**Polymorphism**	**Genotyping Result**				
		Not Deleted		**Deleted**	**Not Available**	
GSTM1	Deletion	42 (41.9%)		61 (58.1%)	8	
GSTT1	Deletion	78 (75.7%)		25 (24.3%)	8	

GST indicates glutathione-S-transferase, *TPMT* indicates thiopurine-S-methyl transferase.

All polymorphisms evaluated respected Hardy-Weinberg equilibrium and their distribution was in accordance with literature data for subjects of Caucasian ethnicity. For the association between genetic variants and azathioprine pharmacokinetics, *TPMT* rs1142345 variant (4.8% of patients) was associated with increased TGN (LME $p = 0.0042$), TGN/dose ratio (LME $p < 0.0001$), decreased azathioprine dose (LME $p = 0.0087$) and MMPN (LME $p = 0.0011$; Figure 2), as well established [2]. Interestingly, all patients with variant *TPMT* were in remission at the first evaluation of thiopurine metabolites, in comparison to 65% of patients with wild-type *TPMT* (LME $p = 0.041$, Figure 2).

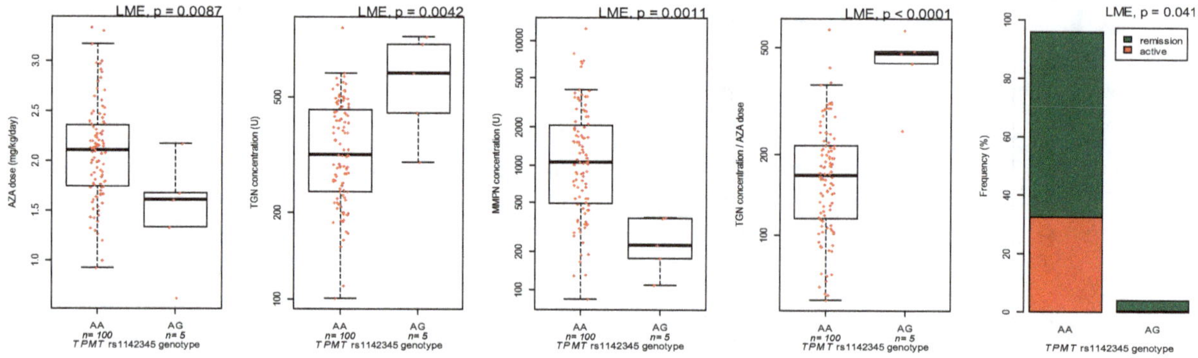

Figure 2. *TPMT* rs1142345 and azathioprine (AZA) dose, thioguanine (TGN) and methylmercaptopurine (MMPN) metabolites and efficacy. Concentration of azathioprine metabolites is expressed as pmol/8 × 10^8 erythrocytes (U). *p*-values are from linear mixed effect model (LME).

GSTM1 deletion (58.1% of patients) was associated with a 18.5% decrease in TGN/dose ratio (LME $p = 0.041$, Figure 3) and 30% decrease in clinical efficacy (LME $p = 0.0031$; Figure 3). Additionally, MMPN was reduced in patients with deletion of *GSTM1* (LME $p = 0.039$; Figure 3).

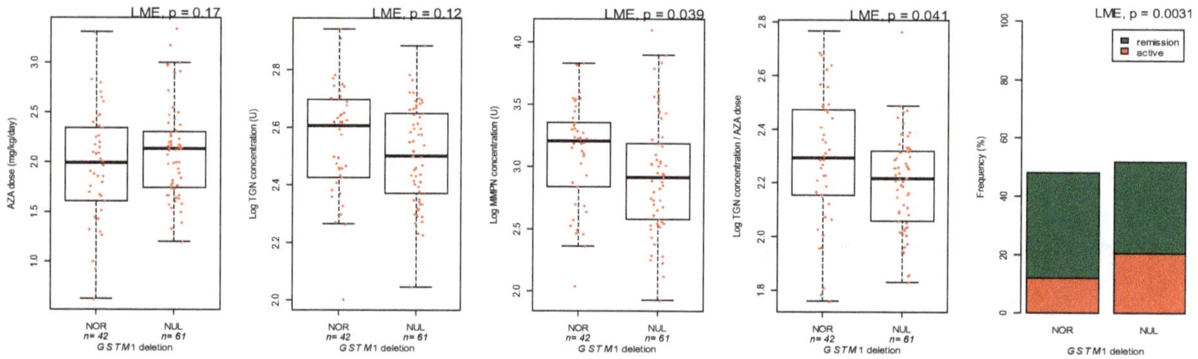

Figure 3. *GSTM1* deletion and azathioprine (AZA) dose, thioguanine (TGN), and methylmercaptopurine (MMPN) metabolites and efficacy. Concentration of azathioprine metabolites is expressed as pmol/8 × 10^8 erythrocytes (U). *p*-values are from linear mixed effect model (LME).

GSTA1 variant (12.8% of patients) showed a trend for an association with decreased clinical efficacy (LME $p = 0.046$, Figure 4); however, no significant effect on azathioprine pharmacokinetics could be detected (Figure 4).

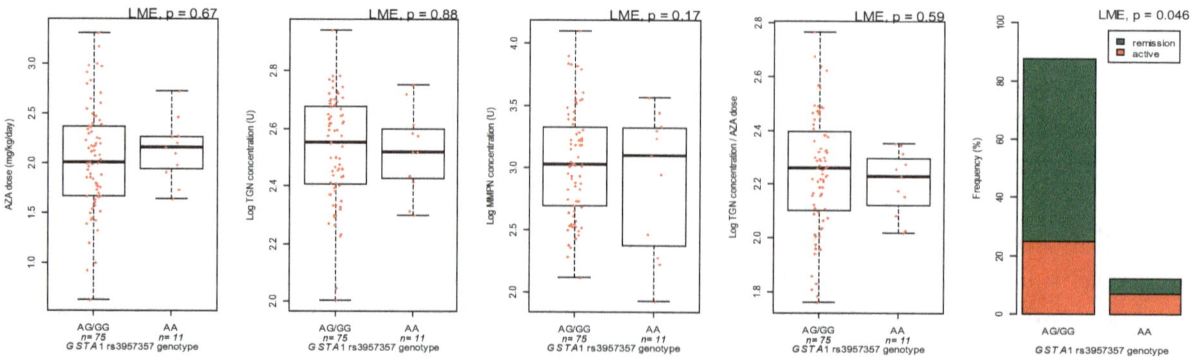

Figure 4. *GSTA1* rs3957357 variant and azathioprine (AZA) dose, thioguanine (TGN) and methylmercaptopurine (MMPN) metabolites and efficacy. Concentration of azathioprine metabolites is expressed as pmol/8 × 10^8 erythrocytes (U). *p*-values are from linear mixed effect model (LME).

GSTT1 deletion was not associated with azathioprine pharmacokinetics and efficacy (data not shown). Multivariate analysis supported the results of the univariate analysis (Table 5).

Table 5. Multivariate analysis considering for each pharmacological dependent variable covariate significant in the univariate analysis.

Azathioprine Related Pharmacological Phenotype (Dependent Variable)	Independent Variable in Multivariate Generalized Linear Model	Comparison	Effect	*p*-Value
Efficacy of azathioprine at the first metabolite measurement	IBD type	UC versus CD	1.96	0.0019
	GSTM1 genotype	Deletion versus Normal	−1.49	0.019
	GSTA1 genotype	AA versus GG/GA	−1.30	0.095
	TPMT genotype	AG versus GG	24.7	0.43
TGN metabolites concentrations	IBD type	UC versus CD	0.061	0.074
	TPMT genotype	AG versus GG	0.23	0.0049
MMPN metabolites concentration	*GSTM1* genotype	Deletion versus Normal	−0.21	0.014
	TPMT genotype	Heterozygous versus wild-type	−0.72	0.0004
Azathioprine dose	Age	Each year	−0.035	<0.0001
	TPMT genotype	Heterozygous versus wild-type	−0.58	0.0056
Ratio TGN/dose	*TPMT* genotype	Heterozygous versus wild-type	0.41	0.0001
	GSTM1 genotype	Deletion versus Normal	−0.072	0.055

GST: glutathione-S-transferase, IBD: inflammatory bowel disease, UC: ulcerative colitis, CD: Crohn's disease, MMPN: methylated nucleotides, TGN: thioguanine nucleotides, *TPMT*: thiopurine-S-methyl transferase. The effect size represents the increase (positive value) or decrease (negative value) in the value of the dependent variable for each independent variable listed. *p*-values are from linear mixed-effect models.

4. Discussion

Despite the introduction of new and effective biologics in the therapy of IBD, the thiopurine drugs azathioprine and mercaptopurine continue to be frequently used for maintaining remission in these diseases. The problem with these drugs is that they are ineffective in a significant percentage of patients, and also induce side effects that can be severe [2]. The reasons for this variability are not clear; however, a number of studies have suggested that variations in enzymes involved in their metabolism can be involved.

For azathioprine, this agent is the prodrug of mercaptopurine, and has to be converted to produce its pharmacological activity. This conversion can occur spontaneously, but is also catalyzed by the enzymes GST, in particular the A and M isoforms [16]. In rat liver homogenates, Kaplowitz et al. have demonstrated that, while at high pH (pH = 8.0) the nonenzymatic and enzymatic reactions occur at similar levels, at pH closer to physiological values, the enzymatic reaction prevails [17]. In addition, in homogenates of human livers obtained from transplant donors, treatment with furosemide, an inhibitor of soluble GSTs [18], inhibited the conversion of azathioprine to mercaptopurine [19]. Additional evidence of a role of GSTs in azathioprine metabolism has been obtained in animal models; indeed, pretreatment of rats with the GST inhibitor probenecid increased the proportion of azathioprine in rat liver and reduced GSH consumption. Similarly, less hepatic GSH depletion was observed after azathioprine treatment in Gunn rats, a model of hyperbilirubinemic rat [17]. Of interest, bilirubin is also a GST inhibitor, with some studies indicating a stronger inhibitory effect of bile acids on GSTM1 in comparison to other isoforms [20].

We previously showed that the frequency of *GSTM1* deletion was significantly lower in patients that developed an adverse event in comparison to patients that tolerated azathioprine treatment, in agreement with a model in which patients with *GSTM1* deletion are less sensitive to the effects of azathioprine, putatively because of the contribution of this enzyme on the conversion of azathioprine to mercaptopurine [13]. Moreover, in a recent previous study [21], we evaluated the effects of GST polymorphisms on azathioprine biotransformation in a cohort of young patients with IBD, tolerant to azathioprine therapy and taking the drug for more than 3 months. Patients with the deletion of *GSTM1* tolerated a dose of azathioprine significantly higher in comparison to patients with normal

GSTM1. Moreover, the amount of active TGNs generated in patients with the deletion of *GSTM1* was significantly decreased in comparison to patients with a normal genotype. Multivariate analysis confirmed that this effect was independent from that of other genes with a significant effect, such as *TPMT*, the main gene known to influence mercaptopurine metabolism [22].

The present study is the first report of an association between azathioprine efficacy and *GSTM1* and *GSTA1* variants in young patients with IBD. Moreover, we confirmed the reduced TGN/azathioprine dose ratio in patients with *GSTM1* deletion we previously reported, which may be associated with the described lower efficacy of azathioprine in patients with this genotype. This could support the need for genotype adjusted tailored therapy, possibly testing the efficacy of strategies leading to higher TGN concentration in patients with *GSTM1* deletion, such as increased azathioprine dose or co-treatment with an aminosalycilate [23], even if prospective studies are needed to further support these strategies.

Therefore, all these studies support a role of *GSTM1* on azathioprine efficacy, mediated by an increased conversion of azathioprine to mercaptopurine. The reaction catalyzed by GSTM1 likely occurs after oral administration mainly in the intestine and the liver, modulating the amount of mercaptopurine and TGNs that are released in the main circulation [24].

Azathioprine dose is strongly associated with patients' age in the present study, an observation consistent with our previous results in children with IBD, showing that these patients require higher doses of azathioprine to achieve similar therapeutic efficacy and TGN concentration [25]. *TPMT* activity indeed is significantly higher in children than in adults [26]; interestingly, in pediatric patients (age less than 18 years), we could observe a lower ratio of TGN/azathioprine dose, as in our previous report. However, when the analysis was extended to young adults (age less than 30 years), the correlation between age and the TGN/dose ratio was lost. This may be related to environmental factors, including epigenetic determinants, even if more studies are needed to elucidate the mechanisms underlying these observations [27].

Considering studies by other groups, our results are in agreement with a recently published paper describing a lower efficacy of azathioprine in patients with *GSTM1* deletion, even if the results were not fully significant [28]. Moreover, in our study, we observed reduced concentration of MMPN nucleotides during azathioprine treatment in patients with *GSTM1* deletion: this result is consistent with a recent study by Broekman et al. [29]; this study also supports a lack of effect of *GSTA1* variants on azathioprine TGN and MMPN concentrations. The clinical implications of these observations need to be further explored. Additionally, age may affect the association of GSTs variants with thiopurine effects; indeed, studies in adult patients could not identify a consistent effect of *GSTM1* variants on thiopurines induced adverse effects [30], and therefore, other studies in the pediatric population are needed.

A recent study investigated the association among *GST* polymorphism, enzyme activity and azathioprine-related adverse drug reactions in Chinese Han patients with IBD, finding that the patients who became neutropenic had a significantly higher GSTs activity when compared with patients who did not develop toxicity [31]. The authors found, in the univariate analysis, that *GSTM1* wildtype genotype had a relationship with leukopenia and flue like symptoms, while *GSTP1* variant was strongly associated with leukopenia. Following adjustment for other potential risk factors, it was shown that *GSTP1* variants only were associated with increased risks of leukopenia. In our current study, we did not consider the effect of *GSTP1* polymorphisms on azathioprine effects and metabolism, since in our previous studies no significant association with adverse effect [13] or biotransformation [21] could be detected. The lack of association may be due to the tissue distribution of *GSTP1* and *GSTT1*, which are not highly expressed in the liver, but even to the lack of specific activity of these enzymes toward the catalysis of the reaction of azathioprine with glutathione [9,16]. Since the GSTP isoform does not catalyze the biotransformation of azathioprine to mercaptopurine [16], other mechanisms could be involved in the association observed by Liu and collaborators, such as induction of oxidative stress or modulation of apoptosis [24]. The study by Liu et al. reporting an effect of *GSTP1* variants on azathioprine induced adverse events, with a milder effect of *GSTM1*, seems to underline that the effects of GSTs on azathioprine pharmacogenetics may be influenced by ethnicity. Indeed, it is already known that variants frequent in Asian patients but uncommon in other ethnic groups, are associated with increased sensitivity to thiopurines, such as *MRP4* and *NUDT15* [32,33].

One limitation of our study is its retrospective design and the consequent difficulty of properly assessing phenomena such as drug interaction, which should rely on data collection from patients' charts. Drug interactions between azathioprine and other agents employed in IBD have been described; in particular, a significant decrease in TGN levels after discontinuation of aminosalicylates has been previously reported [23]. Moreover, for *GSTA1*, a marginal effect on thiopurine efficacy was observed but this was not supported by an effect on thiopurine pharmacokinetics: this may be related to the limited number of patients homozygous for the *GSTA1* variant enrolled. Another limitation is the fact that the current assay for thiopurine metabolites quantifies two main species (thioguanine nucleotides and methyl-mercaptopurine nucleotides), without distinguishing between monophosphate, diphosphate, and triphosphate nucleotides. Innovative mass spectrometry based assays are now available to quantify thiopurine metabolites [34], allowing quantification of phosphorylation of thionucleotides [35] and they could be applied to evaluate differences in thiopurine biotransformation in patients with various GST genotypes. Evaluation of the combined effects of genotypes in this study is limited. Indeed, multivariate analysis indicates independency in the effects of the candidate genotypes considered on the pharmacological variables in the present cohort. A larger cohort is needed to detect significant effects by combined genotypes. For demographic covariates, in particular gender, no significant effect was identified in the univariate analysis; to further evaluate interactive effect of gender and the considered genotypes, a larger cohort is needed.

In conclusion, GSTs variants were associated with azathioprine efficacy and pharmacokinetics; more studies, both clinical and molecular are still needed to apply this evidence to improve outcomes of therapy with azathioprine in young patients with IBD.

Author Contributions: Conceptualization, M.L., G.S., E.C., G.T., A.V., and G.D.; Data curation, M.L., G.S., A.L., M.B., S.N., E.C., and G.D.; Formal analysis, M.L., G.S., D.F., N.M., E.C., and G.D.; Funding acquisition, S.M., M.B.; Methodology, M.L., S.M., D.F., R.F., N.M., A.L., M.B., S.N., and E.C.; Supervision, S.M., N.M., E.C., G.T., A.V., and G.D.; Writing—original draft, M.L., G.S. and G.D.; Writing—review & editing, M.L., G.S., S.M., E.C., A.V., and G.D.

References

1. Ponder, A.; Long, M.D. A clinical review of recent findings in the epidemiology of inflammatory bowel disease. *Clin. Epidemiol.* **2013**, *5*, 237–247. [CrossRef]
2. Louis, E.; Irving, P.; Beaugerie, L. Use of azathioprine in IBD: Modern aspects of an old drug. *Gut* **2014**, *63*, 1695–1699. [CrossRef] [PubMed]
3. Barabino, A.; Torrente, F.; Ventura, A.; Cucchiara, S.; Castro, M.; Barbera, C. Azathioprine in paediatric inflammatory bowel disease: An Italian multicentre survey. *Aliment. Pharmacol. Ther.* **2002**, *16*, 1125–1130. [CrossRef] [PubMed]
4. Prefontaine, E.; Macdonald, J.K.; Sutherland, L.R. Azathioprine or 6-mercaptopurine for induction of remission in Crohn's disease. *Cochrane Database Syst Rev.* **2010**, *6*, CD000545. [CrossRef]
5. Colombel, J.F.; Sandborn, W.J.; Reinisch, W.; Mantzaris, G.J.; Kornbluth, A.; Rachmilewitz, D.; Lichtiger, S.; D'Haens, G.; Diamond, R.H.; Broussard, D.L.; et al. Infliximab, azathioprine, or combination therapy for Crohn's disease. *N. Engl. J. Med.* **2010**, *362*, 1383–1395. [CrossRef]

6. Chouchana, L.; Narjoz, C.; Beaune, P.; Loriot, M.A.; Roblin, X. Review article: The benefits of pharmacogenetics for improving thiopurine therapy in inflammatory bowel disease. *Aliment. Pharmacol. Ther.* **2012**, *35*, 15–36. [CrossRef] [PubMed]
7. Lucafò, M.; Franca, R.; Selvestrel, D.; Curci, D.; Pugnetti, L.; Decorti, G.; Stocco, G. Pharmacogenetics of treatments for inflammatory bowel disease. *Expert Opin. Drug Metab. Toxicol.* **2018**, *14*, 1209–1223. [CrossRef]
8. Stocco, G.; De Iudicibus, S.; Franca, R.; Addobbati, R.; Decorti, G. Personalized therapies in pediatric inflammatory and autoimmune diseases. *Curr. Pharm. Des.* **2012**, *18*, 5766–5775. [CrossRef] [PubMed]
9. Modén, O.; Mannervik, B. Glutathione transferases in the bioactivation of azathioprine. *Adv. Cancer Res.* **2014**, *122*, 199–244. [CrossRef]
10. Zaza, G.; Cheok, M.; Krynetskaia, N.; Thorn, C.; Stocco, G.; Hebert, J.M.; McLeod, H.; Weinshilboum, R.M.; Relling, M.V.; Evans, W.E.; et al. Thiopurine pathway. *Pharm. Genom.* **2010**, *20*, 573–574. [CrossRef] [PubMed]
11. Turner, D.; Otley, A.R.; Mack, D.; Hyams, J.; de Bruijne, J.; Uusoue, K.; Walters, T.D.; Zachos, M.; Mamula, P.; Beaton, D.E.; et al. Development, validation, and evaluation of a pediatric ulcerative colitis activity index: A prospective multicenter study. *Gastroenterology* **2007**, *133*, 423–432. [CrossRef] [PubMed]
12. Dervieux, T.; Boulieu, R. Simultaneous determination of 6-thioguanine and methyl 6-mercaptopurine nucleotides of azathioprine in red blood cells by HPLC. *Clin Chem.* **1998**, *44*, 551–555. [PubMed]
13. Stocco, G.; Martelossi, S.; Barabino, A.; Decorti, G.; Bartoli, F.; Montico, M.; Gotti, A.; Ventura, A. Glutathione-S-transferase genotypes and the adverse effects of azathioprine in young patients with inflammatory bowel disease. *Inflamm. Bowel Dis.* **2007**, *13*, 57–64. [CrossRef] [PubMed]
14. Whirl-Carrillo, M.; McDonagh, E.M.; Hebert, J.M.; Gong, L.; Sangkuhl, K.; Thorn, C.F.; Altman, R.B.; Klein, T.E. Pharmacogenomics knowledge for personalized medicine. *Clin. Pharmacol. Ther.* **2012**, *92*, 414–417. [CrossRef] [PubMed]
15. De Mattia, E.; Cecchin, E.; Polesel, J.; Bignucolo, A.; Roncato, R.; Lupo, F.; Crovatto, M.; Buonadonna, A.; Tiribelli, C.; Toffoli, G. Genetic biomarkers for hepatocellular cancer risk in a caucasian population. *World J. Gastroenterol.* **2017**, *23*, 6674–6684. [CrossRef] [PubMed]
16. Eklund, B.I.; Moberg, M.; Bergquist, J.; Mannervik, B. Divergent activities of human glutathione transferases in the bioactivation of azathioprine. *Mol. Pharmacol.* **2006**, *70*, 747–754. [CrossRef]
17. Kaplowitz, N.; Kuhlenkamp, J. Inhibition of hepatic metabolism of azathioprine in vivo. *Gastroenterology* **1978**, *74*, 90–92.
18. Ahokas, J.T.; Davies, C.; Ravenscroft, P.J.; Emmerson, B.T. Inhibition of soluble glutathione S-transferase by diuretic drugs. *Biochem. Pharmacol.* **1984**, *33*, 1929–1932. [CrossRef]
19. Von Bahr, C.; Glaumann, H.; Gudas, J.; Kaplowitz, N. Inhibition of hepatic metabolism of azathioprine by furosemide in human liver in vitro. *Biochem. Pharmacol.* **1980**, *29*, 1439–1441. [CrossRef]
20. Singh, S.V.; Leal, T.; Awasthi, Y.C. Inhibition of human glutathione S-transferases by bile acids. *Toxicol. Appl. Pharmacol.* **1988**, *95*, 248–254. [CrossRef]
21. Stocco, G.; Cuzzoni, E.; De Iudicibus, S.; Franca, R.; Favretto, D.; Malusà, N.; Londero, M.; Cont, G.; Bartoli, F.; Martelossi, S.; et al. Deletion of glutathione-s-transferase m1 reduces azathioprine metabolite concentrations in young patients with inflammatory bowel disease. *J. Clin. Gastroenterol.* **2014**, *48*, 43–51. [CrossRef] [PubMed]
22. Relling, M.V.; Gardner, E.E.; Sandborn, W.J.; Schmiegelow, K.; Pui, C.H.; Yee, S.W.; Stein, C.M.; Carrillo, M.; Evans, W.E.; Hicks, J.K.; et al. Clinical pharmacogenetics implementation consortium guidelines for thiopurine methyltransferase genotype and thiopurine dosing: 2013 update. *Clin. Pharmacol. Ther.* **2013**, *93*, 324–325. [CrossRef] [PubMed]
23. Stocco, G.; Cuzzoni, E.; De Iudicibus, S.; Favretto, D.; Malusà, N.; Martelossi, S.; Pozzi, E.; Lionetti, P.; Ventura, A.; Decorti, G. Thiopurine metabolites variations during co-treatment with aminosalicylates for inflammatory bowel disease: Effect of N-acetyl transferase polymorphisms. *World J. Gastroenterol.* **2015**, *21*, 3571–3578. [CrossRef] [PubMed]
24. Stocco, G.; Pelin, M.; Franca, R.; De Iudicibus, S.; Cuzzoni, E.; Favretto, D.; Martelossi, S.; Ventura, A.; Decorti, G. Pharmacogenetics of azathioprine in inflammatory bowel disease: A role for glutathione-S-transferase? *World J. Gastroenterol.* **2014**, *20*, 3534–3541. [CrossRef] [PubMed]
25. Stocco, G.; Martelossi, S.; Arrigo, S.; Barabino, A.; Aloi, M.; Martinelli, M.; Miele, E.; Knafelz, D.; Romano, C.; Naviglio, S.; et al. Multicentric Case-Control Study on Azathioprine Dose and Pharmacokinetics in Early-onset Pediatric Inflammatory Bowel Disease. *Inflamm. Bowel Dis.* **2017**, *23*, 628–634. [CrossRef] [PubMed]

26. Serpe, L.; Calvo, P.L.; Muntoni, E.; D'Antico, S.; Giaccone, M.; Avagnina, A.; Baldi, M.; Barbera, C.; Curti, F.; Pera, A.; et al. Thiopurine S-methyltransferase pharmacogenetics in a large-scale healthy Italian-Caucasian population: Differences in enzyme activity. *Pharmacogenomics* **2009**, *10*, 1753–1765. [CrossRef] [PubMed]
27. De Iudicibus, S.; Lucafò, M.; Vitulo, N.; Martelossi, S.; Zimbello, R.; De Pascale, F.; Forcato, C.; Naviglio, S.; Di Silvestre, A.; Gerdol, M.; et al. High-Throughput Sequencing of microRNAs in Glucocorticoid Sensitive Paediatric Inflammatory Bowel Disease Patients. *Int. J. Mol. Sci.* **2018**, *19*, 1399. [CrossRef]
28. Al-Judaibi, B.; Schwarz, U.I.; Huda, N.; Dresser, G.K.; Gregor, J.C.; Ponich, T.; Chande, N.; Mosli, M.; Kim, R.B. Genetic Predictors of Azathioprine Toxicity and Clinical Response in Patients with Inflammatory Bowel Disease. *J. Popul. Ther. Clin. Pharmacol.* **2016**, *23*, e26–e36.
29. Broekman, M.M.T.J.; Wong, D.R.; Wanten, G.J.A.; Roelofs, H.M.; van Marrewijk, C.J.; Klungel, O.H.; Verbeek, A.L.M.; Hooymans, P.M.; Guchelaar, H.J.; Scheffer, H.; et al. The glutathione transferase Mu null genotype leads to lower 6-MMPR levels in patients treated with azathioprine but not with mercaptopurine. *Pharm. J.* **2018**, *18*, 160–166. [CrossRef]
30. Mazor, Y.; Koifman, E.; Elkin, H.; Chowers, Y.; Krivoy, N.; Karban, A.; Efrati, E. Risk factors for serious adverse effects of thiopurines in patients with Crohn's disease. *Curr. Drug Saf.* **2013**, *8*, 181–185. [CrossRef]
31. Liu, H.; Ding, L.; Zhang, F.; Zhang, Y.; Gao, X.; Hu, P.; Bi, H.; Huang, M. The impact of glutathione S-transferase genotype and phenotype on the adverse drug reactions to azathioprine in patients with inflammatory bowel diseases. *J. Pharmacol. Sci.* **2015**, *129*, 95–100. [CrossRef] [PubMed]
32. Moriyama, T.; Nishii, R.; Perez-Andreu, V.; Yang, W.; Klussmann, F.A.; Zhao, X.; Lin, T.N.; Hoshitsuki, K.; Nersting, J.; Kihira, K.; et al. NUDT15 polymorphisms alter thiopurine metabolism and hematopoietic toxicity. *Nat. Genet.* **2016**, *48*, 367–373. [CrossRef] [PubMed]
33. Ban, H.; Andoh, A.; Imaeda, H.; Kobori, A.; Bamba, S.; Tsujikawa, T.; Sasaki, M.; Saito, Y.; Fujiyama, Y. The multidrug-resistance protein 4 polymorphism is a new factor accounting for thiopurine sensitivity in Japanese patients with inflammatory bowel disease. *J. Gastroenterol.* **2010**, *45*, 1014–1021. [CrossRef] [PubMed]
34. Hofmann, U.; Heinkele, G.; Angelberger, S.; Schaeffeler, E.; Lichtenberger, C.; Jaeger, S.; Reinisch, W.; Schwab, M. Simultaneous quantification of eleven thiopurine nucleotides by liquid chromatography-tandem mass spectrometry. *Anal. Chem.* **2012**, *84*, 1294–1301. [CrossRef] [PubMed]
35. Pelin, M.; Genova, E.; Fusco, L.; Marisat, M.; Hofmann, U.; Favretto, D.; Lucafò, M.; Taddio, A.; Martelossi, S.; Ventura, A.; et al. Pharmacokinetics and pharmacodynamics of thiopurines in an in vitro model of human hepatocytes: Insights from an innovative mass spectrometry assay. *Chem. Biol. Interact.* **2017**, *275*, 189–195. [CrossRef] [PubMed]

Permissions

All chapters in this book were first published by MDPI; hereby published with permission under the Creative Commons Attribution License or equivalent. Every chapter published in this book has been scrutinized by our experts. Their significance has been extensively debated. The topics covered herein carry significant findings which will fuel the growth of the discipline. They may even be implemented as practical applications or may be referred to as a beginning point for another development.

The contributors of this book come from diverse backgrounds, making this book a truly international effort. This book will bring forth new frontiers with its revolutionizing research information and detailed analysis of the nascent developments around the world.

We would like to thank all the contributing authors for lending their expertise to make the book truly unique. They have played a crucial role in the development of this book. Without their invaluable contributions this book wouldn't have been possible. They have made vital efforts to compile up to date information on the varied aspects of this subject to make this book a valuable addition to the collection of many professionals and students.

This book was conceptualized with the vision of imparting up-to-date information and advanced data in this field. To ensure the same, a matchless editorial board was set up. Every individual on the board went through rigorous rounds of assessment to prove their worth. After which they invested a large part of their time researching and compiling the most relevant data for our readers.

The editorial board has been involved in producing this book since its inception. They have spent rigorous hours researching and exploring the diverse topics which have resulted in the successful publishing of this book. They have passed on their knowledge of decades through this book. To expedite this challenging task, the publisher supported the team at every step. A small team of assistant editors was also appointed to further simplify the editing procedure and attain best results for the readers.

Apart from the editorial board, the designing team has also invested a significant amount of their time in understanding the subject and creating the most relevant covers. They scrutinized every image to scout for the most suitable representation of the subject and create an appropriate cover for the book.

The publishing team has been an ardent support to the editorial, designing and production team. Their endless efforts to recruit the best for this project, has resulted in the accomplishment of this book. They are a veteran in the field of academics and their pool of knowledge is as vast as their experience in printing. Their expertise and guidance has proved useful at every step. Their uncompromising quality standards have made this book an exceptional effort. Their encouragement from time to time has been an inspiration for everyone.

The publisher and the editorial board hope that this book will prove to be a valuable piece of knowledge for researchers, students, practitioners and scholars across the globe.

List of Contributors

Maaike van der Lee, Henk-Jan Guchelaar and Jesse J. Swen
Department of Clinical Pharmacy and Toxicology, Leiden University Medical Center, 2333ZA Leiden, The Netherlands
Leiden Network of Personalized Therapeutics, 2333ZA Leiden, The Netherlands

Marjolein Kriek
Department of Clinical Genetics, Leiden University Medical Center, 2333ZA Leiden, The Netherlands

Victoria Rollinson, Richard Turner and Munir Pirmohamed
Wolfson Centre for Personalised Medicine, Institute of Systems, Molecular and Integrative Biology, University of Liverpool, Liverpool L69 3GL, UK

Heejin Kam and Hotcherl Jeong
College of Pharmacy, Ewha Womans University, Seoul 03760, Korea

Abdelrahman H. Elsayed and Jatinder K. Lamba
Department of Pharmacotherapy and Translational Research, Center for Pharmacogenomics, University of Florida, Gainesville, FL 32610, USA

Neha S. Bhise
Department of Pharmacotherapy and Translational Research, Center for Pharmacogenomics, University of Florida, Gainesville, FL 32610, USA
Department of Experimental and Clinical Pharmacology, University of Minnesota, Minneapolis, MN 55455, USA

Xueyuan Cao
Department of Acute and Tertiary Care, University of Tennessee Health Science Center, Memphis, TN 38163, USA

Stanley Pounds
Department of Biostatistics, St. Jude Children's Research Hospital, Memphis, TN 38105, USA

Carin A. T. C. Lunenburg and Hans Gelderblom
Department of Medical Oncology, Leiden University Medical Center, 2333 ZA Leiden, The Netherlands

Linda M. Henricks and Jan H. M. Schellens
Department of Clinical Pharmacology, Division of Medical Oncology, The Netherlands Cancer Institute, 1066 CX Amsterdam, The Netherlands
Division of Pharmacology, The Netherlands Cancer Institute, 1066 CX Amsterdam, The Netherlands

André B. P. van Kuilenburg
Department of Clinical Chemistry, Amsterdam University Medical Centre, 1105 AZ Amsterdam, The Netherlands

Ron H. J. Mathijssen
Department of Medical Oncology, Erasmus MC Cancer Institute, 3015 GD Rotterdam, The Netherlands

Matteo Dugo, Andrea Devecchi, Loris De Cecco and Marialuisa Sensi
Platform of Integrated Biology, Department of Applied Research and Technological Development, Fondazione IRCCS Istituto Nazionale dei Tumori, 20133 Milan, Italy

Erika Cecchin
Experimental and Clinical Pharmacology Unit, Centro di Riferimento Oncologico, IRCCS National Cancer Institute, 33081 Aviano, Pordenone, Italy

Delia Mezzanzanica and Marina Bagnoli
Molecular Therapy Unit, Department of Research, Fondazione IRCCS Istituto Nazionale dei Tumori, 20133 Milan, Italy
Rossana Roncato, Lisa Dal Cin, Silvia Mezzalira, Francesco Comello, Elena De Mattia, Alessia Bignucolo, Michela Guardascione, Giuseppe Toffoli and Erika Cecchin
Clinical and Experimental Pharmacology, Centro di Riferimento Oncologico di Aviano (CRO) IRCCS, 3081 Aviano, Italy

Lorenzo Giollo, Simone D'Errico and Antonio Gulotta
GPI, Società per Azioni (SpA), 38123 Trento, Italy

Luca Emili and Vincenzo Carbone
InSilicoTrials Technologies società a responsabilità limitata (s.r.l.), 34148 Trieste, Italy

Luisa Foltran
Department of Medical Oncology, Centro di Riferimento Oncologico di Aviano (CRO), IRCSS, 33081 Aviano, Italy

Ayah Y. Almasri
Department of Applied Biological Sciences, Jordan University of Science and Technology, Irbid 22110, Jordan

Laith N. AL-Eitan
Department of Applied Biological Sciences, Jordan University of Science and Technology, Irbid 22110, Jordan
Department of Biotechnology and Genetic Engineering, Jordan University of Science and Technology, Irbid 22110, Jordan

Rame H. Khasawneh
Department of Hematopathology, King Hussein Medical Center (KHMC), Jordan Royal Medical Services (RMS), Amman 11118, Jordan

Cathelijne H. van der Wouden and Paul C. D. Bank
Department of Clinical Pharmacy and Toxicology, Leiden University Medical Center, 2333 ZA Leiden, The Netherlands
Leiden Network for Personalised Therapeutics, 2333 ZA Leiden, The Netherlands

Kübra Özokcu
Division of Pharmacoepidemiology and Clinical Pharmacology, Utrecht Institute for Pharmaceutical Sciences (UIPS), Utrecht University, 3584 CG Utrecht, The Netherlands

Susanne J. H. Vijverberg and Anke H. Maitland-van der Zee
Department of Respiratory Medicine, Amsterdam University Medical Centers, University of Amsterdam, 1105 AZ Amsterdam, The Netherlands

Zulfan Zazuli
Department of Respiratory Medicine, Amsterdam University Medical Centers, University of Amsterdam, 1105 AZ Amsterdam, The Netherlands
Department of Pharmacology-Clinical Pharmacy, School of Pharmacy, Bandung Institute of Technology, Bandung 40132, Indonesia
Division of Pharmacology, Utrecht Institute for Pharmaceutical Sciences, Utrecht University, 3512 JE Utrecht, The Netherlands

Leila S. Otten and Rosalinde Masereeuw
Division of Pharmacology, Utrecht Institute for Pharmaceutical Sciences, Utrecht University, 3512 JE Utrecht, The Netherlands

Britt I. Drögemöller and Colin J. D. Ross
British Columbia Children's Hospital Research Institute, Vancouver, BC V5Z 4H4, Canada
Faculty of Pharmaceutical Sciences, The University of British Columbia, Vancouver, BC V6T 1Z4, Canada

Jose G. Monzon
Department of Medical Oncology, Tom Baker Cancer Centre, Calgary, AB T2N 4N2, Canada

Mara Medeiros
Nephrology Research Unit, Hospital Infantil de México Federico Gómez, Mexico City 06720, Mexico
Departamento de Farmacología, Facultad de Medicina, Universidad Nacional Autónoma de México, Mexico City 04510, Mexico

Galen E. B. Wright
British Columbia Children's Hospital Research Institute, Vancouver, BC V5Z 4H4, Canada
Department of Medical Genetics, University of British Columbia, Vancouver, BC V6T 1Z4, Canada

Christian K. Kollmannsberger and Karen A. Gelmon
BC Cancer Agency and University of British Columbia, Vancouver, BC V6T 1Z4, Canada

Philippe L. Bedard
Princess Margaret Cancer Centre and University of Toronto, Toronto, ON M5S, Canada

Zhuo Chen and Geoffrey Liu
Medical Oncology and Hematology, Department of Medicine, Princess Margaret Cancer Centre-University Health Network and University of Toronto, Toronto, ON M5S, Canada

Nicole McGoldrick
Pharmaceutical Outcomes Programme, BC Children's Hospital, Vancouver, BC V6H 3N1, Canada

Abhijat Kitchlu
Division of Nephrology, Department of Medicine, University Health Network and University of Toronto, Toronto, ON M5S, Canada

Bruce C. Carleton
Pharmaceutical Outcomes Programme, BC Children's Hospital, Vancouver, BC V6H 3N1, Canada
Division of Translational Therapeutics, Department of Pediatrics, Faculty of Medicine, University of British Columbia, Vancouver, BC V6T 1Z4, Canada

Cristina Lucía Dávila-Fajardo, Xando Díaz-Villamarín, Ana Estefanía Fernández-Gómez, Paloma García-Navas and José Cabeza Barrera
Department of Clinical Pharmacy, San Cecilio University Hospital, Institute for Biomedical Research, ibs.GRANADA, 18016 Granada, Spain

Alba Antúnez-Rodríguez and Luis Javier Martínez-González
Genomics Unit, Centro Pfizer-Universidad de Granada-Junta de Andalucía de Genómica e Investigación Oncológica (Genyo), 18016 Granada, Spain

José Augusto Dávila-Fajardo
English Department, Official Language School Leganes, 28915 Leganés, Madrid, Spain

Yingqi Xu, Shuting Lin, Hongying Zhao, Jingwen Wang, Chunlong Zhang, Qun Dong, Congxue Hu, Desi Shang, Li Wang and Yanjun Xu
College of Bioinformatics Science and Technology, Harbin Medical University, Harbin 150081, China

Erika Cecchin and Giuseppe Toffoli
Centro di Riferimento Oncologico, IRCCS, 33081 Aviano, Italy

Marianna Lucafò
Centro di Riferimento Oncologico, IRCCS, 33081 Aviano, Italy
Institute for Maternal and Child Health IRCCS Burlo Garofolo, 34137 Trieste, Italy

Stefano Martelossi, Diego Favretto, Matteo Bramuzzo and Samuele Naviglio
Institute for Maternal and Child Health IRCCS Burlo Garofolo, 34137 Trieste, Italy

Gabriele Stocco
Department of Life Sciences, University of Trieste, 34127 Trieste, Italy

Raffaella Franca
Department of Medical, Surgical and Health Sciences, University of Trieste, 34149 Trieste, Italy

Angela Lora, Alessandro Ventura and Giuliana Decorti
Institute for Maternal and Child Health IRCCS Burlo Garofolo, 34137 Trieste, Italy
Department of Medical, Surgical and Health Sciences, University of Trieste, 34149 Trieste, Italy

Noelia Malusà
Sanitary Services Agency 1, 34129 Trieste, Italy

Index

www.ingramcontent.com/pod-product-compliance
Lightning Source LLC
LaVergne TN
LVHW082221200926
848484LV00008B/2281
9798887403748